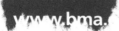

Principles of Exposure Measurement in Epidemiology

Principles of Exposure Measurement in Epidemiology

Collecting, Evaluating, and
Improving Measures of
Disease Risk Factors

SECOND EDITION

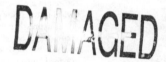

Emily White
University of Washington and
Fred Hutchinson Cancer Research Center, Seattle, USA

Bruce K. Armstrong
The University of Sydney, Sydney, Australia

Rodolfo Saracci
National Research Council, Pisa, Italy

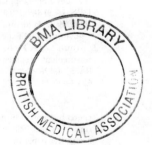

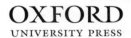

OXFORD
UNIVERSITY PRESS

OXFORD
UNIVERSITY PRESS

Great Clarendon Street, Oxford OX2 6DP

Oxford University Press is a department of the University of Oxford.
It furthers the University's objective of excellence in research, scholarship,
and education by publishing worldwide in

Oxford New York

Auckland Cape Town Dar es Salaam Hong Kong Karachi
Kuala Lumpur Madrid Melbourne Mexico City Nairobi
New Delhi Shanghai Taipei Toronto

With offices in

Argentina Austria Brazil Chile Czech Republic France Greece
Guatemala Hungary Italy Japan Poland Portugal Singapore
South Korea Switzerland Thailand Turkey Ukraine Vietnam

Oxford is a registered trade mark of Oxford University Press
in the UK and in certain other countries

Published in the United States
by Oxford University Press Inc., New York

British Library Cataloguing in Publication Data

Data available

Library of Congress Cataloging-in-Publication Data

White, Emily, 1946–
  Principles of exposure measurement in epidemiology : collecting, evaluating, and improving
measures of disease risk factors / Emily White, Bruce K. Armstrong, Rodolfo Saracci.— 2nd ed.
    p. ; cm.
  Rev. ed. of: Prinicples of exposure measurement in epidemiology / Bruce K. Armstrong, Emily
White, Rodolfo Saracci. 1992.
  Includes bibliographical references and index.
  ISBN-13: 978–0–19–850985–1 (alk. paper) 1. Epidemiology—Methodology.
  [DNLM: 1. Epidemiologic Research Design. 2. Risk Assessment—methods.
3. Environmental Exposure. 4. Environmental Monitoring—methods. WA 950 W583p 2008]
I. Armstrong, B. K. II. Saracci, Rodolfo, 1936– III. Armstrong, B. K. Principles of exposure
measurement in epidemiology. IV. Title.
  RA652.4.A28 2008
  614.4—dc22

                                                                                      2007043092

Typeset by Cepha Imaging Private Ltd., Bangalore, India
Printed in Great Britain
on acid-free paper by
Ashford Colour Press Ltd., Gosport, Hampshire

ISBN 978–0–19–850985–1

10 9 8 7 6 5 4 3 2 1

Preface

Accurate measurement of exposure to putative causes of disease is essential to the validity of epidemiological research. Yet most of the training and books on epidemiological methods cover study design and/or data analysis, but give little emphasis to the actual conduct of epidemiological studies, including ascertaining the data on exposures. We attempted to fill that gap with publication of the first edition of this book in 1992 (paperback 1994), with Bruce Armstrong as the lead author.

This book covers principles and methods that can be applied to measuring a wide range of exposures, including demographic, anthropometric, nutritional, medical, reproductive, genetic, metabolic, and environmental factors. We cover the methods and quality control approaches for the most commonly used data collection methods in epidemiology, including personal interviews, self-administered questionnaires, abstraction of records, keeping of diaries, measurements in blood and other body products, and measurements of the environment. We do not discuss measurement of exposure to infectious agents, and we only provide principles, general methods, and examples, but not detailed reviews, of measurement methods for specific exposures.

This book also covers three other major topics relevant to exposure measurement. The first is methods to design, analyse, and interpret validity and reliability studies which quantify the degree of exposure measurement error. This topic is included because such ancillary studies are important in understanding the effects of exposure measurement error on the 'parent' epidemiological study. The second topic is methods to maximize response rates. While this topic falls under the construct of reducing selection bias, and most of the rest of the book is focused on reducing misclassification bias, it is included because it is an important aspect of the data collection phase of most epidemiological studies. The third additional topic—ethical issues in the conduct of epidemiological research—is included for the same reason.

A large amount of research relating to exposure measurement has been conducted over the last 15 years, and this second edition of the book has given us the opportunity to add information from newer studies on a range of topics covered in the first edition. We have also added several new topics, including approaches to dose–time modelling, information on newer and more automated ways of collecting data such as computer-assisted interviewing and electronic diaries, new approaches to pre-testing questionnaires such as use of cognitive interviews, current approaches to quality control, internal consistency reliability (Cronbach's α), sample size calculations for validity and reliability studies, terminology and issues in collecting specimens for genotyping, calculation of response rates, ways to maximize follow-up in cohort studies, and ethical issues relating to the development of bio-repositories within long-term cohort studies and to ways of informing study participants of personal risks, as derived from genetic tests for example.

We have written this book primarily as a text for graduate courses in epidemiology (instructors may contact Emily White (ewhite@fhcrc.org) for sample course outline and course assignments), and as a reference book for use by graduate students and practising epidemiologists in the planning of their research. Because our target audience comes from a range of backgrounds, the statistical treatment of the subject has been kept to a fairly basic level. Specifically, derivations of equations have not been given, although the assumptions and models used have generally been stated so that those with a strong statistical background could arrive at the derivations for themselves. Where possible, references to derivations have also been given. Also, to facilitate the use of this book by non-epidemiologists with an interest in the topic, we have limited use of epidemiological jargon as far as possible.

We would like to thank those who helped with the first and/or second editions. Noel Weiss, former Chairman of the Department of Epidemiology, University of Washington, encouraged and provided support for the course on which much of this book is based, and read and commented on the first edition. We also thank our other colleagues who contributed ideas, encouragement, and criticism in the preparation of this book. In this respect, we would especially acknowledge the assistance given by Shirley Beresford, Harvey Checkoway, Janet Daling, Dallas English, D'Arcy Holman, Julie Hunt, John Kaldor, Tom Koepsell, Ann Kolar, Alan Kristal, Sonia Maruti, Margaret Pepe, Ross Prentice, Bruce Psaty, Judith Straton, Harri Vainio, and Jan Watt in reading and commenting on chapters at various stages in their production and, in some cases, the whole book. We also thank Alyson Littman, Jennifer Marino, Tabitha Harrison, and Linda Massey who provided research and technical assistance. The students who have taken the course on which the book has been based have also, by their interest, questions, and observations, contributed much to its development; they have our thanks.

While the preparation of the book has been a team effort, each of us contributed most to certain chapters. The primary chapter authors were as follows: Chapter 1 (EW, BKA, RS), Chapter 2 (BKA and EW), Chapter 3 (EW),

Chapter 4 (EW), Chapter 5 (EW), Chapter 6 (BKA and EW), Chapter 7 (BKA and EW), Chapter 8 (EW and BKA), Chapter 9 (RS), Chapter 10 (RS), Chapter 11 (EW and BKA), and Chapter 12 (BKA and RS).

Seattle   E.W.
Sydney   B.K.A.
and Pisa   R.S.
June 2007

Contents

1

Exposure measurement

The first step facing an epidemiologist ... is to specify the conceptual 'true' exposure. The answer will often be less than obvious since, in one sense, every measure is a surrogate for a more proximal cause of disease. ... Even when a specific step in the causal sequence of events is selected as the 'true' exposure, the dimension of time will usually need to be considered since most epidemiologic exposures fluctuate and/or drift within persons.
(*Willett 1989*)

Introduction

Epidemiology is a comparatively new science. Its methods were first developed when the study of diseases due to infectious organisms was the field's main focus. The measurement of exposure was then grounded in microbiology, and most epidemiologists had substantial training or experience in this area. Interest in non-infectious determinants of disease was commonly confined to the more readily measurable host factors such as age, sex, education, etc. Measurement of the microbiological determinants was simplified by the possibility of isolation and culture of a specific organism that was the presumed agent of disease, the short interval that commonly separated exposure from onset of clinical symptoms, and the possibility of serological documentation of exposure that had occurred in the past.

Exposure measurement has become substantially more complex with the growth of the study of non-infectious diseases over the past 60 years. There are several reasons for this complexity.

- There may be no *necessary* cause for the disease under study, and any single component cause may make only a small contribution to aetiology
- The interval from onset, and perhaps cessation, of exposure to appearance of disease is more often measured in years than in days, weeks, or months

- The agent of disease may leave no easily measurable indicator of past exposure
- The range of agents of interest has increased greatly, and includes complex exposures such as diet, psychosocial factors, and metabolic factors.

With the increasing multiplicity and complexity of exposures studied in epidemiology, there is a growing interest in the general principles and methods of exposure measurement, as well as in the accuracy of measuring specific exposures. While epidemiologists realize that inaccurate exposure measurements are one of the main sources of bias in epidemiological studies, the magnitude of this bias is generally under-appreciated. For example, for an exposure that is measured so well that it correlates with the true exposure of interest with a correlation coefficient of 0.7, this could bias a true risk ratio of 3.0 to become an observed risk ratio of 1.7! This suggests that even greater attention should be paid to the process of exposure measurement.

This chapter covers the initial steps in exposure measurement that occur during the planning of an epidemiological study of the relationship between an exposure and a disease (or other outcome). The planning process for exposure measurement begins with conceptualizing the true exposure hypothesized to cause the disease (Figure 1.1). Key issues related to the true exposure are discussed, including specifying the active agent and determining where in the exposure–disease biological sequence to measure the exposure. Since the true aetiological exposure is often not measurable, the researcher needs to create an operational way to measure the exposure. This involves an iterative process of determining the appropriate exposure variable, the individual items to be measured, and the measurement instrument(s) (Figure 1.1). The *exposure variable* is the variable that will be used in the statistical analysis of the exposure–disease relationship after the epidemiological study has been completed (e.g. cumulative dose). We discuss the issues and terminology around defining and/or selecting the most appropriate dose representation and the most critical time window during which the exposure has the greatest effect on disease risk. Once a dose variable has been defined, the researcher would create a list of the items needed for its computation and other items important for its valid analysis. For example, if the true exposure of interest were the actual lifetime quantity of cigarettes smoked, the exposure variable in the analysis might be lifetime pack-years based on self-report, which would be computed from two items asked of each subject: number of years the subject smoked cigarettes and average packs per day smoked. The last step in the planning process depicted in Figure 1.1 is the selection or development of

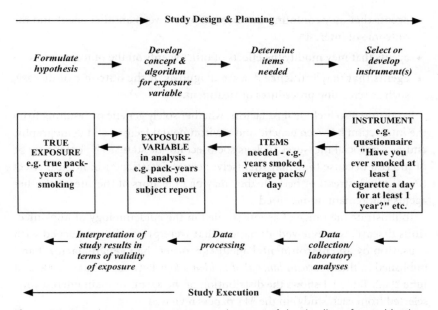

Figure 1.1 Steps in exposure measurement in terms of the timeline of an epidemiological study.

the instrument(s) to be used, for example an interviewer-administered questionnaire, use of medical records, and/or analysis of human specimens. This topic is only briefly mentioned in this chapter, but is covered in detail in other chapters.

We conclude by outlining the contents of the entire book, and where the topics covered fit within the design, conduct, and interpretation of an epidemiological study.

Exposure

Range of exposures studied in epidemiology

In epidemiology, the word *exposure* is a very broad term used to denote any of a subject's attributes or any agent which may be a cause or predictor of the outcome under study. Another common term for exposure is *risk factor*. The term exposure encompasses:

◆ agents that may cause physiological effects (e.g. food as determining body growth)

◆ agents that may cause or protect from disease

- agents that may confound the association between another agent and the outcome of interest
- agents that may modify the effects of other agents on the outcome
- agents that may influence disease diagnosis or the outcome of disease, such as screening procedures or treatment.

Exposures also include host factors, whether solely genetic or resulting from the interaction between genetic and environmental factors, and demographic and psychosocial measures such as socio-economic status. The latter may be of interest because they may themselves cause a particular biological effect (e.g. through stress) or because they may be indicators of the effects of other agents that remain unmeasured.

To illustrate the range of agents studied in the epidemiology of non-infectious disease, we reviewed all papers that were primarily concerned with causation by an environmental agent (i.e. other than genetic factors) and published in the *American Journal of Epidemiology* between January 2000 and June 2002. Table 1.1 shows the distribution of the agents of main interest (one selected from each study) in the 311 papers reviewed.

The most common exposures studied over this time period were factors related to diet, anthropometrics, and physical activity (30 per cent of the papers). Almost 20 per cent of the papers had medical factors as the main exposure, including medication use and measures from biospecimens not classifiable to a single external exposure, such as HDL cholesterol. Other common exposures studied were demographic factors (5 per cent), reproductive and sexual history (6 per cent), tobacco and alcohol use (10 per cent), psychosocial factors (8 per cent), occupational exposures (8 per cent), and exposures in the environment (14 per cent).

Within one epidemiological study, many types of exposures will be measured. In this book, we assume that a study has a primary exposure of interest, and we often present the principles and methods of exposure measurement in terms of the main exposure, which is generally measured in the most detail. However, these principles and methods would apply to other study exposures (covariates) as well. We also assume that the study is observational, i.e. that the main exposure is not randomly assigned by the investigator. In randomized trials, the measurement of the main exposure (the intervention or treatment) is simply the group assignment. For randomized trials, the principles and methods presented in this book would apply primarily to the covariates to be measured.

Objective of exposure measurement

The objective of exposure measurement in an epidemiological study is to measure the exposure(s) of interest as accurately as possible, within the

Table 1.1 Distribution of the exposures of main interest (one selected from each study) in 311 papers on the aetiology of non-infectious disease published in the *American Journal of Epidemiology* between January 2000 and June 2002[a]

Exposures	Distribution (%)
Demographic factors	5.1
Socio-economic status	2.9
Race	1.6
Other demographic factors	0.6
Diet, anthropometrics, and physical activity	30.3
Nutrients, foods and, supplements	15.4
Caffeine use	1.0
Anthropometrics	9.7
Physical activity and fitness	4.2
Medical factors and use of medications	18.4
Oral contraceptive and hormone replacement use	2.0
Other medications	2.6
Other medical factors[b]	13.8
Reproductive and sexual history	6.4
Tobacco, alcohol, and illicit substance use	9.6
Active smoking	4.5
Environmental tobacco smoke	1.0
Alcohol drinking	3.5
Illicit substance use	0.6
Psychosocial factors	8.4
Mainly social factors	4.2
Other psychosocial factors	4.2
Occupation	8.0
Specific occupations or exposures	6.4
Occupation in general	1.6
Exposures in the environment	13.8
Ionizing radiation	1.6
Non-ionizing radiation	2.9
Contaminants and pollutants of water	1.9
Pollutants of air	3.5
Other exposures in the environment	3.9

[a] Excludes genetic and infectious exposures.

[b] Includes measures in the human body not classifiable to a single specific external exposure (e.g. HDL cholesterol).

practical constraints of limiting subject burden and study costs. The accuracy or validity of the exposure measure is the closeness of the exposure as measured on each subject in the study to each subject's true exposure. The *true exposure* is the agent of interest, for example the amount of exposure to the hypothesized casual agent under study over the relevant time period of life.

Active biological agent

As noted in the introduction, the researcher should first consider what the true underlying exposure of interest is, before attempting to define its measurement. One issue in conceptualizing the true exposure is to hypothesize what the *active agent* is, i.e. the component of the exposure (e.g. a chemical compound or biological activity) which causes (or prevents) the disease of interest. This aids in selecting or developing an exposure variable that will accurately reflect the true underlying exposure. By specifying the active agent, the researcher can attempt to make the exposure measure *specific*, in the sense that the measure isolates the putative causal component(s) from a broader class of exposures. The exposure variable should also be *sensitive*, in the sense that it includes all sources of the active agent of interest. For example, if aluminium is the hypothesized active agent in a study of Alzheimer's disease, for the exposure to be specific, the researcher must be able to separate drugs, such as analgesics and antacids, that contain aluminium from those that do not. For the exposure measurement to be sensitive, other sources of aluminium should also be included, such as aluminium ingested from foods and possibly even aluminium that may be absorbed though the skin from antiperspirants.

For some types of exposures, the active agent differs depending on the disease. For example, coffee intake has been found to be associated with reduced risk of both diabetes and Parkinson's disease. However, the active agent in the protection from Parkinson's disease appears to be caffeine (Ross *et al.* 2000), while some other nutrient in coffee, and not caffeine, appears to be responsible for the reduced risk of diabetes (Pereira *et al.* 2006).

Exposure–disease biological pathway

Traditionally, 'exposure' and 'disease' were considered to be separate concepts. However, modern molecular epidemiology acknowledges that the exposure–disease relationship is actually a *biological pathway*, with a sequence of causal events or states between the external exposure and disease. This has implications for exposure measurement. Exposures can be measured at one or more points on this pathway, as the available, administered, absorbed, or active dose, as shown in Figure 1.2.

The *available dose* is the amount of the exposure measured in the subject's external environment. An example of available dose is the concentration of asbestos fibres per millilitre of ambient air in a person's workplace over the time he/she was employed. Sometimes the available dose measurements in the external media do not relate to a specific person but rather to a group or

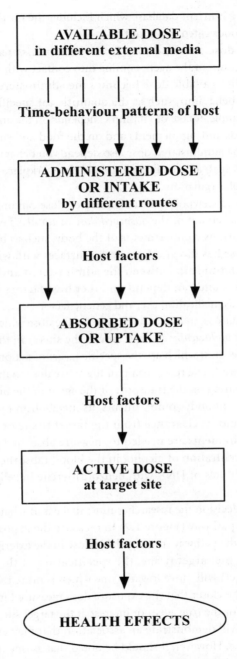

Figure 1.2 Exposure dose concepts in the exposure–disease pathway.

population (e.g. a nutrient database which includes the nutrient composition of hundreds of foods eaten in a country).

The available dose usually differs from the *administered dose* or *intake*, i.e. the actual amount of the agent coming into contact with the human body. How much of the available dose becomes the administered dose depends on the subject's behaviour, such as the quantities of specific foods actually ingested. For example, intake of vitamin C depends on the amount of vitamin C in various foods and supplements and on the food and supplement intake of the subject. The administered dose also depends on behaviours that protect against exposure, such as use of respirators in the workplace or sunscreens to protect against solar radiation.

From a biological viewpoint, the administered dose can only be regarded as a surrogate measurement of the *absorbed dose* or *uptake*, i.e. the dose which actually enters various compartments of the body, such as blood (unless the administered dose has direct effects at the surfaces with which it comes in contact). The relationship between the administered and absorbed dose is usually complex and can depend on other host factors including other behaviours, such as medication use, and genetic factors.

The absorbed dose is, in turn, a surrogate for the dose which really matters, the *active dose* or *biologically effective dose* at the site(s) in the body (organs, tissues, cells, molecules) which are the specific target of action of the agent on the disease of interest. The relationship of the active dose to the absorbed dose is complex, depending on the transport of the agent in the body, its distribution among different body compartments, its metabolism to both active and inactive forms, and its clearance from the target tissue or from the body. Biological measurements are needed to measure absorbed or active doses, for example concentration of alcohol in the blood (absorbed dose) or concentrations of adducts of DNA with benzo(a)pyrene in cells from the lung (active dose).

Therefore one decision the researcher must make is at what point(s) on the biological causal pathway (Figure 1.2) to measure the exposure. Usually, as one moves down the pathway from available dose in the external environment to active dose at the target tissue, the specification of the agent (and its amount per subject) will move towards one which is more relevant to causation of disease. The closer that the exposure dose measured in a study can be to the active dose of the true agent of interest at the target site, the more likely it is that a study will demonstrate an association that may exist between an agent and a disease. However, it should be noted that as one moves down the exposure–disease pathway, the objectives of the epidemiological study move from the public health perspective of understanding how environmental factors and human behaviours affect disease to a more biological perspective of elucidating exposure–disease mechanisms. These perspectives are both valid and offer different insights into disease prevention modalities.

Of course, the four exposure steps in the pathway in Figure 1.2 do not apply to all exposure–disease relationships. Some causal pathways would be simpler than the diagram, for example hysterectomy in relation to uterine cancer risk, while others would be more complex, such as the role of physical activity in cardiovascular disease risk, which probably acts through several mechanistic pathways.

Finally, the exposure–disease pathway also includes a sequence in the subsequent health effects. This begins with the early biological effects on the target tissue, then altered structure or function, then clinical disease, and, when appropriate, outcome of disease (Schulte 1993). As these are all measures of disease (or its precursors or outcomes), they are beyond the scope of this book. However, many measurement principles in this book would also apply to measures of these health effects.

Measurement and scales of measurement

Once the researcher has clarified what the true exposure of interest is, he/she needs to develop an operational way to measure the exposure. This involves an iterative process of determining the appropriate representation of the exposure variable in terms of dose and time, the individual items to be measured and the measurement instrument(s) (Figure 1.1). One consideration in the measurement process is the determination of the scale of measurement of the exposure variable and of the individual items. In this section, we first define measurement and then discuss the various scales of measurement.

Definition of measurement

Measurement is generally defined as the assignment of numbers or labels to objects and events according to rules (Stevens 1951; Goude 1962), although in epidemiology the 'objects and events' are more commonly behaviours, molecules (in the environment and in the human body), and abstract concepts such as socio-economic status. A key part of this definition is the existence of rules that determine the assignment, as this is essential to scientific rigour. Anderson and Mantel (1983) have drawn attention to the need for measurement 'rules' in epidemiology:

> One conspicuous cause of instability in survey data is the failure of field workers … to follow operational methods of measurement. A method of measurement is considered operational if two requirements are satisfied. First, instructions for use of the method must [exist and] be understandable to other investigators who may wish to

follow them. Second, there should be a demonstration (at least a pilot study) to show that measurements resulting from this method are reproducible.

Scales of measurement

Four scales of measurement have been defined traditionally, ordered according to the implied degree of sophistication of the measurement (Stevens 1951).

In a *nominal scale*, the numbers, words, or signs are used only as labels and do not tell us anything about an individual's ranking. Examples of nominal scales commonly used in epidemiology are sex, occupation (if not ordered in some way to reflect level of exposure), and class of medication used for a specific condition such as diabetes.

In contrast, in an *ordinal scale*, numbers are used to indicate a rank ordering of classes of the variable, but differences between them cannot be taken to indicate the actual size of differences between the classes in the value of the underlying measurement. Examples of ordinal scales used in epidemiology include socio-economic status and crude or non-uniformly distributed categories of exposure, for example when the subject is asked to indicate his/her usual recreational activity as 'daily', '4–6 times a week', '1–3 times a week', '1–3 times a month', or 'less than once a month'.

On an *interval scale*, the relative values of the numbers assigned to different individuals reflect true differences in the values of the underlying measurements. However, the zero point for the scale may be arbitrary (as it is, for example, in the Fahrenheit and celsius scales of temperature measurement). Examples of interval scale measurements in common use in epidemiology include year of birth and other variables measured in calendar time.

A *ratio scale* of measurement permits the valid comparison of measurements by calculation of both true differences and ratios, i.e. one measurement may be said to be some multiple of another. This means that the zero point of the scale is the 'true' zero. For example, a subject who consumes 500 mg of supplemental vitamin C per day can be considered to consume twice as much supplemental vitamin C as someone who consumes 250 mg. Most exposure variables in epidemiological studies can be measured on a ratio scale.

These scales of measurement were originally defined as a way of identifying the types of statistical procedure that were permissible in the analysis of particular kinds of data (Stevens 1951). Nominal and ordinal data were considered susceptible only to simple counts, identification of the mode, and contingency table procedures. Interval or ratio scale measurements were considered necessary before means and standard deviations could be calculated and linear regression techniques applied. While this approach has been criticized (see Stevens 1968) and statistical methods have advanced substantially since the scales were defined, it remains true that the options for analysis are greater when more sophisticated scales of measurement are used.

These observations have practical implications for the design and numerical coding of measurement instruments. Specifically, when exposures can be quantified, they should be collected as actual numerical values rather than in broader ordinal categories. For example, in the collection of data on cigarette smoking, it is better to record the subject's estimate of the actual number of cigarettes smoked in a day, rather then an indicator of a predefined category (e.g. <14, 15–24, 25–34, etc.) Even if the category intervals are of equal width, the mean value of observations in each category, and therefore the distance between categories, cannot be estimated accurately. Thus, in this circumstance, only statistics that apply to ordinal scales of measurement can be used validly (although equality of 'distance' between interval categories is often assumed to test for linear trend). Moreover, collection of exposure information from subjects in its most detailed form allows the researcher the greatest flexibility at the time of study data analysis. Even if the exposure will ultimately be analysed as an ordinal variable (which has the advantages of being easy to understand and of not making assumptions about the shape of the dose–response curve), collecting the exposure information on a more detailed numerical scale (interval or ratio) allows the researcher great flexibility in defining the exposure variable(s) that will be used at the time of data analysis.

The way scales of measurement are described in this book is more in line with current practice. The primary division in the classification is between *continuous variables* which in theory can take on an infinite number of values (but in practice have a large number of values) and *categorical variables* which take on a smaller finite number of values. Categorical variables are further classified as nominal categorical, ordered categorical, or dichotomous. *Nominal and ordered categorical variables* are as described above for nominal and ordinal scale variables. *Dichotomous* (also called binary) variables are variables which take on only two values, and so the distinction between nominal and ordinal is immaterial. The most commonly used statistical models in epidemiology for analysis of a binary disease or outcome, the linear logistic model for case–control and cross-sectional studies and the Cox proportional hazards model for cohort studies, can be applied to nominal, ordinal, and continuous exposure variables.

Exposure dose

Because the hypothesized true exposure generally cannot be perfectly measured (e.g. lifetime alcohol intake), the measurement process usually begins with creating an operational definition of exposure that *can* be measured, albeit with error. Issues that need to be considered are the best way to represent the dose (amount) of exposure as its relates to disease causation, the most critical time period during which the exposure is likely to cause disease and the actual algorithm to calculate the exposure dose variable over that time period that will be used in the statistical analysis of the epidemiological study.

Measurement of the *exposure dose*, i.e. the level or quantity of exposure, as opposed to simply the fact of exposure does not just provide the opportunity for a more detailed and informative description of the relationship between an exposure and a disease. It is also important in inferring the presence, or absence, of a cause and effect relationship, because the presence or absence of a dose–response relationship (increasing incidence of disease with increasing or decreasing exposure to the agent) is part of the evidence considered when making inferences about aetiology (Weiss 1981). In addition, the power of a study to detect an association may be increased if a particular functional form of dose–response (e.g. linear) is expected and quantitative dose data are collected to permit expression of the results in that form.

Some exposures lend themselves to a very simple measure of 'dose', such as history of gall bladder removal or genotype at a specific single nucleotide. However, many exposures are more complex to quantify in that they can vary between individuals in years of exposure, frequency of exposure (e.g. times per week) in those years, and/or intensity of exposure at each exposure event. Complex exposures can be expressed by simple variables such as ever/never exposed, years of exposure, or current frequency of exposure, and these might sometimes be useful at the time of data analysis. However, these simplified measures of exposure dose often may not sufficiently measure the amount of exposure as it relates to disease causation, i.e. the simpler measures often have substantial measurement error. This error, if non-differential by disease status, leads to attenuation of the magnitude of the exposure–disease association and loss of study power to detect an association.

Cumulative dose

The most common and useful concept of dose is cumulative dose. *Cumulative dose* is a summary of the level or quantity of exposure over a person's lifetime or over a specific time period. While each type of exposure is unique, the calculation of cumulative dose, for exposures measured by behaviours, generally takes a form similar to the following equation (for each person in the study):

$$\text{cumulative dose} = \sum_i (\text{years}_i \times \text{frequency}_i \times \text{intensity}_i)$$

where years is the number of years the person was exposed, frequency is the frequency of exposure episodes (e.g. times or hours per day, week, or month) for the person in those years, and *intensity* is the amount of the active agent per exposure episode (i.e. the dose of active agent per episode). The summation is over each type of exposure *i* which has the active agent. For example, to compute the cumulative dose of supplemental vitamin C over a 10-year period (if supplement use as opposed to food intake was the main interest), the algorithm should include the two main sources of supplemental vitamin C: multivitamins (m) and individual vitamin C supplements (c). For each source, the number of years the supplement was taken over the last 10 years, the days per week the supplement was used (in those years), and the dose per day (on the days taken) are multiplied and then summed across the two sources for each subject:

$$\text{cumulative dose of supplemental vitamin C over 10 years}$$
$$= (\text{years}_m \times \text{days}_m \times \text{dose}_m) + (\text{years}_c \times \text{days}_c \times \text{dose}_c).$$

Often the information on intensity (dose per episode) comes from an external (environmental) source. For example, the intensity (dose per day) of vitamin C from individual supplements could be asked of the subject, but the dose per day from multivitamins could be ascertained by asking the subject what brand of multivitamin was taken and then applying the information from a database of the composition of multivitamins by brand. Other examples of external databases of intensity are energy expenditure per hour per kilogram body weight (METs or metabolic equivalents) for various physical activities (Ainsworth *et al.* 2000) and nutrient compositions of foods (Schakel *et al.* 1997).

Dividing or multiplying cumulative dose by a constant for all subjects does not change the concept of cumulative dose. In the example of supplemental vitamin C above, a quantitatively accurate cumulative dose would need to be multiplied by 52 (because frequency was expressed as times per week not times per year), but that is not necessary for the interpretation. In fact, the estimated cumulative dose of supplemental vitamin C from the above equation would be easiest to interpret if it were divided by 70 for each subject, to yield the average daily dose of vitamin C over the 10-year period. Although this would be labelled 'average dose per day over 10 years', it would still be a measure of cumulative dose, since multiplying or dividing by the same constant for all subjects does not change its interpretation. Thus *average dose*, if it covers the same time period (e.g. the same number of years) for all subjects, is the same concept as cumulative dose.

The appropriate cumulative dose equation will vary by the exposure. Some exposures vary so little in frequency between persons (e.g. oral contraceptive use is typically taken as one pill per day) that years × intensity (where intensity is dose per pill of the active agent of interest) would be sufficient to measure cumulative dose. If the intensity also varies little between subjects, then years alone would be a good measure of cumulative dose. On the other hand, some exposures would require equations that are more complex. Often frequency needs to include two factors: frequency of episodes of exposure, and the number of exposure 'units' per episode. For example, for cumulative energy expenditure from recreational activity, frequency would need to be established by two questions for each type of activity: sessions per week and minutes per session. In these cases, the cumulative dose equation above would have both these frequency factors, and intensity in the equation would be the dose of the active agent per unit of exposure (e.g. energy expenditure per minute associated with a specific activity).

Another complexity is that sometimes the summation would need to be over each change in frequency or intensity of exposure. For example, if the dose per day for individual vitamin C supplements for a subject was 250 mg/day for the first four years of the 10-year period and 500 mg for the next six years, these would need to be separate elements in the summation.

Some exposures may vary too much over time within individuals to compute cumulative dose over a long time period. Ascertaining diet over even one year is so complex—usually requiring asking portion size and frequency of intake of over 100 foods—that it is not feasible to ascertain cumulative dose over many years. Therefore nutrient intake from food might need to be ascertained by reference to only one specific year in a person's life.

For exposures measured in the environment or the human body, cumulative dose might be best expressed as the average of the measure of interest over the relevant time period. For example, the cumulative (absorbed) dose of vitamin C over a 10-year period could be calculated as the average plasma vitamin C measured several times over the 10 years, if it is feasible to collect multiple blood samples over time.

Other dose representations

Cumulative dose is a way to summarize exposure into a single variable, but, as it is a summary, the specific information on duration, frequency, and intensity of exposure is obscured. For example the cumulative dose of alcohol over some time period would be the same for a person who consistently drank one bottle of beer per day as for another person who consistently drank seven beers every Saturday night, but abstained for the rest of the week. These two exposure profiles may have substantially different health effects. Therefore cumulative dose may not always be the best representation of exposure as a predictor of the disease of interest. Other exposure dose representations are discussed in this section. As with cumulative dose, all these exposure variables can be derived for the whole lifetime or for a particular time period. See Checkoway *et al.* (2004) for a review of more advanced biologically based methods.

Separate variables for duration, frequency, and intensity

Separate variables for duration, frequency, and intensity of exposure might better fit a model of disease risk. In several carcinogenic processes, duration has been shown to carry more weight than other aspects of exposure. For example, lung cancer risk in lifelong smokers increases with about the second power of the number of cigarettes smoked per day, but with the fourth power of duration of smoking (Doll and Peto 1978).

Dose rate or exposure rate

Frequency and intensity can be multiplied to yield the *dose rate* or *exposure rate* in the years exposed, and this variable could then be considered separately in the data analysis from duration. For example, for supplemental vitamin C, a person who took 500 mg of vitamin C for 3–4 days per week for five years would have a dose rate of 250 mg/day, and this could be a separate variable from duration (five years) in the data analysis.

Cumulative dose above some level of intensity

An understanding of the biological relationship between exposure and disease could lead to more appropriate approaches to the representation of the exposure variables. For some diseases, causation may not be a function of cumulative dose, but rather a function of cumulative dose of only those exposures above some level of intensity. This could occur, for example, when prolonged exposure to an agent at low exposure rate can stimulate detoxification processes which would become saturated and ineffective at higher rates. In such cases, only exposures above some intensity level would lead to disease. For example, in a study of orofacial clefts in newborns in relation to maternal periconceptional alcohol consumption (1 month before to 3 months after conception), even daily drinking did not increase the risk of this birth defect (Shaw and Lammer 1999). However, weekly or more frequent episodes of consuming five or more drinks per drinking occasion was associated with risk ratios of 3–7 for various orofacial cleft syndromes.

The equation for cumulative dose above some intensity level would be similar to the equation for cumulative dose given above, except that only those exposure episodes above some level of intensity would be summed. For example, if it were hypothesized that a particular health benefit only accrued for higher-intensity physical activities, then cumulative dose of energy expenditure from physical activity would be calculated by summing only over moderate- and high-intensity activities.

Peak exposure

Finally, some diseases may be most influenced by *peak exposure*, i.e. the highest exposure level (exposure rate) experienced by a subject for some minimal amount of time (e.g. one year).

Evaluating multiple representations of dose

When the best representation of exposure dose is not known, several types of dose variables can be calculated from the data items collected and tested (alone or in combination) in models during data analysis of the epidemiological study. The model with the best fit (e.g. using a goodness of fit statistic such as −2 log likelihood) would indicate how to represent the exposure variable in terms of disease risk.

The importance of correct representation of dose was underlined in a study of different approaches to representation of exposure to formaldehyde in a cohort study of formaldehyde workers in the USA (Blair and Stewart 1990). The variables used were:

- duration of employment
- duration of exposure
- exposure rate (average exposure over years exposed)
- level for job with the highest 8-hour time-weighted average exposure
- estimated highest peak exposure
- cumulative exposure.

Duration of employment and duration of exposure were highly correlated, as were highest 8-hour time-weighted average exposure and exposure rate. Exposure rate showed little correlation with duration of employment, duration of exposure, or peak exposures. Other correlations between the variables studied were moderate. These correlations clearly show that different representations of dose will rank subjects differently according to their exposure and therefore are likely to give quite different results for the relationship between exposure and disease.

The effect of representation of exposure on results of analyses was illustrated by Lee-Feldstein (1989), who examined the effect of different representations of arsenic exposure on risk of lung cancer in several cohorts of men exposed to arsenic in copper smelting. In none of the cohorts was simple duration of employment a significant risk factor for lung cancer. In the cohort employed in the earliest time period (before 1925), the jobs with maximum level of exposure to arsenic and cumulative exposure were significantly associated with risk of cancer. For a later cohort (first employed 1925–1947), neither duration of employment nor cumulative exposure was significantly associated with risk of cancer. These studies indicate that the choice of the representation of exposure can substantially influence the results obtained.

In summary, the correct representation of the exposure dose variable is essential to valid exposure measurement. Even if the individual items collected (e.g. years and frequency of exposure) are highly accurate, an incorrect choice for the exposure dose variable could obscure the relationship of exposure to disease. Whenever the biological effects of a particular exposure and its linkage to the disease under study are not well understood, it is wise to examine the effects of several representations of exposure, within the limits of what is possible in terms of data collection. This underlines the need for adequately specified and comprehensive measurements of exposure variables.

Timing of exposure

Aetiological exposure time window

Although one notion of time, the duration of exposure, is included in the concept of dose of exposure, in this section *exposure time* refers to when the exposure occurred. Thus dose, the quantity or level of exposure, and time, when the exposure occurred, are separate concepts.

For many (if not all) diseases, it is likely that an *aetiological exposure time window* (see Figure 1.3) exists, during which a particular exposure is most relevant to causation of the disease of interest (Rothman 1981). Inclusion of episodes of that exposure before or after that time window in the exposure variable used in the data analysis would lead to exposure measurement error and its adverse effects on the results of an epidemiological study.

The time window is generally expressed by counting backwards in time from the diagnosis of disease. For example, exposures might be most critical in the time period 5–20 years before disease diagnosis. The width of the time window can represent the range of time during which a single exposure event (e.g. tubal ligation) causes or prevents disease in a population (e.g. ovarian cancer). It can also be thought of as the time window during which episodic or chronic exposures accumulate (in an individual and in the population) to complete the action of that exposure in causing the disease. For example, Pearce (1988) examined asbestos exposure during various time periods in

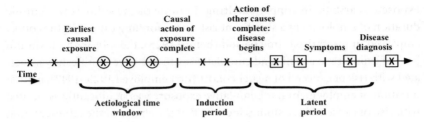

Figure 1.3 Time periods in the exposure–disease time sequence: **X** times of the exposure of interest; Ⓧ exposure episodes that cause the disease; X̄ exposure episodes that could be influenced by the disease.

relation to lung cancer mortality. He found that high cumulative asbestos exposure over the time window 20–25 years prior to death was clearly associated with the greatest risk (almost five-fold), after adjustment for exposure in other time windows.

While timing of exposure is often measured backwards from diagnosis, the critical time period when the exposure has its greatest pathological effects for some exposure–disease associations may be more related to age or to certain physiological states. These include the following time periods:

- *in utero* (or specific months *in utero*)
- childhood
- adolescence
- time in relation to pregnancy or childbirth
- time in relation to menopause
- calendar years.

For example, hormone therapy may be associated with a reduced risk of coronary heart disease for the first 10 years after menopause, while it may have an adverse effect after that time period (Salpeter *et al.* 2006). Examination of exposure time windows defined by calendar year may be important when the nature of the exposure has changed owing to secular trends. For example, the manufacturing processes and protective measures from occupational exposures may change over time.

Induction and latent periods

Rothman (1981) proposed a theory of sequential component causes of disease which states that causes must arise in a certain sequence for the disease to occur. According to this theory, after the aetiological time window for an exposure of interest, there is an induction period during which any remaining component causes in the aetiological sequence occur. The *induction period* is the interval from the time that the action of the exposure of interest is complete to the onset of disease (Figure 1.3). Further exposure to the agent of interest during the induction period does *not* contribute to disease risk. For example, adenocarcinoma of the vagina is caused by *in utero* exposure to diethylstilbestrol (DES), although the disease is usually diagnosed at about age 15–30. During the years after exposure, the other component causes occur (probably hormonal activity during adolescence) to complete the sequence of causation.

The length of the induction period depends on the specific exposure under study as well as on the disease. If the exposure of interest is early in the causal sequence, then there is a long induction period. If the exposure is late in the sequence, there is a short induction period. If it is the final cause in the sequence, there is no induction period. For example, animal models of cancer have shown that there are at least two types of causative agents: initiators which increase the risk of disease, and promoters which only increase risk if administered after the initiators. Initiators will have long induction periods and promoters shorter induction periods.

The *latent period* is the time interval from the onset of the disease until it is diagnosed (Figure 1.3). For example, for cancer, this would be the time from when one cell or clone of cells has irreversibly started the path to cancer until it has progressed to a sufficient number of cells or tumour size to be diagnosed. The length of the latent period depends on factors influencing the speed of disease progression and on factors affecting time of disease detection, such as screening. Exposures during the latent period *do not* contribute to disease aetiology, and including them will lead to misclassification of exposure (except of course, when the focus of the study is on an exposure that is hypothesized to speed disease progression). Moreover, as discussed in the next section, exposures during the latent period could be influenced by the disease.

Since the time disease begins is rarely known, the induction and latent period are often treated as a single entity, and labelled the induction period, latent period, or induction/latent period.

Excluding exposures that could be influenced by disease during the latent period

Since the disease is present in some form during the latent period, exposures during this period could be influenced by the disease (Figure 1.3). Therefore when exposures are measured during the latent period, an interpretation of an observed exposure–disease association as the exposure causing the disease could, in fact, be in the opposite direction, i.e. *reverse causality*. There are two main situations which can lead to reverse causality of the exposure–disease relationship. First, for physical or biological measures in the human body taken at any time during the latent period (or after disease diagnosis), except for fixed characteristics such as genotype, the biological effects of the disease could influence the measure of the exposure. For example, in a study of iron status and colon cancer risk, if serum iron levels were measured within the year before diagnosis, one might observe an inverse association due to occult blood loss from the tumour among cases, when in reality long-term iron levels may have no effect on or may increase colorectal cancer risk. The second situation occurs when measures of behavioural exposures are ascertained for the time period after symptoms of the disease begin. For example, in a study of colon cancer and fibre supplement intake, asking questions about fibre supplement intake for the year before diagnosis could lead to reverse causality. Those with constipation as a symptom of colon cancer might have starting taking fibre supplements, leading to a positive association of fibre supplement use and colon cancer, when in fact there may be no association or a protective effect of long-term fibre supplement use.

Therefore, when computing cumulative dose, it is important to exclude exposure episodes which occur during the time period when they could be influenced by pre-clinical disease. In case–control studies, it may be best to avoid even *collecting* information about exposures during the time period when the disease could influence the exposure. Since specimens are collected after diagnosis in case–control studies, generally only biomarkers of fixed characteristics (e.g. genotype) are appropriate for study. Information about behaviours should only be collected during a time period before symptoms are likely. This is usually handled by establishing a *reference date*, after which no exposure information is collected. This is usually the diagnosis date or some fixed time period before diagnosis for cases and an assigned date for controls. For example, for colon cancer, it could be two years before diagnosis for cases and an assigned date for controls. The assigned date for controls should be such that the distributions of calendar year of the reference year, of age at reference date, and of recall period (time from the interview date back to the reference date) are all similar for cases and controls. This is best implemented by recruiting and interviewing cases and controls simultaneously.

A reference date does not apply in cohort studies because study data and specimens are collected before the disease of interest has been diagnosed in any participants. Nonetheless, it is important to exclude exposures that could have been influenced by the biological effects of the disease or by its symptoms. When information on current exposure or a specimen for analysis is collected at a data collection point (e.g. baseline), the disease events occurring soon after the data collection point should be dropped from analysis for the time period during which the pre-clinical effects of the disease could have influenced the exposure. For example, for a study of colon cancer and fibre supplements, colon cancer cases occurring within two years after data collection could be dropped. The concern that disease could influence exposures is less of a concern if information on long-term exposure has been collected (e.g. 10-year use of fibre supplements).

Exposure variables which include timing of exposure

Although it is most important to exclude exposure episodes during that part of the latent period during which disease could influence exposure, it is also beneficial to exclude *all* exposure episodes which occurred outside the aetiological exposure window, to make the results of the epidemiological study more accurate (Figure 1.3). Unfortunately, the lengths of the aetiological window and the induction/latent period are not usually known with any certainty. However, collection of the details of the timing and dose of exposure over a long time period will at least permit analyses that examine the length of the induction/latent period and of the aetiological time window.

Several types of variable can be used to express how the timing of exposure is related to disease risk. These are described below.

Time since first/last exposure

For exposures with finite durations (e.g. medication use or occupational exposures), an analysis of the effect of timing of exposure usually begins with an examination of the effects of time since first exposure (or age at first exposure) and time since last exposure on risk of disease. *Time since first exposure* is the time from the first exposure to diagnosis for cases and from first exposure to a similar date assigned to controls (see above for how reference dates are assigned). For early-stage causes, the exposure–disease association will be strongest for those where many years have elapsed since exposure began. For example, studies from Australia (English and Armstrong 1988), Europe (Autier *et al.* 1997), and Hawaii (Le Marchand *et al.* 2006) report that early age of migration from a low-UV to a high-UV exposure area is a risk factor for melanoma.

The *time since last exposure* is the time from the last exposure to diagnosis for cases and from the last exposure to a similar assigned date for controls. For late-stage causes, those individuals exposed within some recent period would experience the greatest increased risk, while those whose last exposure was in the more distant past might have not have had the other necessary subsequent causes and their risk has returned to close to that of unexposed individuals. If only recent exposures increase risk, then there is a short induction/latent period, and the exposure is a late-stage cause. For example, a study in Italy found that current smokers had an approximate threefold increased risk of acute myocardial infarction, while those whose last exposure was two years or more in the past had risks close to those of non-smokers (Negri *et al.* 1994).

Latency analysis

Another approach to considering timing of exposure is to count only distant exposures before disease when computing the cumulative dose (or other dose variable) in order to exclude more recent exposure episodes which occurred during the presumed induction/latent period. This is called *latency analysis* (or *exposure lagging* in cohort studies), and it increases study power to detect an early stage cause because exposures during the induction/latent period would not have contributed to disease risk. For example, in an analysis of asbestos exposure and lung cancer mortality (Checkoway *et al.* 1990), a model with a cumulative exposure variable which excluded the most recent 10 years of asbestos exposure showed a steeper dose–response gradient compared with a model which included all exposure (Table 1.2).

Recency analysis

One can also consider only recent exposures in computation of dose; this is sometimes called *recency analysis*. The aim is to remove exposures which

Table 1.2 Relative risks for asbestos exposure and lung cancer mortality using latency and exposure window methods[a]

	Exposure in model		
Cumulative exposure[b]	**Cumulative exposure : no latency**	**Cumulative exposure: 10 year latency**	**Cumulative exposure in time window 10–25 years[c]**
1 (ref.)–low	1.0	1.0	1.0
2	2.1	2.3	2.6
3	1.5	2.4	2.0
4	3.4	5.2	3.3
5	4.3	4.0	6.0
6	5.7	6.9	9.8
7–high	11.2	15.3	17.0

[a] Adapted from Checkoway *et al.* 1990, with permission.
[b] Strata defined so that each contains five lung cancer deaths; stratum boundaries vary between models.
[c] Years prior to death.

occurred before the aetiological time window in order to increase study power to detect late-stage causes, because earlier exposures would not have contributed to disease risk. For example, based on the study of myocardial infarction cited above, including smoking dose for only a year before diagnosis for cases (and a similar time period for controls) might be the most accurate representation of smoking in relation to myocardial infarction.

Exposure time window analysis

A final approach would be only to count exposures during the hypothesized aetiological time window by removing exposure episodes which occurred both before and after that window. If such a window exists, this type of analysis will have the most power to detect an exposure–disease association. For example, in the models from the study of lung cancer mortality shown in Table 1.2, the dose–response gradient of risk was steepest for the model in which the asbestos cumulative exposure variable only included asbestos exposure during the period 10–25 years before lung cancer death.

Timing of exposure in cohort studies

The above approaches have been described within the context of a case–control study. In a prospective cohort study, during which subjects complete one or several exposure assessments and are followed up for outcomes, the approach would be different. The risk of disease in each follow-up year would be based on each subject's exposure counted backwards from that year, i.e. exposure would be time dependent. For example, in the analysis presented in the last column of Table 1.2, the exposure was calculated for each subject for each follow-up year as the cumulative dose of asbestos for the time window 10–25 years before that follow-up year.

Statistical issues and more advanced methods

Although this book does not cover data analysis of epidemiological studies (except for validity and reliability studies), in this section we provide some guidance for analyses of dose and timing of exposure in relation to disease risk.

As noted above, the lengths of the induction/latent period and the aetiological exposure window are usually not known, but the investigator could investigate different lengths of these two time periods to see which model best fits the study data. This can be done by including cumulative exposure variables for non-overlapping time windows in the same model in order to look for the exposure time period with the greatest strength of association or statistical significance within the model. This approach was taken in an analysis of non-steroidal anti-inflammatory drug use and colorectal cancer (Collet *et al.* 1999) which considered exposure in five discreet time windows. They found that cumulative dose over the 11–15 years before diagnosis was associated with a much greater risk reduction than the other periods. Another approach is to examine multiple (overlapping) induction/latent periods or exposure time windows, each in a separate model, and compare the models for goodness of fit. This was the approach taken by Longstreth *et al.* (2004) in a study of dental X-rays and intracranial meningioma. They examined 10-year exposure time windows with a latency (induction/latent period) which varied from 10 to 35 years before diagnosis, by one-year increments. They found that, among women, an induction/latent period of 28 years led to the greatest association; specifically, the number of full-mouth dental X-rays during the 10-year window 28–37 years before diagnosis showed the strongest association with disease risk.

Exploratory modelling, such as that described earlier to select the best dose variable or that described above to determine the most critical exposure time period, must be interpreted with caution. When one selects from several models based on the one with the greatest effect size, significance, or goodness of fit, the one selected will tend to overestimate the effect size or significance due to chance.

Another statistical concern is that certain components of dose and time are correlated and need to be modelled simultaneously. For example, cumulative dose and age at first exposure would generally be correlated; for example, those who began drinking daily at a young age would generally also have higher life-time cumulative dose of alcohol. Thus, when examining the effect of one, the other would need to be adjusted for in the model. Similarly when considering cumulative exposure dose during one time period, one would need to adjust for cumulative dose of the exposure during other time periods, as exposure to the same agent in different time periods in life would be correlated.

Finally, the above approaches of latency, recency, and exposure time window analyses make the assumption that exposures in any given time period either do or do not contribute to disease risk. In reality, some form of weighted cumulative exposure may be more appropriate, with different time windows carrying different weights. This approach has been used for silica crystals and asbestos, which have long retention times (e.g. Dement *et al.* 1983). Seixas *et al.* (1993) describe a general model to determine the optimal weights for different exposure time periods.

A more comprehensive account of the representation and/or modelling of the relationships between exposure, time, and response can be found in Breslow and Day (1987), Thomas (1988), Rothman and Greenland (1998), and Checkoway *et al.* (2004).

Items to measure in a study

After the issues discussed above have been considered, the next step is to determine the individual items to measure in the study. The researcher begins by creating a comprehensive list of the items required to compute the dose variable for the main exposure(s) of interest plus the items needed for its valid analysis, including known or suspected confounding factors and factors hypothesized to modify the effects of the main exposure on the outcome.

To ensure that all required items are included, the researcher should have:

◆ a statement of the complete research objectives

◆ a detailed algorithm for the main exposure dose variable(s)

◆ a data analysis plan.

It is tempting to create a list of items before the last two steps have been formulated. However, without full planning, the researcher can find at the time of data analysis that a key item needed to compute exposure dose or an important confounding factor was not collected. Therefore it is important to have thought through the exposure dose variables and the other variables that will be needed at the end of data collection *before* creating the list of items to measure at the beginning of a study.

In creating the list of data items to collect, there is often a conflict between the desire to collect information considered to be necessary to the objectives of the study and the need to not overburden participants. Increased burden can lead to study refusal or withdrawal, or inaccuracy of measurements. For this reason, the aim of an epidemiological study may need to be quite focused, to allow complete measurement of one or a few primary exposures. Inclusion of each additional item should be judged against the aims of the study.

Table 1.3 gives a list of items to consider for data collection; these are discussed in more detail below.

Items needed to compute dose and evaluate timing of exposure

To compute the cumulative exposure dose, one needs to collect information on duration, frequency, and intensity (dose per episode) for each type of exposure with the active agent. Thus one of the first steps is to clarify which external exposures have the active agent. As noted above, it is important to have the exposure variable be specific to that agent to avoid mixing it with other similar exposures that do not have the activity. For example, if caffeine is the likely active agent in coffee that reduces the risk of Parkinson's disease, then separate questions on caffeinated and decaffeinated coffee would need to be asked. The exposure variable also needs to be sensitive, i.e. it needs

Table 1.3 Types of items collected in epidemiological studies

Items needed to compute exposure dose (for each type of exposure with the active agent)
Age began and age ended (or age at each event if exposure is infrequent)
Frequency of exposure during that time:

Episodes per day/week/month
Units (e.g. number of minutes of exercise, number of pills) per episode

Intensity (dose of active agent per unit) directly for each subject (e.g. dose of active agent per pill) or indirectly by asking details about exposure (e.g. brand name of drug) to link to an external database of intensity
External database of intensity by type of exposure (e.g. energy expenditure by activity, drug formulation by brand)

Items needed to evaluate effect of timing of exposure
Age began and age ended for each type of exposure (as above)
Ages at physiological states which may define aetiologically important time periods (e.g. menarche, childbirth, menopause)

Other features of exposure
Route of exposure
Protective factors (e.g. sunscreen, respirator use)

Potential confounders of behavioural exposure–disease associations
Risk factors for the disease
Factors associated with initiation or duration of exposure, e.g. indications for use of drug (ascertained for both exposed and non-exposed)
Factors associated with avoidance or discontinuation of exposure, e.g. contraindications for a drug
Demographic and behavioural correlates of exposure

Potential confounders of biomarker–disease associations
Body mass
Current health
Behavioural and endogenous factors associated with production, transport, or clearance of biomarker
Factors in handling and analysis, e.g. time from specimen collection to freezing, time in freezer, laboratory batch in which specimen was analysed

Other factors
Potential effect modifiers of exposure–disease association
Factors related to the biological mechanism(s)
Screening for the disease (ascertained for both cases and controls)

Factors to describe the study population
Age
Sex
Race
Education and/or socio-economic status
Other factors used in subject selection

to include the full range of exposures which have the active agent. Therefore for caffeine exposure, one would need to collect information on consumption of caffeinated tea, carbonated beverages containing caffeine, and use of analgesics by brand or type, to separate those analgesics that contain caffeine from those that do not.

Information on duration and frequency of each type of exposure with the active agent also needs to be collected. For infrequent exposures such as major medical X-rays, one could ascertain the age (or year) of each exposure. For chronic exposures, one could assess age begun, age ended, and frequency (per day, week, or month) of exposure. Frequency sometimes needs to be assessed by two (or more) questions: frequency of the exposure episodes and 'units' of exposure per episode. For example, for medications, one may need to ascertain days per week and pills per day, or for food intake, one could ask subjects about frequency of consumption of each type of food and portion size.

Intensity (dose of active agent per episode or per unit of exposure, depending on how one asks about frequency) can be ascertained directly for each subject (e.g. by asking questions or from pharmacy records), or enough detail about the exposure should be collected so that the researcher can link the exposure type to intensity codes from an external source. For example, for a study of caffeine exposure, if each subject is asked about the brand(s) or type(s) of analgesics used, the researcher can use this information to determine the amount of caffeine per pill. Before data collection begins, the researcher should gather the information on intensity that comes from these external sources, such as formulations of a specific class of drug or tables of energy expenditure by type of activity. By scrutinizing these tables before a study begins, the researcher will know what level of detail is needed for each subject. For example, the calendar year that a specific drug was taken might be needed to determine its formulation, if that formulation has changed over time. For recreational activity, determining energy expenditure might require not just knowledge of the type of activities each subject engaged in (e.g. walking), but also, for some activities, the level of intensity the subject put into the activity (e.g. pace of walking).

If frequency or intensity of exposure commonly changes over time within subjects, then one would need to ascertain age began, age ended, frequency, and intensity for each change in pattern of exposures. For example, one could ask about the age begun and the age ended for each brand of oral contraceptives taken.

If the aetiologically important time window is related to a physiological state rather than years before diagnosis (assessed via age), then the study also needs information on the age of the physiological state (e.g. age at menarche, age of first pregnancy, age at menopause).

Other features of an exposure may also be important to collect. One aspect is the route of exposure to the agent. For example, oral but not nasal use of snuff may cause cancer of the mouth. Another is behaviours that may protect against exposure. For example, in a study of the relationship of sun exposure to skin cancer, it would be important to record the use of protective clothing and sunscreens as well as the amount, pattern, and duration of outdoor exposure. Protective factors could be incorporated into the computation of cumulative dose, or treated as separate variables that are potential effect modifiers.

Other items

The other items to be collected include potential confounders, effect modifiers, and general descriptive data about the population.

Confounders are factors associated with the disease (independent of exposure) and associated with the exposure (independent of disease). Confounding is one of the major sources of bias in epidemiological studies, and information on potential confounding factors must be collected to assure a valid data analysis.

A detailed review of the epidemiology of the disease will lead to a list of disease risk factors that may be confounders. Typically, information on all major risk factors for the disease under study are collected (within the limits imposed by participant burden and study costs), even factors that are unlikely to confound the specific exposure–disease relationship under study.

In preparing a list of potential confounders, the factors associated with the exposure are less often considered but are an important group. These include factors related to the initiation or duration of exposure and factors associated with its avoidance or discontinuation. For example, for drugs, it is important to consider the reasons for use. If a condition that is an indication for use is also a risk factor for the disease, then failure to control for that condition would lead to *confounding by indication*. For example, in a study of oral contraceptive use during adolescence and breast cancer risk, it is possible that some of the indications for use at an early age (dysmenorrhoea or acne) are markers of endogenous hormone levels that are related to breast cancer risk. Therefore, for drug exposures, one should ascertain for all subjects (both users and non-users of the drug) the medical conditions that are the indications and contraindications for the drug to be able to control for them in the analysis.

Demographic and behavioural correlates of the main exposures of interest should also be considered. Healthy behaviours tend to be correlated;

for example, one study found that long-term users of calcium supplements exercised more, ate more fruits and vegetables, and participated more often in cancer screening than those who did not take calcium supplements (White *et al.* 2004). Unhealthy behaviours (e.g. cigarette smoking and excessive alcohol intake) are also often correlated.

Consideration of confounding is needed even with the use of measures in human specimens. For instance, a biomarker may be correlated with body mass, with acute and chronic illnesses, and with current behaviours (e.g. diet and medication use) and endogenous factors (e.g. genetic factors and other biomarkers) associated with its production, transport, and/or clearance. The level of a biomarker can also be influenced by variations between subjects in specimen handling and analysis, for example the time from specimen collection to freezing, the time in the freezer, and the laboratory batch in which the specimen was analysed. These factors should be recorded, because if they differ between cases and controls, they can be confounders.

Other types of covariates that the researcher should consider measuring are potential effect modifiers of the exposure–disease relationship, measures related to the biological mechanism(s), and measures of screening for the disease. Effect modifiers that are often considered are demographic factors, other risk factors for the disease, and factors related to the exposure–disease causal pathway.

Finally, certain universal factors are always collected in a study to describe the population fully for comparison with other studies and to help understand the generalizability of the study results. These include age, sex, race, education or socio-economic status, and other factors used in the selection of the population(s) for study.

The measurement instrument

The final step in planning for exposure measurement is the selection or development of a measurement instrument (Figure 1.1). In this book, we use the term *measurement instrument* or *measurement method* to refer to a procedure designed to measure one or several of the variables of interest in an epidemiological study. Examples of measurement instruments include:

- self-administered questionnaires
- personal interviews
- abstraction of medical records
- diaries, such as food diaries
- biochemical analysis of blood or other specimens from the subjects
- physical or chemical analysis of the environment.

We use the term measurement instrument in its broadest sense to include all aspects of the measurement process involving individual subjects:

- instructions for application of the measurement method
- the method itself
- specification of procedures that follow application of the main method, up to the point of presentation of a 'clean' data file for analysis.

For example, in the case of a personal interview, it will include:

- specifications for the training of interviewers and instructions given to them
- instructions or explanations given by interviewers to subjects
- the questionnaire used to elicit data from the subjects
- the subsequent editing of the completed interview by the interviewer, by the supervisor, and/or by computer
- other quality control procedures.

In the case of the measurement of the concentration of some analyte in blood, it will include:

- procedures for the preparation of subjects
- procedures for the collection, transport, and storage of the specimen
- analytical procedures in the laboratory
- attendant quality control procedures.

A measurement instrument deserves to be so called only when all the procedures outlined above are written down in such detail that one set of investigators could, within the limits of biological or physical variability, reproduce the measurements obtained by another using only this written description.

Summary

In epidemiology, the word exposure is used as a broad term to denote any of a subject's attributes or any agent which may be a cause or predictor of the disease (or outcome) under study. The objective of exposure measurement is to measure the exposure(s) of interest as accurately as possible, within the practical constraints of limiting subject burden and study costs.

Issues that need to be considered early in the process of exposure measurement include the following.

- What is the active agent, i.e. the component of the exposure (e.g. a chemical compound or biological activity) which causes (or prevents) the disease of interest?

- What exposures have and do not have the active agent? An exposure measure needs to be specific, i.e. it should isolate exposures with the causal agent from similar exposures that do not. An exposure measure also needs to sensitive, i.e. it needs to include all sources of the active agent of interest.

- Where on the biological exposure–disease pathway (from available dose in the external environment to active dose at the target site in the body) should the exposure be measured to best meet the study aims?

- On what scale will the measurements be made: continuous, ordered categorical, nominal categorical, or dichotomous? It is best to collect the individual data items from each subject in the most detailed form possible; this allows the researcher the greatest flexibility at the time of study data analysis.

Except for the simplest exposures, the most important exposure variable is the exposure dose, i.e. the amount of exposure. Analysis of exposure dose increases study power compared with only considering the presence or absence of exposure, and demonstration of a dose–response gradient is part of the evidence for causality. The following issues need to be considered in creating an algorithm for exposure dose.

- What is the best representation of exposure dose in terms of disease causality? This is often cumulative dose, which generally takes the form:

$$\text{duration} \times \text{frequency} \times \text{intensity}$$

where intensity is the dose of the active agent per episode of exposure and the above equation is summed over each type of exposure that has the active agent. However, other representations such as cumulative dose summed over only high-intensity exposures (e.g. only high-intensity activities) or use of separate variables for duration and dose rate (frequency × intensity) might better express the relation of the exposure to the disease of interest.

- During what time period is the exposure most likely to cause the disease (the aetiological exposure time window)? By excluding exposure episodes which occur before that time window (recency analysis), after that time period (latency analysis) or both before and after (exposure window analysis), the exposure dose variable will be more accurate and therefore the study will have more power to detect an exposure–disease association. The time period is usually measured backward from disease diagnosis, but instead there could be a specific critical exposure time period in life, such as childhood.

- Could the disease have influenced the exposure in some subjects? Exposures that could be influenced by the disease, i.e. behaviours that are measured for times when the cases might have had symptoms or biomarkers that are not fixed and that were measured during the latent period of the disease, should *not* be included in the exposure dose variable. To do so could lead to reverse causality.

After the above issues have been considered, the researcher should then prepare a list of individual items to be measured in the study. These include the items to assess duration and frequency of exposure and enough information about the exposure (e.g. type of recreational activity or brand name of drug) to impute an intensity for that exposure type. Confounders must also be measured; correlates of the exposure should be considered as potential confounders as well as other risk factors for the disease. A final step in planning for exposure measurement is the selection or development of the measurement instrument(s), i.e. the procedure(s) designed to measure the items of interest, such as an interviewer-administered questionnaire. It is essential to the reproducibility of exposure measurements that these procedures be documented fully in writing.

About this book

We describe the scope of this book by discussing how the topics covered fit within the context of designing, conducting, and interpreting an epidemiological study. Some of these steps are shown in Figure 1.1.

A study begins with the researcher formulating the study hypothesis, aims, and significance. As discussed earlier in this chapter, this should include a conceptualization of the true exposure and the time period over which it might cause disease.

The next step is study design, which is an iterative process as follows.

(a) Selecting the type of study (e.g. case–control), the study populations(s), the sampling scheme, and sample size. These topics are well covered in most books on epidemiological methods, and are not included in this book.

(b) Formulating an operational definition of the exposure variable (e.g. cumulative dose) and an algorithm for its computation, and determining the items needed for the dose variable(s), confounders and effect modifiers. These topics have been covered in this chapter.

(c) Selecting the type of instrument(s) to be used to collect the exposure information (e.g. an in-person interview, use of records, or analysis of human specimens). In Chapter 2, we introduce the methods of exposure measurement commonly used in epidemiology and outline the considerations that go into deciding which method, or methods, to use in a particular study. For the researcher to understand if the exposure variable as measured by a specific instrument is sufficiently accurate to meet the aims of the study, he/she must read the literature on, or conduct a study of, the accuracy of the exposure measure. Chapters 3 and 4 deal extensively with the design, analysis, and interpretation of validity and reliability studies of exposure measures.

(d) Formulating study outcomes and how they will be defined. This topic tends to be specific to the disease or condition to be studied and is not covered in this book, although many of the principles of measurement discussed here would apply to outcomes as well as to exposures.

Once the study has been designed (and funded!), there is a period of detailed planning and refinement. This involves, for example, the actual construction of the wording and format of the questionnaire and the development of the procedures for collecting and analysing specimens. During this time, study staff are hired and trained, a detailed study procedure manual is written, procedures are pre-tested, and quality control approaches are developed. In Chapter 5, we cover general quality control procedures for development of instruments and procedures, staff training and supervision, pre-testing, and data processing, as well as other general methods of reducing exposure measurement error. Then we discuss these topics in the specific context of design of questionnaires in Chapter 6; the personal interview in Chapter 7; the use of diaries, proxy respondents, and records in Chapter 8; measurements in human subjects themselves in Chapter 9; and measurements in the environment in Chapter 10.

As part of the study planning, issues relating to recruitment of the study participants must also be considered. We discuss strategies to maximize response rates in epidemiological studies in Chapter 11, which departs from the preceding theme of accurate measurement of exposure *in individuals* to accurate measurement of exposure in *whole populations*. Finally, in Chapter 12, the ethical issues raised by the methods of exposure measurement are discussed and advice is given regarding ethical practice in epidemiology.

After a study is planned, the study implementation begins. As shown in Figure 1.1, during study execution, the instrument is used to collect the data items needed, with the associated quality control procedures and methods to enhance subject participation. Then, during data processing, the data items collected are used to create the exposure variable(s) needed in the data analysis. After the statistical analysis is completed, study report(s) are written. One important topic discussed in any study report is the potential biases that impact on the validity of the results of the study. Two aspects of this are addressed in this book: misclassification bias due to the measured exposure not accurately representing the true exposure of interest (covered in Chapters 3 and 4), and selection bias introduced by failing to include all those who were eligible for the study (discussed in Chapter 11).

Although much of this book is about *conducting* epidemiological studies, we have primarily presented the content in terms of *planning* epidemiological studies. This is to emphasize the point that the more thought and effort that goes into study planning, the fewer problems will occur during the often lengthy time period over which epidemiological studies are conducted and analysed.

We do not deal with the measurement of specific exposures in epidemiology except by way of illustration of general principles. Some recent books which cover the measurement of specific exposures include the following: for diet, Willett (1998); for physical activity and fitness, Welk (2002); for medication use, Strom and Kimmel (2006); for psychosocial measures related to health, McDowell and Newell (1996) and Bowling (1997); for sexually related behaviours and attitudes, Davis *et al.* (1997); and for occupational and environmental exposures, Nieuwenhuijsen (2003) and Checkoway *et al.* (2004). The overall aim of this book is to provide general principles and methods to help advance these areas and less studied or new areas of exposure measurement.

References

Ainsworth, B.E., Haskell, W.L., Whitt, M.C., *et al.* (2000). Compendium of physical activities: an update of activity codes and MET intensities. *Medicine and Science in Sports and Exercise*, **32**, S498–504.

Anderson, D.W. and Mantel, N. (1983). On epidemiologic surveys. *American Journal of Epidemiology*, **118**, 613–19.

Autier, P., Dore, J.F., Gefeller, O., *et al.* (1997). Melanoma risk and residence in sunny areas. *British Journal of Cancer*, **76**, 1521–4.

Blair, A. and Stewart, P.A. (1990). Correlation between different measures of occupational exposure to formaldehyde. *American Journal of Epidemiology*, **131**, 510–16.

Bowling, A. (1997). *Measuring Health: A Review of Quality of Life Measurement Scales* (2nd edn). Open University Press, Philadelphia, PA.

Breslow, N.E. and Day, N.E. (1987). *Statistical Methods in Cancer Research*. Vol. II, *The Design and Analysis of Cohort Studies*, pp. 232–70. International Agency for Research on Cancer, Lyon.

Checkoway, H., Pearce, N., Hickey, J.L.S., and Dement, J.M. (1990). Latency analysis in occupational epidemiology. *Archives of Environmental Health*, **45**, 95–100.

Checkoway, H., Pearce, N.. and Kriebel, D. (2004). *Research Methods in Occupational Epidemiology* (2nd edn). Oxford University Press.

Collet, J.-P., Sharpe, C., Belzile, E., Boivin, J.-F., Hanley, J., and Abenhaim, L. (1999). Colorectal cancer prevention by non-sterodal anti-inflammatory drugs: effects of dosage and timing. *British Journal of Cancer*, **81**, 62–68.

Davis, C.M., Yarber, W.L., Bauserman, R., Scheer, G., and Davis, S.L. (1997). *Handbook of Sexually-Related Measures*. Sage, Thousand Oaks, CA.

Dement, J.M., Harris, R.L., Symons, M.J., and Shy, CM. (1983). Exposures and mortality among chrysotile asbestos workers. II: Mortality. *American Journal of Industrial Medicine*, **4**, 421–33.

Doll, R. and Peto, R. (1978). Cigarette smoking and bronchial carcinoma: dose and time relationships among regular smokers and lifelong non-smokers. *Journal of Epidemiology and Community Health*, **32**, 303–13.

English, D.R. and Armstrong, B.K. (1988). Identifying people at high risk of cutaneous malignant melanoma: results from a case–control study in Western Australia. *British Medical Journal*, **296**, 1285–8.

Goude, G. (1962). *On Fundamental Measurements in Psychology*. Almqvist and Wiksell, Stockholm.

Lee-Feldstein, A. (1989). A comparison of several measures of exposure to arsenic: matched case–control study of copper smelter employees. *American Journal of Epidemiology*, **129**, 112–24.

Le Marchand, L., Saltzman. B.S., Hankin, J.H., *et al.* (2006). Sun exposure, diet, and melanoma in Hawaii Caucasians. *American Journal of Epidemiology*, **164**, 232–45.

Longstreth, W.T., Jr, Phillips, L.E., Drangsholt, M., *et al.* (2004). Dental X-rays and the risk of intracranial meningioma: a population-based case–control study. *Cancer*, **100**, 1026–34.

McDowell, I. and Newell, C. (1996). *Measuring Health* (2nd edn). Oxford University Press.

Negri, E., La Vecchia, C., D'Avanzo, B., Nobili, A., and La Malfa, R.G. (1994). Acute myocardial infarction: association with time since stopping smoking in Italy. *Journal of Epidemiology and Community Health*, **48**, 129–33.

Nieuwenhuijsen, M. J. (ed.) (2003). *Exposure Assessment In Occupational and Environmental Epidemiology*. Oxford University Press.

Pearce, N. (1988). Multistage modeling of lung cancer mortality in asbestos textile workers. *International Journal of Epidemiology*, **17**, 747–52.

Pereira, M.A., Parker, E.D., and Folsom, A.R. (2006). Coffee consumption and risk of type 2 diabetes mellitus: an 11-year prospective study of 28 812 postmenopausal women. *Archives of Internal Medicine*, **166**, 1311–16.

Ross, G.W., Abbott, R.D., Petrovitch, H., *et al.* (2000). Association of coffee and caffeine intake with the risk of Parkinson disease. *Journal of the American Medical Association*, **283**, 2674–9.

Rothman, K.J. (1981). Induction and latent periods. *American Journal of Epidemiology*, **114**, 253–9.

Rothman, K.J. and Greenland, S. (1998). *Modern Epidemiology* (2nd edn). Lippincott–Williams & Wilkins, Philadelphia, PA.

Salpeter, S.R., Walsh, J.M., Greyber, E., and Salpeter, E.E. (2006). Coronary heart disease events associated with hormone therapy in younger and older women: a meta-analysis. *Journal of General Internal Medicine*, **21**, 363–366.

Schakel, S.F., Buzzard, I.M., and Gebhardt, S.E. (1997). Procedures for estimating nutrient values for food composition databases. *Journal of Food Composition and Analysis*, **10**, 102–14.

Schulte, P.A. (1993). A conceptual and historical framework for molecular epidemiology. In *Molecular Epidemiology: Principles and Practices* (ed. P.A. Schulte and F.P. Perera), pp. 3–44. Academic Press, San Diego, CA.

Seixas, N.S., Robins, T.G., and Becker, M. (1993). A novel approach to the characterization of cumulative exposure for the study of chronic occupational disease. *American Journal of Epidemiology*, **137**, 463–71.

Shaw, G.M. and Lammer, E.J. (1999). Maternal periconceptional alcohol consumption and risk for orofacial clefts. *Journal of Pediatrics*, **134**, 298–303.

Stevens, S.S. (1951). Mathematics, measurement and psychophysics. In *Handbook of Experimental Psychology* (ed. S.S. Stevens), pp. 1–49. Wiley, New York.

Stevens, S.S. (1968). Measurement, statistics and the schemapiric view. *Science*, **161**, 849–56.

Strom, B.L. and Kimmel, S.F. (ed.) (2006). *Textbook of Pharmacoepidemiology*. Wiley, Chichester.

Thomas, D.C. (1988). Models of exposure–time–response relationships with applications to cancer epidemiology. *Annual Review of Public Health*, **9**, 451–82.

Welk, G.J. (2002). *Physical Activity Assessments for Health-Related Research*. Human Kinetics, Champaign, IL.

Weiss, N.S. (1981). Inferring causal relationships: elaboration of the criterion of 'dose–response'. *American Journal of Epidemiology*, **113**, 487–90.

White, E., Patterson, R.E., Kristal, A.R., *et al.* (2004). VITamins And Lifestyle cohort study: study design and characteristics of supplement users. *American Journal of Epidemiology*, **159**, 83–93.

Willett, W. (1989). An overview of issues related to the correction of non-differential exposure measurement error in epidemiologic studies. *Statistics in Medicine*, **8**, 1031–40.

Willett, W. (1998). *Nutritional Epidemiology* (2nd edn). Oxford University Press.

2

Methods of exposure measurement

Accuracy and 'practicability' (of data collection methods) are often inversely correlated. A method providing more satisfactory information will often be a more elaborate, expensive or inconvenient one ... Accuracy must be balanced against practical considerations, and that method chosen which will provide the maximal accuracy within the bounds of the investigator's resources and other practical limitations.
(Abramson 1984)

Introduction

Methods used for the measurement of exposure in epidemiology range from objective methods of measurement of fixed human attributes (e.g. blood type) that are as precise and valid as any in biomedical science, to methods that depend totally on the imperfect capacity of human beings to recall information. Furthermore, past exposures are often important in epidemiological studies, and typically neither objective methods (e.g. laboratory assays) nor subjective methods (e.g. interview) can accurately capture past exposures.

In this chapter, we provide a classification of and a brief introduction to the methods of measurement of exposure that are used in epidemiology. The issues that must be considered in choosing a method for a particular study are outlined. The choice between face-to-face interview, telephone interview, and self-administered questionnaire is dealt with in detail because of the importance of self-report of information about exposure.

Classification of exposures

Exposures can be classified in a number of ways which determine different approaches to their measurement.

Personal attribute or environmental agent?

The measurement of personal attributes implies access to data about individual subjects. On the other hand, it is possible to document *potential* exposure to environmental agents without any specific information about individual subjects except that they were resident in the environment measured and could have been exposed to the agent of interest. Measurements of environmental agents without knowledge of individual exposure to them is the hallmark of ecological studies of disease aetiology.

Subjective or objective data?

Whether recording an individual attribute or contact with an agent in the environment, we commonly depend on subjective statements about the attribute or contact. The person providing the subjective data may be either the subject of our study or a proxy respondent. Subjective responses are prone to manifold sources of error including, among others:

- lack of understanding of the task by the subject
- failure in recall of the required data
- the effects of the perceived threat of a topic of questioning on the subject's response to it.

The alternatives to subjective data are reference to records of exposure, observation by the investigator, or chemical or physical measurements on the subject or the environment. Subjectivity cannot be eliminated entirely from any of these alternatives, but responsibility for its control is moved away from the research subject towards the investigator and, to that extent, they are more 'objective' measurements.

Present or past exposure?

Data on present exposure (i.e. exposure at the time of data collection for the study) may be of limited usefulness in chronic disease epidemiology. First, present exposure may not correlate highly with aetiologically relevant exposure that occurred some time in the past (Rothman 1981) and, secondly, there could be uncertainty, in some situations, over whether exposure preceded disease or disease preceded exposure. The documentation of past exposure is inevitably more difficult than the documentation of present exposure. It usually requires either records of the exposure or recourse to human memory. Of course, in prospective cohort studies 'present' exposure data from questionnaires and/or biological specimens collected years before diagnosis of the disease of interest would provide more accurate information on earlier exposures than questionnaires and specimens collected closer to diagnosis.

However, even in long-term cohort studies, past exposures would often be needed to capture the aetiologically important time period for the cases that occur early in the follow-up period.

Methods overview

Table 2.1 lists the methods available for the measurement of exposure in epidemiology and classifies them according to the types of measurements that they can make in the terms that have been described above. These methods are introduced briefly below; they are described in more detail in Chapters 6–10.

Personal interview

The personal interview, whether face-to-face or by telephone, is the most commonly used method of obtaining data about subjects themselves or their environments. It permits the collection of data on past as well as present exposure, although both are subject to numerous sources of errors in recall. There is a tendency for subjects to over-report socially desirable behaviours and under-report socially undesirable behaviours. This is called *social desirability bias*. Over-reporting may also occur when recall is requested for a particular period in the past. Subjects tend to recall instances of exposure that occurred outside the exposure period, and report them as occurring within the exposure period. This is called *telescoping*. Low-impact exposures may have been forgotten. Also, present exposures (e.g. present diet) may influence recall about past exposures (e.g. past diet). The health, mood, and motivation of the respondents at the time of the interview may also influence their responses. Moreover, these sources of recall error could differ between those with and without the disease under study; this form of differential measurement error is called *recall bias*.

The involvement of an interviewer in the data collection process has several advantages. The interviewer helps secure the subject's cooperation, reduces misunderstanding about the meaning of questions, and maximizes, by prompting, the collection of usable data. More data, and more detailed and complex data, can be collected in the course of an interview than, say, by means of a self-administered questionnaire. However, it is also possible that the interviewer could introduce error, either through his/her misunderstanding of the tasks or indirectly by influencing the subject's responses. The main disadvantage of personal interviews is their cost.

Telephone interviewing and face-to-face interviews differ in certain respects. In telephone interviews, the use of visual cues, such as 'show cards' with the possible question responses, is impossible, and must be compensated for in

Table 2.1 Methods of exposure measurement in epidemiology classified according to whether they collect mainly subjective or objective data and can measure present or past exposure to personal attributes or environmental agents

Measurement method	Data		Time		Type of exposure	
	Subjective	Objective	Present	Past	Personal attribute	Environmental exposure
Personal interview	+	–	+	+	+	+
Self-administered questionnaire	+	–	+	+	+	+
Diary	+	–	+	–	+	+
Observation by investigator	–	+	+	–	+	+
Reference to records	–	+	+	+	+	+
Physical or chemical measurements on subject	–	+	+	–	+	+
Physical or chemical measurements on environment	–	+	+	+	–	+

questionnaire design. There is evidence that this compensation may lead to response differences, which are described below (section on the method of administration of questionnaires). In addition, certain communication styles differ between telephone and in-person communication. The 'expectant pause', for example, cannot be used as effectively as a probe for additional information on the telephone. One of the few advantages of the telephone over face-to-face interviews is that the presence of others (e.g. the respondent's spouse) is unlikely to influence the subject's responses in telephone interviews.

Most interviewing of subjects for epidemiological studies is now conducted as *computer-assisted interviewing* (CAI). The types of CAI and acronyms for them are listed in Table 2.2. These include *computer-assisted personal interviewing* (CAPI), using a portable computer in the respondent's home, and *computer-assisted telephone interviewing* (CATI). CAI can aid the interviewer in several ways, including the programming of the proper skip pattern for questions and immediate checks for out-of-range or conflicting responses (de Leeuw and Nicholls 1996; Nicholls *et al.* 1997). In addition to these advantages, computer-assisted telephone interviewing (CATI) has the advantage of allowing automated tracking of calls and online monitoring of interviews by a supervisor, who can see the computer screen currently visible to the interviewer as well as hear the interview. The main disadvantages of CAI are the start-up costs for incorporating new technology into a research setting.

Details about questionnaire design and interviewing are covered in Chapters 6 and 7.

Self-administered questionnaires

Self-administered questionnaires are limited by the same sources of recall error (e.g. poor recall of low impact exposures) as the personal interview.

Table 2.2 Types of computer-aided administration of questionnaires and their acronyms

Acronym	Type of questionnaire administration
CAI	Computer-assisted interviewing
CAPI	Computer-assisted personal interviewing
CATI	Computer-assisted telephone interviewing
CASAQ	Computer-assisted self-administered questionnaire
ACASI	Audio computer-assisted self-interviewing
VCASI	Video computer-assisted self-interviewing

They are also limited because less detail and complexity of information can be sought, skip patterns are often not properly followed, and memory aids such as show cards cannot be presented. The main advantage is the lower cost.

Self-administered questionnaires can be administered under supervision (e.g. in a clinic or in a person's home after an interview) or can be dropped off or mailed and completed without supervision. Supervision has the advantage that questions can be answered or problems dealt with during the course of the questionnaire or on completion. Historically, mailed self-administered questionnaires have been considered to have low response rates. Nevertheless, gradual trends towards lower response rates in surveys involving personal interview and improvements in follow-up and other procedures for maximization of response to mail surveys have led to smaller, although still significant, differences.

Technology has also increased the options for completion of self-administered questionnaires beyond the traditional pencil-and-paper mode. If the subject is to complete a self-administered questionnaire under supervision, *computer-assisted self-administered questionnaires* (CASAQ) can be used, via a desktop computer, portable computer, or tablet computer. When audio or video reading of the questions is added, these are termed *audio or video computer-assisted self-interviewing* (ACASI or VCASI). Finally, web-based questionnaires are another option for participants who have access to the internet (Dillman 2000). The main disadvantages of computer-assisted techniques are the need for some computer skills by the respondent and, in the case of web-based questionnaires, the need for the respondent to have computer access to the internet. Computer-assisted self-interviews have the same advantages as other forms of computer-assisted interviewing listed above. For example, computer based questionnaires would eliminate the problem of respondents' failure to follow skip patterns correctly that is common for paper-and-pencil questionnaires.

Use of proxy respondents

The use of proxy or surrogate respondents, i.e. people who provide information on exposure in place of the subjects themselves, is an important variation on the subjective methods of exposure measurement so far outlined. Proxy respondents are used in epidemiology when the subjects of study are for some reason (youth, death, dementia) unable to provide the data required. They are used most commonly in case–control studies of fatal disease when the only alternative to proxies may be a series of cases potentially biased by survival.

Data on exposure provided by proxies are prone to all the errors of data provided by the subjects themselves and some additional ones. The proxy may never have known the facts sought. In addition, when death is the reason for the subject's unavailability for interview, the fact of his/her death may alter the proxy's recall of the relevant facts. However, in some circumstances the proxy may be at least as likely to know of the exposure as the subject (as when a parent responds on behalf of a child in respect of exposures in early life).

Practical aspects of the use of proxy respondents and the validity of data obtained from them are dealt with in more detail in Chapter 8.

Diaries

Diaries can only be used for the collection of present personal behaviour or experiences. However, they are more accurate for this purpose than recall methods (Verbrugge 1980; McKeown *et al.* 2001). Diaries are also limited to frequent behaviours. For example, diaries have been used to collect diet, exercise, and medication use in epidemiological studies.

Diaries are better than interviews for recording experiences that are transient or of low impact. They minimize recall error, including errors due to poor memory and telescoping. In addition, for the comparatively short periods of life that they cover, they can present a more comprehensive picture of the exposure than is possible by recall methods; for example, they allow weighing of foods for diet diaries. However, subjects may modify their behaviour when recording a diary to be more socially desirable or to simplify recording, so that the recorded behaviours do not accurately reflect usual behaviours.

For diaries to represent exposure over a fairly long period there must be reasonably long recording periods distributed over the period of interest, especially if the behaviour recorded is highly variable. Diaries generally cost more than collecting the same data by personal interview, are more expensive to process, and are more difficult to analyse. The subject burden is high, and this makes it difficult to recruit a representative sample of the population of interest and to obtain a high response rate (Verbrugge 1980). These disadvantages have led to limited use of diaries in epidemiology. They have been used primarily as a comparison method for validation studies of questionnaires or other methods.

Automated methods of collecting behaviour data in real time, such as physical activity monitors, share some of the properties of diaries. They also have some of the properties of observation and of physical measures (e.g. they are objective).

More information about the use of diaries in epidemiological studies is given in Chapter 8.

Observation of the subject by the investigator

Like diary methods, observation by the investigator can be applied only to the measurement of present exposure. Attributes such as sex and race are commonly measured by observation. Some other attributes, such as eye colour and hair colour, may be recorded entirely subjectively by a field worker or more objectively by comparison with a set of standards. In the latter situation, the distinction between what is an observation by the investigator and what is a physical measurement on the subject becomes blurred.

The direct observation of variable attributes or behaviours of subjects requires that the observer 'participate' in the life of the subject during the period of observation. Such *participant observation* methods have been little used in epidemiology. One example is a dietitian or nutritionist observing mealtimes in the subject's household, and recording or even sometimes sampling (for analysis!) what the subject eats. Other examples include observation of infection control practices (Kelen *et al.* 1989) and measurement of physical activity (Patterson *et al.* 1988). Direct observation of behaviour has been used not so much as a primary method in epidemiology as for the validation of other methods of measurement (e.g. recall of diet (Karveti and Knuts 1985) and self-reported seat-belt use at the population level (CDC 1988)).

In the measurement of behaviour, direct observation of subjects has a number of strengths and weaknesses. On the positive side, it is more objective, can be used for low-impact behaviours, and allows for a substantial amount of detail. On the negative side, it can be applied to present behaviour only, is restricted generally to a comparatively short sampling period, and can be applied only to quite frequent behaviours. Other limitations of observation are that it can only be implemented with a fairly highly selected group of subjects, requires extensive training of observers, and is time consuming and expensive.

There are also some important sources of error, including inadequate sampling of time periods, biased sampling of time periods (for instance in dietary observation, only meals may be observed and food eaten between meals may not be recorded), too many events to record accurately, observer fatigue with 'drift' in recording, and an effect of the observation on the behaviour being observed.

Observation techniques will not be dealt with further in this book. A detailed treatment from the perspective of studies in psychology can be found in Reis (2000).

Reference to records

In this context 'records' means records that have not been collected specifically for the purpose of exposure measurement for an epidemiological study, and include paper records and electronic databases. Occupational, medical, birth, and death records are those most commonly used in epidemiological studies. Sometimes they are simply records of the subject's recall of the exposure, obtained nearer to the time that it occurred, or they may be records made by others who were associated with the exposure (e.g. dose of ionizing radiation given for treatment of disease, as recorded by the therapist) or records of measurements made on the subject or the subject's environment.

One advantage of the use of records is that they can provide prospectively recorded information, collected on exposures in the past, and so are less subject to the biases associated with recall of exposures. In particular, differential exposure measurement error between those with and without disease is unlikely to affect records recorded before disease onset. Other advantages are that the data collection costs are usually low, and the study time is reduced because some or all of the data collection has been carried out by others. The accuracy of selected data items can be better than that obtained by personal interview (see Chapter 8). Finally, if a study using records does not require contact with the subjects, then the response rate can be quite high.

The main limitation of records is that they do not exist for most exposures of interest, and when they do exist, they may not cover the entire time period of interest. Moreover, records rarely contain information on all the potential confounding and modifying factors of interest. Most records have had multiple recorders, which often leads to inconsistent definitions of terms and even different sets of items collected. In addition, as in the case of prescriptions, intended exposures may be recorded, but the subject may not have complied. Similarly, when records are used in ecological studies, the data collected may relate to certain geographical areas or population subgroups, but may not be relevant to each subject in the study.

The use of records in epidemiology is covered in Chapter 8.

Physical or chemical measurements on the subject

The usefulness of physical or chemical measurements for epidemiology depends largely on whether they relate to fixed or variable attributes of the subject or the environment and how variable the attributes are. At one extreme are measurements of genotypes, which remain fixed throughout life and can be measured at any time. At the other extreme are measurements of carbon monoxide in expired air which, strictly speaking, relate only to intake of cigarette smoke (or another carbon monoxide source) within the preceding few hours. Only the present status of variable attributes can be measured by physical or chemical methods. Anthropometric variables (e.g. height, weight, and skinfold thicknesses), blood lipid levels, and the concentrations of trace elements in hair or nails, are examples of moderately stable attributes that can be measured physically or chemically. Occasionally, past environmental contacts can be inferred from present measurements on the subject (e.g. presence of DNA adducts in cells as an indicator of past, as well as present, exposure to certain carcinogens).

A particular problem for physical and chemical measurements, and, to a lesser extent, all measurements made after the onset of disease, is the possibility that the presence of disease may alter the values obtained by measurement. This is a major limitation of the use of physical or chemical measurements of variable exposures in cross-sectional and case–control studies. An example is the inverse relationship between plasma cholesterol concentration and incidence of colorectal cancer, which may be due to an effect of the cancer in lowering plasma cholesterol (McMichael *et al.* 1984).

Physical or chemical measurements on the environment

Physical or chemical measurements of the environment present similar problems, except that they are unlikely to be influenced by disease in the subject. Unless records exist, they can usually only relate to the current environment. It may sometimes be possible to make present measurements that reflect the past environment of subjects (e.g. lead in the water supplies of their former homes), but the use of such data to represent the existence or levels of exposure over periods in the distant past is very uncertain. In epidemiology, they have been used most commonly in the analysis of retrospective cohort studies of occupation and disease, in order to add measurement of exposure to the agent of specific interest to data on the place, nature, and duration of employment. Chapters 9 and 10 cover the use of physical and chemical measurements on subjects and in the environment.

Experience of use of different methods

Table 2.3 summarizes the main methods used for measurement of exposure in the 311 epidemiological studies referred to in Table 1.1. Personal interview was the predominant method, and 90 per cent of these were face-to-face interviews rather than by telephone. Physical or chemical measurements on the subject or the environment were the second most important source of exposure data (and this would have been an even greater proportion had we not excluded studies of genetic and infectious exposures). Self-administered questionnaires were the third most common method, delivered by mail in about two-thirds of these studies and administered in a supervised setting in one-third. Use of records, primarily non-medical records, was fourth. Diaries or direct observation of subjects by the investigators were not the main method of exposure measurement in any of the studies. In four studies the method of measurement of exposure was so inadequately described as to defy classification under any of the headings of Table 2.3!

Table 2.3 Distribution of the main methods of exposure[a] measurement (one selected from each study) in 311 papers on the aetiology of non-infectious disease published in the *American Journal of Epidemiology* between January 2000 and June 2002

Method	Distribution (%)
Personal interview	30.5
Face-to-face	26.7
Telephone	3.2
Unclassifiable type	0.6
Self-administered questionnaire	24.4
By mail	16.7
Under supervision	7.7
Reference to records	16.4
Medical records	2.3
Other records	14.1
Physical or chemical measurements	27.4
On subject	19.0
On environment	8.4
Unclassifiable	1.3

[a] Excludes genetic and infectious exposures.

Choice of method

The first principle in choosing a method for measuring an exposure in an epidemiologic study is that it must be the same method, applied in an identical way, to those with and without the disease under study. Any differences in the method between cases and controls (e.g., telephone vs. in person interview), the source of information (e.g., medical records vs. cancer registry) or the application of the protocol (e.g., handling of biologic specimens after collection) could lead to spurious differences between the case and control groups (i.e, differential measurement error, see Chapter 3).

For most situtations, there is no simple way of choosing the best method of measurement of exposure. As often as not, the choice will depend on practical rather than theoretical considerations. In particular, the costs of different possible methods relative to the funds available will influence the choice.

Apart from the practical considerations, the following factors all influence the choice of a method:

- ◆ type of study
- ◆ type, amount, and detail of data required by the study's objectives
- ◆ frequency and impact of the exposure on the subjects' lives
- ◆ variability in the frequency or level of exposure over time

♦ availability of records or physical or chemical methods for measuring the exposure

♦ accuracy of the method of measuring the exposure.

These issues are discussed in this section. In the section following this one, we discuss the issues to consider after a questionnaire has been selected as the method, specifically whether the mode of administration should be face-to-face interview, telephone interview, or self-administration.

Type of study

Prospective cohort studies or *randomized controlled trials* (for exposures other than the experimental exposure) are amenable to all the methods discussed, including those for present and past exposures and objective and subjective methods. While it is tempting to think of prospective studies as only needing collection of data on present exposures, information on past exposures may be needed to meet the aims of the study. Past exposures are particularly important in studies of chronic diseases, when the exposures of interest may act over many years to cause the disease of interest, and when cases occurring soon after data collection will be included in the analysis. In addition, if the exposure is highly variable over time, it may be necessary to measure it again at intervals during the course of follow-up. Although all methods of exposure measurement are applicable to prospective studies, records of past exposure are rarely used in such studies, and diaries and observation may be too costly for large cohort studies.

Almost by definition, *retrospective cohort studies* depend on records for their measurements of exposure. Examples include the study of disease following exposure to workplace hazards, using records of employment, occasionally supplemented by measurements of the work environment, and the study of prescription drugs in conditions other than the one they were prescribed to treat, using pharmacy databases.

The logic of *case–control studies* requires that the exposure measurements permit inferences about past exposure, at least in the period before onset of disease and often in periods long before that. Thus personal interviews, self-administered questionnaires, and reference to records about subjects or their environment have been the methods most commonly used in these studies. Since the disease and its treatment or sequelae could influence present behaviour or metabolism, diaries, observation, or physical or chemical measurements on subjects for exposures that are not fixed characteristics would not be appropriate (i.e. the error would be differential). Measurements in the environment of the subjects are also sometimes used in case–control studies, but this assumes stability of the exposure over time.

Cross-sectional studies are similar to case–control studies in that measurement of past exposure is usually required. However, in some situations the study hypothesis may relate directly to the effects of *present* exposure on a rapidly responsive outcome variable such as blood pressure; in this case, any of the methods applicable to past or present exposure may be chosen.

Amount and detail of data required

The personal interview is often the best method when large amounts of detailed data are required, particularly if past exposure must be documented. A diary can provide very detailed data, for example a complete list of all foods eaten and, for each food, a portion size estimate or actual weight, but only for present behaviours. Records vary in their completeness and amount of detail, but for some exposures they may provide more detail than the subjects themselves can recall. For example, the pharmacy records of subjects in a closed medical care system can give exact drug name, dose per pill, prescribed pills per day, and total number of pills dispensed (although not necessarily taken). If physical or chemical measurements are available for the exposure, they might provide precise information, but only on current exposure.

Impact and frequency of the exposure

In selecting a method to measure the exposure, the impact and frequency of the exposure need to be considered together. Low-impact exposures (eating a carrot) are more difficult to measure than exposures with a high impact on the subjects' lives (major surgery). If an exposure is both low impact and infrequent, it will be almost impossible to measure. The subject will be unable to recall such exposures, it is unlikely that they will have been measured and recorded in the past, and any practical programme of sampling of the subject's present experience of them (e.g. by diary) or their concentration in the internal or external environment is unlikely to provide measurements that are sufficiently free of variability *within* individuals to be useful.

Diary methods are ideal for low-impact frequent exposures, and observation may also be applicable. Physical or chemical measurements are also suitable for low-impact exposures, subject to the availability of such measurements. However, all these methods generally only measure present but not past exposure and generally only capture a short time period which could lead to substantial error if the frequency or level of exposure varies over time (see next section). One example of the measurement of a low-impact but frequent exposure is measurement of the consumption of aflatoxin in food, which has essentially no 'impact' for impoverished residents of tropical countries. Thus measurement of its intake has depended on the sampling of foods eaten and measurement of aflatoxin concentration in the food or the concentration of aflatoxin or its reaction products in body fluids. However, for these measurements to be useful epidemiologically, it must be assumed that the sampling period chosen is representative of the generality of past (or future) exposure. Records are also sometimes useful for the measurement of low-impact exposures. For example, in the occupational environment an exposure variable such as ionizing radiation may have been measured and recorded even though the subjects were unaware of their exposure to it.

Frequent exposures of moderate or high impact (e.g. recreational physical activity) will be measurable by recall methods and may be the subject of records. They can also be sampled by diary methods, observation by the investigator, or physical or chemical measurements where appropriate, but as noted above are limited in only measuring present exposure over a short time period. Low-frequency exposures of high impact (e.g. major illnesses) are best measured by subjective recall or by reference to records (if available).

Variability of the exposure over time

All the methods of measurement of exposure listed in Table 2.1 can be used for the measurement of exposures that do not vary much over time. For exposures that vary day to day, month to month, or year to year in frequency or intensity (dose per exposure event), the method of measurement needs to be able to reflect the exposure in the period of time thought to influence the development of the disease under study. In-person interviews can be used to measure exposures that vary over time, either by asking subjects for their usual exposure (e.g. usual intake of types of foods) or by collecting specific information on how the exposure varied over time (e.g. alcohol consumption over a lifetime). Self-administered questionnaires might also be used if the questions can be kept simple, and records would capture variability over time if they were available. The methods that only measure current exposure (diaries, observation, and physical and chemical measures on the subject) can be used for exposures that vary in frequency or intensity over time, but their accuracy may be poor unless the measures are repeated for each subject over multiple days, over different seasons, or across several years to determine accurately the mean exposure of the subject over the time period of interest (see Chapter 5).

Accuracy and availability of the method

Of course, not all methods of measurement are available for all exposures. Some exposures can only be ascertained by questionnaire (e.g. lifetime alcohol use), while some can only be measured by physical or chemical methods on human specimens (e.g. serum cholesterol concentration or genotype). Records may be available only for certain populations, if at all.

When multiple methods are available for a particular exposure, the accuracy of the various methods needs to be considered. For example, to assess physical activity, the researcher could select among questionnaires, diaries, monitoring devices that measure movement, or objective measures of physical fitness. The researcher should not assume that objective methods are always more accurate than subjective methods, because the objective method may not capture the aetiologically important time period or, in the case of laboratory analyses, may be hampered by specimen degradation or laboratory error. Instead, the researcher needs to understand the validity of each method, either through published validity/reliability studies or by conducting a new validity/reliability study. Then the most accurate method(s), within the constraints of the study, should be selected.

Combinations of methods

It is common to combine a number of different methods of measurement of exposure within a single study. This may be done:

+ for validation purposes on a subset only
+ to combine results of two or more different approaches to measurement into a single, more accurate, measure of exposure (see Chapter 5)
+ because it may be better to use different approaches to collect different parts of the desired data.

For example, the investigator may carry out a personal interview and also collect some data by self-administered questionnaire. This might be done to save money or because of the possible advantage of self-administered questionnaires over interviews in the collection of sensitive data.

The Women's Health Initiative provides a good example of the multiplicity of types of exposure measurement that can be used in a single study (Anderson *et al.* 2003; Ritenbaugh *et al.* 2003). At baseline, participants completed self-administered questionnaires about demographics, medical history, diet and other health-related behaviours, and psychosocial factors. They completed a face-to-face interview on past and current use of hormone replacement therapy because of the complexity of those questions. They were asked to bring all medications including vitamin and mineral supplements to the clinic; information on dose and duration of use of each drug was then ascertained in an interviewer-administered computer-aided medication inventory. Participants had anthropometric and blood pressure measurements taken, had electrocardiograms, and provided blood samples for future analyses of nutrients and other measures. Most of these measures were repeated periodically throughout the study. Women in the dietary modification component also completed a four-day food diary at baseline and, to monitor diet further, selected subsamples of those participants completed telephone-administered 24-hour dietary recalls each year. While records were not used for exposure assessment in this study, medical records were used to verify and classify disease outcomes (cancer, cardiovascular disease).

Choosing method of administration of questionnaires: face-to-face, telephone, or self-administered

Questionnaires were the main method of exposure measurement in 55 per cent of the 311 epidemiological studies summarized in Table 2.3. As shown in the table, the most common modes of administration were face-to-face interview (27 per cent of all studies) and self-administration (24 per cent), while telephone interview only accounted for 3 per cent.

One common study design decision that the researcher often needs to make is to choose among these three methods of questionnaire administration. Table 2.4 summarizes the performance characteristics of face-to-face interviews, telephone interviews, and mailed self-administered questionnaires (Dillman 1978; de Leeuw 1992; Aday 1996; Bowling 2005). Of course, not all self-administered questionnaires are sent through the mail; about one-third of the self-administered questionnaires used in the recent epidemiological studies summarized in Table 2.3 were completed under supervision (e.g. in a clinic or in a person's home in conjunction with an interview). Some of the disadvantages of self-administered questionnaires highlighted in Table 2.4 relate to distribution by mail, and some of these limitations would be mitigated by administration under supervision or via computer.

Overall, the face-to-face interview rates as high as or higher than the other two approaches on all the characteristics listed, except with respect to the probability of social desirability bias, the possibility of the effects of others present on the accuracy of the data, and the practical issues of hiring personnel, time needed to complete the study, and costs. The particular strengths of face-to-face interviews lie in the length and complexity of the interview that is possible. Self-administered questionnaires have a few advantages (and a number of disadvantages) compared with the other two methods. They may promote more truthful responses to sensitive questions and usually cost less to administer than either method of personal interview and require fewer expert staff. Their particular disadvantages are the comparative simplicity of the questionnaires that can be used, and the lower expected response rate if sent by mail. More details about the issues in Table 2.4 are discussed below.

Table 2.4 Comparison of face-to-face interviews, telephone interviews, and mailed self-administered questionnaires with respect to performance characteristics[a]

Performance characteristics	Method		
	Face-to-face interviews	Telephone interviews	Self-administered (mail) questionnaires
Obtaining a representative sample			
Opportunity for all members of population to be included in sample			
Completely listed populations	High	High	High
Populations not completely listed (e.g. household occupants)	High	Medium	Medium
Control over selection of respondents within sampling units	High	High	Medium
Response rates	High	Medium	Low
Questionnaire content and construction			
Allowable length of questionnaire	High	Medium	Medium
Allowable complexity of questions	High	Low	Low
Success with open-ended questions	High	Medium	Low
Use of visual aids (show cards, pictures, calendars)	High	Low	Low
Success with skip patterns	High	High	Low
Success with controlling sequence in which questions are asked	High	High	Low
Success with tedious or boring questions	High	Medium	Low
Insensitivity to questionnaire design	High	High	Low
Obtaining accurate and complete answers			
Clarification and probing by interviewer	High	Medium	Low
Avoidance of social desirability bias in sensitive questions	Low	Low	Medium
Avoidance of contamination by others	Medium	High	Medium
Ability to consult records, pill bottles, etc.	Medium	Low	Medium
Avoidance of item non-response	High	Medium	Low
Avoidance of early termination	High	Medium	Low
Respondent burden			
Cognitive ease	High	Medium	Low
Respondents' preference/ satisfaction	High	Medium	Low

Table 2.4 (continued) Comparison of face-to-face interviews, telephone interviews, and mailed self-administered questionnaires with respect to performance characteristics[a]

	Method		
Performance characteristics	Face-to-face interviews	Telephone interviews	Self-administered (mail) questionnaires
Practical issues			
Likelihood that personnel requirements can be met	Low	Medium	High
Speed of data collection	Low	Medium	High
Overall potential for low-cost interviews	Low	Medium	High
Reduced marginal costs with increasing numbers of participants	Low	Medium	High
Insensitivity of costs to increasing geographical dispersion	Low	Medium	High

[a] Dillman 1978; de Leeuw 1992; Aday 1996; Bowling 2005.

Obtaining a representative sample and high response rates

When a list of all potential study subjects is available, the choice of questionnaire administration method does not impact on the ability to obtain a representative population sample. However, when the method of questionnaire *administration* (face-to-face, telephone, mail) is paired with the method of random *sampling* (door-to-door, random digit dialling, and mailing to a population-based mailing list, respectively), obtaining a representative sample is influenced by the method. Door-to-door sampling is more likely to cover the population than the other two. Telephone sampling is limited because some people have no telephone, some have only a mobile phone which may not be part of the random telephone prefix list used, and some have two telephones (which makes them twice as likely to be selected). Sampling the population through mailing lists is limited by the coverage of the mailing list obtained. For example in the USA, drivers' licence lists are sometimes used; these would under-represent the elderly and those who do not own cars (low-income groups, those living in very high density areas).

Often one address or telephone number has multiple eligible subjects, and control of selection of participants among the eligibles should be based on an algorithm defined by the researcher. Control of subject selection within a household is greater for face-to-face and telephone interviews than mailed questionnaires.

Response rates also vary by data collection method. High response rates are important for case–control and cross-sectional studies, as low response increases the likelihood of selection bias (see Chapter 11). Hox and de Leeuw (1994) conducted a meta-analysis of 45 studies which compared the response rates among in-person interviews, telephone interviews, and mailed questionnaires. On average, the response rates were 70 per cent for in-person interviews, 67 per cent for interviews conducted by telephone, and 61 per cent for mailed questionnaires. These response rates reflect what was attained after multiple attempts to contact each potential subject. For self-administered questionnaires, response rates should be higher if the questionnaire is given to the respondent in-person (e.g. after a home interview or in a clinic) rather than sent in the mail.

Questionnaire content and construction

In-person interviews have numerous advantages over the other two methods. An interviewer meeting face to face with the respondent can maintain motivation for completion of a longer questionnaire. Based on practice, an in-person interview could last as long as 2 hours, while a telephone interview longer than 30–40 minutes would probably lead to a high percentage of refusals or early terminations. Compared with the other two methods, in-person interviews also allow greater complexity in terms of the concepts in the questions or responses, and allow the use of visual aids such as show cards, calendars, and pictures. Interviews perform better than self-administered questionnaires for open-ended questions (where answer lists are not provided and the respondent answers in his/her own words) because the interviewer can probe to obtain appropriate answers. However, respondents give less information in response to open-ended questions in telephone interviews than in in-person interviews (de Leeuw 1992). Both in-person and telephone interviews have success with skip patterns and with controlling the sequence in which the questions are asked, while self-administered questionnaires perform poorly in these areas. The physical design is particularly important for self-administered questionnaires to enhance the completion of the questionnaire by the study participants.

For these reasons, Sudman and Bradburn (1984) concluded that mailed questionnaires performed best when they were short, dealt with highly salient topics, did not contain open-ended questions, did not require complex branching, did not contain questions that required probes, and did not require that questions be answered in a strict order (because of the impossibility of controlling the order in which subjects answer questions in mailed questionnaires). On the positive side, if it is desirable that a subject consult records or other people when answering, this is more likely to happen with a mailed questionnaire. A mailed questionnaire also gives the subject more time to reflect on the questions and recall the relevant details. However, both of these advantages may become disadvantages in case–control studies, if they lead to greater efforts by cases than by controls to provide accurate data.

Obtaining accurate answers

There have been numerous studies comparing responses by mode of administration of questionnaires. While most of these report moderate to good concordance across methods, such studies cannot provide information about which mode is most accurate. Only a few studies have compared the different approaches to collecting questionnaire data with respect to their validity against prior records of the information. In studies of Pap smears and pelvic examinations (Hochstim 1967), of ambulatory care and hospital admissions (Weeks et al. 1983), and of physician visits (Siemiatycki et al. 1984), the confirmation rates in comparison with records were similar across the different modes of questionnaire administration. Overall, there appears to be no consistent evidence of better or worse performance of any of the three methods in terms of validity of information (de Leeuw 1992), with the exception of sensitive questions (see below).

Despite this limited evidence that the three methods do not differ in their validity, face-to-face interviews do have certain advantages over the other two modes that should aid in obtaining accurate answers. The interviewer can clarify questions that are not understood and probe when responses are incomplete. Although telephone interviews also have these advantages, there is a concern that responses may be less accurate by telephone because of differences in communication style between in-person and telephone communication. Aday (1996) suggests that the in-person interviewer can make more use of visual cues to determine if the respondent has understood the question, and respondents feel freer to ask questions to clarify their response than over the telephone. Pauses are more uncomfortable on the telephone than in-person, which may lead the respondent to respond before he/she has had time to retrieve the information fully (Bradburn et al. 1987). In a meta-analysis conducted by de Leeuw and van der Zouwen (1988), telephone interviews were found to be shorter on average than face-to-face interviews, the individual utterances were shorter, and subjects responded to fewer items on lists.

There is also evidence that when a list of responses is read on the telephone, subjects are more likely to choose the first or the last one than when they can see the whole list for themselves (Jordan et al. 1980; Sudman et al. 1996). This may be due to difficulties in recall of the list in the telephone setting.

On the positive side, compared with the other two methods, the telephone interview can be private in almost any surroundings because bystanders can only hear one side of the conversation.

Sensitive questions

In contrast with most of the above issues, self-administered questionnaires are superior to the other two methods for sensitive questions. Sensitive questions are questions on topics that are illegal, contra-normative, or not often discussed in public. Examples of sensitive topics are illegal drug use and sexual behaviours that put a person at risk of sexually transmitted diseases. There is also some sensitivity around reporting income, excessive alcohol use, and tobacco use. Sensitive behaviours are most often negative behaviours, and are typically under-reported because of social desirability bias.

There is considerable evidence that more impersonal methods of data collection yield more accurate reporting of sensitive behaviours than interviewer-administered questionnaires. The impersonal methods include self-administered questionnaires, including various techniques of computer-assisted self-interviewing (CASI) (via laptop, palmtop, or audio-CASI), and certain types of automated telephone interviewing. These self-administered approaches have been found to yield higher reporting of alcohol intake (Kraus and Augustin 2001), illegal drug use and drug-related behaviours (Gribble *et al.* 2000; Newman *et al.* 2002; Turner *et al.* 2005), sensitive sexual behaviours (Ghanem *et al.* 2005), urinary symptoms in men (Rhodes *et al.* 1995; Garcia-Losa *et al.* 2001), and risk behaviours during pregnancy (Mears *et al.* 2005) compared with interviewer-administered questionnaires. While higher reporting of sensitive behaviours implies greater accuracy of the impersonal data collection methods, one study was able to directly assess the validity of self-reported drug use by comparison with urine testing. This study confirmed that CASI was superior to interviews (van Griensven *et al.* 2006). There does not appear to be any relative advantage between telephone and in-person interviews in terms of eliciting more accurate information on sensitive behaviours (de Leeuw 1992).

While self-administered questionnaires can be recommended for sensitive questions, it is not recommended that they be delivered by mail. In most studies which compared these methods, the self-administered questionnaire or CASI was introduced in person, sometimes after less sensitive questions had been asked by an interviewer. While mailed questionnaires on tobacco or alcohol use may be acceptable, mailed questionnaires on the most sensitive behaviours (e.g. sexual behaviours or illegal drug use) could be offensive. In fact, a meta-analysis found that inclusion of sensitive questions in mailed questionnaires reduces response rates by a small amount (Edwards *et al.* 2006). Perhaps the best approach for sensitive questions is a mixed mode, using a self-administered questionnaire, CASI or telephone CASI mode for the sensitive questions after an in-person interview or telephone interview on the less sensitive questions has been conducted.

One exception to this may be that psychological problems may be disclosed more often in face-to-face interviews than by other means. Newman *et al.* (2002) found that psychological distress was more often reported in an in-person interview than in audio CASI, and Henson *et al.* (1978) found that psychiatric symptoms were reported more often in in-person than in telephone interviews. In this case, it is possible that rapport with the interviewer during an in-person interview helps elicit physiological problems from the subject.

Another method of assessing certain sensitive behaviours more accurately is to combine questionnaire or interview methods with a biochemical measure of the exposure. When participants know that an objective measure is to be used, they often report the sensitive behaviour more accurately on a questionnaire or interview. This is related to the so-called *bogus pipeline* approach (Jones and Sigall 1971). The term 'pipeline' referred to 'a direct pipeline to the soul', and 'bogus' to the fact that the pipeline was opened by convincing the subject that the investigator had some instrument that could measure (whether in fact or in fiction) the response that the subject was being asked to record. The bogus pipeline approach has been shown to increase the reporting of smoking in children (Evans *et al.* 1977) when saliva samples were taken, and the reporting of alcohol use among pregnant women when blood and urine samples were taken, which they were told would confirm their self-reported use (Lowe *et al.* 1986).

Avoiding item non-response and early termination

Skipping of certain questions by the respondent, or *item non-response*, is also influenced by mode of data collection. In a meta-analysis, de Leeuw (1992) found that self-administered questionnaires had significantly more missing data items than face-to-face interviews, with telephone interviews falling in between. One reason is that respondents often fail to follow the branching (skip) patterns in self-administered questionnaires and therefore miss certain questions, while interviewers (especially if using computer-aided interviewing) guide the respondents through the appropriate questions. However, computer-assisted self-administered questionnaires overcome this problem (de Leeuw and Nicholls 1996).

One exception to the pattern of more missing data on self-administered questionnaires than interviews is for sensitive questions. Not only do self-administered questionnaires yield more accurate data on sensitive behaviours, they also yield less missing data on sensitive questions than interview methods (de Leeuw 1992).

Respondents can also terminate an interview because of boredom, offence, or feeling that the interview is taking too much of their time. This leads to item non-response for the remainder of the questions. (For mailed question-naires, a terminated questionnaire is unlikely to be returned to the study, and so would lead to complete non-response.) Telephone interviews are particularly prone to termination of the interview before it is completed; this is even greater for completely automated voice-activated telephone interviews (Bowling 2005). It is likely that the more personal nature of a face-to-face interview is the reason that that method has fewer early discontinuations.

Respondent cognitive burden and preference

Self-administered questionnaires have the greatest cognitive burden, as they require reading skills and the ability to follow the response and skip instructions. Sudman and Bradburn (1984) noted that mail surveys work especially poorly among the aged and the poorly educated, as these groups find them hard to read or understand and have generally had less experience in completing them. The elderly may also suffer from poorer reading vision. Electronic self-administered questionnaires also require basic computer literacy. However, computer-assisted questionnaires have high acceptability among most respondents (Ryan et al. 2002).

Telephone and in-person interviews only require basic listening and speak-ing skills. While most adults have these capabilities, some groups, such as the very old, may have limited hearing.

In-person interviews may have less cognitive burden than telephone inter-views because understanding an interviewer whom one can see is easier than understanding questions posed by telephone. An in-person interview may also be less monotonous and more varied in format (e.g. by the use of show cards or other memory prompts) than a telephone interview. Perhaps for these reasons or because of greater rapport with an in-person interviewer, partici-pants have reported a preference for face-to-face interviews over telephone interviews (Nicholaas et al. 2000). In one experiment with all three modes, participants were most satisfied with the experience of the face-to-face inter-view, followed by the telephone interview, and least satisfied with completing the mailed questionnaire (de Leeuw 1992).

Practical issues

While face-to-face interviews perform better than the other two modes on almost all the above criteria, they perform the poorest on the practical requirements. Face-to-face interviews generally require more skilled staff and require longer to complete data collection; therefore they have the highest costs. Another administrative problem is that it may be difficult to hire and/or supervise in-person interviewers if the study sample is widely dispersed or the interviewers are required to visit areas that they would not normally enter. Mailed questionnaires and telephones interviews are administratively easier for wide geographical areas in terms of both costs and supervision of staff. A study can be completed more quickly when mailed questionnaires are used than with the other two modes. In addition, with mailed questionnaires, the costs per person (marginal costs) tend to go down with increasing sample size, while the other two modes tend to have little per-person cost savings for very large samples. Although the actual per-subject costs depend on the study protocol, the population being surveyed, and the total sample size, a crude estimate is that face-to-face interviews cost twice as much as those by telephone (Kulka *et al.* 1984), and telephone interviews cost twice as much as mailed surveys (McHorney *et al.* 1994).

Summary

A variety of subjective and objective methods of exposure measurement directed towards present or past personal attributes or environmental contacts are used in epidemiology. They include personal interviews, either face-to-face or by telephone, self-administered questionnaires, diaries of behaviour, reference to records, physical or chemical measurements on the subject, physical or chemical measurements in the environment, and, infrequently, direct observation of the subject's behaviour by the investigator. When the subject is too young, too ill, or deceased, it is also common to obtain data about him/her from a proxy respondent, usually a member of the subject's family. The methods selected must be identical for cases and controls.

In addition to costs, the choice of method is influenced by the type of study to be undertaken, the amount of detail required by the study's objectives, the frequency and impact of the exposure on the subjects' lives, the variability in the frequency and level of exposure over time, and the accuracy of the methods that are available to measure the specific exposure of interest. Combinations of methods are often necessary or desirable for validation purposes, to reduce error in measurement, or because different exposures require different approaches to collection.

Subjective recall of exposure, collected by way of face-to-face or telephone interview or self-administered questionnaire, is the predominant method of collection of exposure data in epidemiology. There appears to be little difference between these methods with respect to the validity of the data obtained. Nonetheless, face-to-face interviews are clearly best for the collection of large amounts of complex data. Where subjects are widely dispersed and the questionnaire can be kept comparatively brief, telephone interviews may be favoured. However, telephone interviews may lead to less complete responses. Self-administered questionnaires may perform better than the other approaches in eliciting sensitive or socially undesirable behaviour, but perform poorly on complex questions, open-ended questions, and questions with branching. Self-administered questionnaires have substantial advantages over in-person or telephone interviews in terms of staff requirements, speed of completion of study, and per-subject costs.

References

Abramson, J.H. (1984). *Survey Methods in Community Medicine* (3rd edn), p. 121. Churchill Livingstone, Edinburgh.

Aday, L.A. (1996). *Designing and Conducting Health Surveys: A Comprehensive Guide* (2nd edn). Jossey-Bass, San Francisco, CA.

Anderson, G.L., Manson, J., Wallace, R., *et al.* (2003). Implementation of the Women's Health Initiative study design. *Annals of Epidemiology*, **13** (Suppl), S5–17.

Bowling, A. (2005). Mode of questionnaire administration can have serious effects on data quality. *Journal of Public Health*, **27**, 281–91.

Bradburn, N.M., Rips, L.J., and Shevell, S.K. (1987). Answering autobiographical questions: the impact of memory and inference on surveys. *Science*, **236**, 157–61.

CDC (Centers for Disease Control) (1988). Comparison of observed and self-reported seat belt use rates- United States. *Morbidity and Mortality Weekly Reports*, **37**, 549–51.

de Leeuw, E.D. (1992). *Data Quality in Mail, Telephone, and Fact to Face Surveys*. TT-Publikaties, Amsterdam.

de Leeuw, E. and Nicholls, W. (1996). Technological innovations in data collection: acceptance, data quality and costs. *Sociological Research Online*, **1**. Available online at: www.socresonline.org.uk/socresonline/1/4/leeuw.html

de Leeuw, E.D. and van der Zouwen, J. (1988). Data quality in telephone and face-to-face surveys: a comparative meta-analysis. In *Telephone Survey Methodology* (ed. R.M. Groves, P.N. Biemer, L.E. Lyberg, J.T. Massey, W.L. Nicholls, and J. Waksberg), pp. 283–99. Wiley, New York.

Dillman, D.A. (1978). *Mail and Telephone Surveys: The Total Design Method*. Wiley, New York.

Dillman, D.A. (2000). *Mail and Internet Surveys: The Tailored Design Method* (2nd edn). Wiley, New York.

Edwards, P., Roberts, I., Clarke, M., *et al.* (2006). *Methods to Increase Response Rates to Postal Questionnaires*. Cochrane Database of Systematic Reviews. Available online at: http://cochrane.org/reviews/en/mr000008.html

Evans, R.I., Hanse, W.B., and Mittelmark, M.B. (1977). Increasing the validity of self-reports of smoking behavior in children. *Journal of Applied Psychology*, **62**, 521–3.

Garcia-Losa, M., Unda, M., Badia, X., *et al.* (2001). Effect of mode of administration on I-PSS scores in a large BPH patient population. *European Urology*, **40**, 451–7.

Ghanem, K.G., Hutton, H.E., Zenilman, J.M., Zimba, R., and Erbelding, E.J. (2005). Audio computer assisted self interview and face-to-face interview modes in assessing response bias among STD clinic patients. *Sexually Transmitted Infections*, **81**, 421–5.

Gribble, J.N., Miller, H.G., Cooley, P.C., Catania, J.A., Pollack, L., and Turner, C.F. (2000). The impact of T-ACASI interviewing on reported drug use among men who have sex with men. *Substance Use and Misuse*, **35**, 869–90.

Henson, R., Cannel, C.F., and Roth, A (1978). Effect of interview mode on reporting of moods, symptoms, and need for social approval. *Journal of Social Psychology*, **105**, 123–9.

Hochstim, J.R. (1967). A critical comparison of three strategies of collecting data from households. *Journal of the American Statistical Association*, **62**, 976–82.

Hox, J.J. and de Leeuw, E.D. (1994). A comparison of non-response in mail, telephone, and face-to-face surveys. *Quality and Quantity*, **28**, 329–44.

Jones, E.E. and Sigall, H. (1971). The bogus pipeline: a new paradigm for measuring affect and attitude. *Psychology Bulletin*, **76**, 349–64.

Jordan, L.A., Marcus, A.C., and Reeder, L.G. (1980). Response styles in telephone and household interviewing: a field experiment. *Public Opinion Quarterly*, **44**, 210–22.

Karveti, R.L. and Knuts, L.R. (1985). Validity of the 24-hour dietary recall. *Journal of the American Dietetic Association*, **85**, 1437–42.

Kelen, G.D., DiGiovanna, T., Bisson, L., Kalainov, D., Sivertson, K.T., and Quinn, T.C. (1989). Human immunodeficiency virus infection in emergency department patients. *Journal of the American Medical Association*, **262**, 516–22.

Kraus, L. and Augustin, R. (2001). Measuring alcohol consumption and alcohol-related problems: comparison of responses from self-administered questionnaires and telephone interviews. *Addiction*, **96**, 459–471.

Kulka, R.A., Weeks, R.A., Lesser, J.T., and Whitmore, R.W. (1984). A comparison of the telephone and personal interview modes for conducting local household health surveys. In National Center for Health Services Research, *Health Survey Research Methods: Proceedings of the 4th Conference on Health Survey Research Methods*, Report No. DHHS PHS 82–3346, NCHSR Proceedings Series, pp 116–27. US Government Printing Office, Washington, DC.

Lowe, J.B., Windsor, R.A., Adams, B., Morris, J. and Reese, Y. (1986). Use of a bogus pipeline method to increase accuracy of self-reported alcohol consumption among pregnant women. *Journal of Studies on Alcohol*, **47**, 173–5.

McHorney, C.A., Kosinski, M. and Ware, J.E., Jr (1994). Comparisons of the costs and quality of norms for the SF-36 health survey collected by mail versus telephone interview: results from a national survey. *Medical Care*, **32**, 551–67.

McKeown, N.M., Day, N.E., Welch, A.A., *et al.* (2001). Use of biological markers to validate self-reported dietary intake in a random sample of the European Prospective

Investigation into Cancer United Kingdom Norfolk cohort. *American Journal of Clinical Nutrition*, **74**, 188–96.

McMichael, A.J., Jensen, A.M., Parkin, D.M., and Zaridze, D.G. (1984). Dietary and endogenous cholesterol and human cancer. *Epidemiologic Reviews*, **6**, 192–216.

Mears, M., Coonrod, D.V., Bay, R.C., Mills, T.E., and Watkins, M.C. (2005). Routine history as compared to audio computer-assisted self-interview for prenatal care history taking. *Reproductive Medicine*, **50**, 701–6.

Newman, J.C., Des Jarlais, D.C., Turner, C.F., Gribble, J., Cooley, P., and Paone, D. (2002). The differential effects of face-to-face and computer interview modes. *American Journal of Public Health*, **92**, 294–7.

Nicholaas, G., Thomson, K., and Lynn, P. (2000). *The Feasibility of Conducting Electoral Surveys in the UK Telephone*. Centre for Research into Elections and Social Trends, London, and National Centre for Social Research and Department of Sociology, University of Oxford.

Nicholls, W.L. II, Baker, R.P., and Martin, J. (1997). The effect of new data collection technologies on survey data quality. In *Survey Measurement and Process Quality* (ed. L. Lyberg, P. Biemer, M. Collins, *et al.*), pp. 221–48. Wiley, New York.

Patterson, T.L., Sallis, J.F., Nader, P.R., *et al.* (1988). Direct observation of physical activity and dietary behaviors in a structured environment: effects of a family-based health promotion program. *Journal of Behavioral Medicine*, **11**, 447–59.

Reis, H.T. (ed.) (2000). *Handbook of Research Methods in Social and Personality Psychology*. Cambridge University Press.

Rhodes, T., Girman, C.J., Jacobsen, S.J., *et al.* (1995). Does the mode of questionnaire administration affect the reporting of urinary symptoms? *Urology*, **46**, 341–5.

Ritenbaugh, C., Patterson, R.E., Chlebowski, R.T., *et al.* (2003). The Women's Health Initiative Diary Modification trial: overview and baseline characteristics of participants. *Annals of Epidemiology*, **13**(Suppl), S87–97.

Rothman, K.J. (1981). Induction and latent periods. *American Journal of Epidemiology*, **114**, 253–9.

Ryan, J.M., Corry, M.E., Attewell, R., and Smithson, M.J. (2002). A comparison of the electronic version of the SF-36 General Health Questionnaire to the standard paper version. *Quality of Life Research*, **11**, 19–26.

Siemiatycki, J., Campbell, S., Richardson, L., and Aubert, D. (1984). Quality of response in different population groups in mail and telephone surveys. *American Journal of Epidemiology*, **120**, 302–14.

Sudman, S. and Bradburn, N. (1984). Improving mailed questionnaire design. In *Making Effective Use of Mailed Questionnaires* (ed. D.C. Lockhart), pp. 33–47. Jossey-Bass, San Francisco, CA.

Sudman, S, Bradburn, N.M., and Schwarz, N. (1996). *Thinking About Answers: The Application of Cognitive Processes to Survey Methodology*. Jossey-Bass, San Francisco.

Turner, C.F., Villarroel, M.A., Rogers, S.M., *et al.* (2005). Reducing bias in telephone survey estimates of the prevalence of drug use: a randomized trial of telephone audio-CASI. *Addiction*, **100**, 1432–44.

van Griensven, F., Naorat, S., Kilmarx, P.H., *et al.* (2006). Palmtop-assisted self-interviewing for the collection of sensitive behavioral data: randomized trial with drug use urine testing. *American Journal of Epidemiology*, **163**, 271–8.

Verbrugge, L.M. (1980). Health diaries. *Medical Care*, **18**, 73–95.

Weeks, M.F., Kulka, R.A., Lessler, J.T., and Whitmore, R. (1983). Personal versus telephone surveys for collecting household health data at the local level. *American Journal of Public Health*, **73**, 1389–94.

3

Exposure measurement error and its effects

The most elegant design of a clinical study will not overcome the damage caused by unreliable or imprecise measurement.
(Fleiss 1986)

Introduction

Measurement error is one of the major sources of bias in epidemiological studies. It can lead to spurious conclusions about the relationship between exposure and disease. In this book we confine our attention to error in the measurement of exposure.

The *exposure measurement error* for an individual can be defined as the difference between the measured exposure and the true exposure. The *true exposure* is the agent of interest, for example the amount of exposure to the hypothesized causal agent of the disease over a specified aetiological time period. *Validity* refers to the capacity of an exposure variable to measure the true exposure in a population of interest. Measures of validity are measures of the exposure measurement error in a population.

Error in measurement of the exposure can be introduced during almost any phase of a study. Possible causes include:

- faulty design of the instrument
- errors or omissions in the protocol for use of the instrument
- poor execution of the protocol during data collection
- limitations due to subject characteristics (e.g. poor memory of past exposures, or day-to-day variability in biological characteristics)
- errors during data entry and analysis.

Examples of each of these are given in Table 3.1.

Table 3.1 Examples of sources of measurement error

Errors in the design of the instrument
   Lack of coverage of all sources of the exposure
   Inclusion of exposures that do not have the actual active agent
   Time period assessed by instrument not the true aetiological time period
   Measure (questionnaire or laboratory measure) not reflective of exposure in target tissue
   Phrasing of questions that lead to misunderstanding or bias

Errors or omissions in the protocol for use of the instrument
   Failure to specify protocol in sufficient detail
   Failure to specify a method to handle unanticipated situations consistently
   Failure to include standardization of instrument periodically throughout data collection

Poor execution of the study protocol
   Failure of data collectors or laboratory technicians to follow protocol in same manner for
      all subjects
   Failure of subjects to read instructions in self-administered questionnaire
   Improper handling and/or analysis of biological specimens
   Influence of the personality, sex, race, or age of interviewer on subject's responses

Limitations due to subject characteristics
   Memory limitations of subjects including poor recall of exposures and influence of recent
      exposures on memory of past exposures
   Limitations of proxy respondents' knowledge and memory of subject's exposures
   Tendency of subjects to over-report socially desirable behaviours and under-report socially
      undesirable behaviours
   Variability in biological char acteristics over time (e.g. day-to-day variations, seasonal
      variation)

Errors during data capture and analysis
   Data entry errors
   Errors in conversion tables used to convert subject responses to units of active agent
   Programming errors in creating variables for analysis

A particular concern is *differential exposure measurement error*, which occurs when exposure measurement error differs according to the disease or outcome being studied. Sources of differential error include:

- *recall bias*, i.e. when cases, for example, report exposures differently from controls because of their knowledge or feelings about the disease
- the influence of the data collector's knowledge of the subject's disease status on the exposure measure
- different distributions of laboratory technicians or interviewers between cases and controls
- differences in specimen handling or storage between cases and controls
- the biological effects of the disease or treatment on the exposure
- the biological effects or symptoms of the pre-diagnostic phase of the disease

♦ the influence of a strong nsk factor for the disease (e.g. family history) on the reporting of the exposure

While differential exposure measurement error is a major concern when studies involve retrospective collection of exposure data, the latter two sources of differential error can occur in prospectively collected data as well.

The most important effect of measurement error in a study is that it leads to bias in the odds ratio (or other measure of association between the exposure and outcome); this is called *misclassification bias* or *information bias*.

This chapter is divided into two main sections, the first on measurement error in continuous exposure variables and the second on measurement error (misclassification) in categorical exposure variables. Within each of these sections, the parameters to quantify the degree of measurement error in an exposure variable are described. These parameters are computed by comparing the mismeasured exposure with a perfect measure of the true exposure in a population. In this chapter, it is assumed that a measure of the true exposure exists (even though sometimes it does not), and that measurements of the true exposure are known on the entire population. In actual practice, measurement error would be ascertained in a validity study, which would be conducted on a small sample of subjects who would be measured with both the imperfect and perfect measure of exposure. The two main sections each include a discussion of how the parameters that quantify the exposure measurement error can be used to estimate the effects of this degree of error on the bias in the odds ratio in the parent epidemiological study, and on power and sample size. The *parent epidemiological study* refers to the study that will use (or has used) the mismeasured exposure to estimate the odds ratio for the exposure–disease relationship. The odds ratio from the parent epidemiological study is called the *observable odds ratio* because it is the odds ratio that will be obtained (on average) that differs from the true odds ratio due to exposure measurement error.

Further ways of estimating measurement error, including techniques which do not require a perfect measure of the true exposure, are given in Chapter 4.

Continuous Exposure Measures

The theory of measurement error in a continuous variable and its effects on studies of a continuous outcome were first developed in the fields of psychometrics, survey research, and statistics (Hansen *et al.* 1961; Lord and Novick 1968; Cochran 1968; Nunnally 1978; Allen and Yen 1979; Bohrnstedt 1983; Fuller 1987). The effects of measurement error have since been derived in the context of epidemiological studies of a continuous exposure variable and a dichotomous disease outcome (Prentice 1982; Whittemore and Grosser 1986; Armstrong *et al.* 1989). See Thürigen *et al.* (2000) for a review.

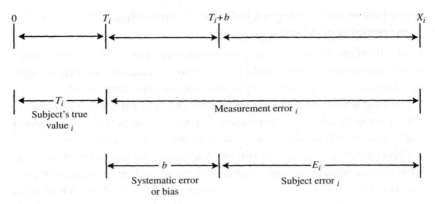

Figure 3.1 Measurement error in the measurement of X_i.

A model of measurement error

A simple model of measurement error in a population is

$$X_i = T_i + b + E_i$$

where $\mu_E = 0$ and $\rho_{TE} = 0$. This model is illustrated in Figure 3.1. In it, the observed measure X_i for a given individual i differs from the true value T_i for that individual as a consequence of two types of measurement error. The first is systematic error or *bias b* which would occur (on average) for all measured subjects. The second, E_i, is the additional error in X_i for subject i. E is referred to as the *subject error*, to indicate that it varies from subject to subject. It does not refer to error due to subject characteristics, but rather may include all of the sources of error outlined in Table 3.1.

For the population of potential study subjects, X, T, and E are variables with distributions; for example, the distribution of E is the distribution of subject measurement errors in the population of interest. X, T, and E have expectations (population means over an infinite population) denoted by μ_X, μ_T, and μ_E, respectively, and variances denoted by σ_X^2, σ_T^2, and σ_E^2. Because the average measurement error in X in the population is expressed in the model as a constant b, it follows that μ_E, the population mean of the subject error, is zero. The assumption of the model that the correlation coefficient of T with E, ρ_{TE}, is zero implies that the true values of exposure are not correlated with the subject errors in the population. In other words, subjects with high true values are assumed not to have systematically higher (or lower) errors than subjects with lower true values.

> *Example.* Suppose that a portable scale is used to weigh subjects for a study of weight and hip fracture among a population of elderly women. Although current weight (X) will be measured, the true

exposure of interest (T) is the subject's average weight over the previous 5 years. (The true exposure could be measured in theory by averaging multiple weighings over the 5-year period.) Measures of weight in the population of interest would yield observations for X that would differ from each subject's true weight T because of measurement error, as shown in the example in Table 3.2.

The measurement error can be broken down into two components:

- the systematic bias b which would affect all members of the study population
- the remainder E of the error which varies from subject to subject.

In this example, suppose that the bias in X (in the population to be studied) is 1 kg. The sources of systematic bias in X might be:

- the scale is miscalibrated so that it reads on average 0.5 kg too heavy
- subjects currently weigh on average 0.5 kg more than their average weight over the previous 5 years.

The sources of subject error might include:

- randomness in the mechanics of the scale beyond the scale's usual 0.5 kg overestimation
- the difference between each individual's current weight and her average 5-year weight (beyond the average 0.5 kg increase).

Other sources of error which could contribute to bias and subject error include:

- the weight of the subject's clothes
- misreading of the scale by the interviewer
- random hour-to-hour and day-to-day fluctuations in 'current' weight.

Table 3.2 Example of measurement error in observations of body weight in a series of subjects where X_i represents the observed weight, T_i the true weight, b the bias, and E_i the remainder of the error

	Subject (i)			
	1	2	3	4 ...
X_i (kg)	61	50	70	63
T_i (kg)	59	52	69	60
Measurement error	2	-2	1	3
b (kg)	1	1	1	1
E_i (kg)	1	-3	0	2

Measures of measurement error

Two measures of measurement error are used to describe the validity of X, i.e. the relationship of X to T in the population of interest, based on the above model and assumptions. One is the bias or the average measurement error in the population, which is the difference between the population mean of X and the population mean of T:

$$b = \mu_X - \mu_T.$$

A positive b means that X overestimates the amount of exposure on average, whereas a negative b means that X underestimates exposure.

The other is a measure of the *precision* of X, i.e. a measure of the variation in the measurement error in the population. One measure of precision is the variance σ_E^2 of E. (Note that the model is formulated in such a way that the variance σ_E^2 is the variance of the measurement error; b, a constant, does not contribute to the variance.)

The measure of precision we adopt here is the correlation ρ_{TX} of T with X, termed the *validity coefficient* of X. Under the above model, it can be shown that the square of ρ_{TX} is 1 minus the ratio of the variance of E to the variance of X (Allen and Yen 1979):

$$\rho_{TX}^2 = 1 - \frac{\sigma_E^2}{\sigma_X^2} = \frac{\sigma_T^2}{\sigma_X^2}. \qquad [3.1]$$

ρ_{TX}^2 is also the proportion of the variance of X explained by T. From Equation 3.1 it can be seen that the smaller the error variance, the greater ρ_{TX}^2. ρ_{TX} can range between 0 and 1, with a value of 1 indicating that X is a perfectly precise measure of T. ρ_{TX} is assumed to be zero or greater, i.e. for X to be considered to be a measure of T, X must be positively correlated with T.

To further understand the separate concepts of bias and precision, consider a situation in which X only has a systematic bias, with $E_i = 0$ for all subjects (i.e. $\rho_{TX} = 1$ and $\sigma_E^2 = 0$). For example, suppose that the only source of error in a measurement of weight (X) is that the scale weighs each subject exactly 1 kg too heavy. Then, despite this systematic bias, the variable X could be used to order each person correctly in the population by his/her value of T. X would be perfectly precise. However, if E_i varied from person to person (around the mean $\mu_E = 0$), the ordering would be lost. The greater the variance of E, relative to the variance of X, the less precise is X as a measure of T. In this case the scale lacks precision ($\rho_{TX} < 1$) even though it is correct on average ($b=0$).

Example. Continuing the preceding example, the bias would be measured as the difference between the population mean of X and the population mean of T, i.e. 1 kg. The precision could be measured by the correlation of T with X. Suppose that ρ_{TX} were 0.8; this would mean that only 64 per cent (0.8^2) of the variance in X is explained by T, with the remainder of the variance being due to error.

Measurement error is not an inherent property of an instrument, but rather a property of the instrument applied in a particular manner to a specific population. Therefore the error can vary not only between two instruments which measure the same exposure, but also for a single instrument when applied differently or when applied to different population groups which vary by, say, level of education. Importantly, measurement error could also differ between the population of cases and the population of controls to be studied in an epidemiological study. In addition, the validity coefficient is dependent on the variance of the true exposure in the population σ_T^2. Therefore even if the error variance σ_E^2 were the same for two populations, ρ_{TX} would differ if σ_T^2 differed.

The terminology used in measurement error varies between fields of study. We will use the terms validity, accuracy, and measurement error as general terms describing the accuracy of X as a measure of T, including both the concepts of bias and precision. Some authors use the terms validity and accuracy to refer to lack of bias only. In addition, 'true value' can have various meanings. We define T as the underlying variable of interest. Our definition of the 'true value' is similar to what is termed a 'construct' or 'latent variable' in other fields, although these terms imply that the true value is unmeasurable.

Effects of measurement error on the population mean and variance of exposure

In a study population, both the mean and variance of the measured exposure X differ from the true exposure mean and variance because of measurement error. Under the above model, the population mean of X differs from the true mean (the population mean of T) by b:

$$\mu_X = \mu_T + b.$$

The population variance of X, based on the model and assumptions, is (Allen and Yen 1979):

$$\sigma_X^2 = \sigma_T^2 + \sigma_E^2 = \frac{\sigma_T^2}{\rho_{TX}^2}. \qquad [3.2]$$

Thus the variance of X in the population is greater than the variance of T, because of the addition of the variance of the measurement error.

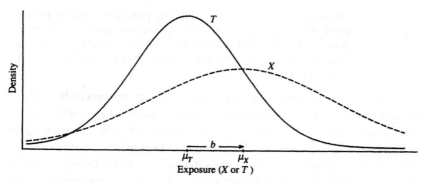

Figure 3.2 The effect of measurement error on the distribution of a normally distributed exposure. T, true exposure; X, exposure measured with error; μ_T, population mean of T; μ_X, population mean of X.

From the example given above, if the validity coefficient (ρ_{TX}) were 0.8, then the variance of measured weight X would be 56 per cent greater than the variance of T ($\sigma_X^2 = \sigma_T^2 / 0.8^2 = 1.56\,\sigma_T^2$ by Equation 3.2).

Figure 3.2 demonstrates the effect of measurement error on the distribution of X in a population assuming, for the purposes of the example, a normally distributed exposure and normally distributed error. The bias in the measure causes a shift in the distribution of X compared with T. The imprecision of X (measured by ρ_{TX}) causes a greater variance or dispersion of the distribution of X compared with that of T. Even if a measure were correct on average ($b = 0$), there could still be substantial effects of measurement error because of lack of precision which would lead to a greater dispersion in the measured exposures.

Effects of differential measurement error on the odds ratio

Measurement errors have an effect on the observable mean and variance of an exposure variable within a population, but of greater concern is the effect of exposure measurement error on the measure of association (e.g. an odds ratio or a correlation) between an exposure and an outcome in a study. In the next few sections of this chapter, examples of such effects of measurement errors will be given.

The equations given in this chapter are based on the assumption that the only source of error in the measure of association between the exposure and disease is measurement error in the exposure. The other sources of bias, including measurement error in the disease, selection bias, confounding, or the error due to sampling a finite number of subjects, are assumed to be absent.

It is common in epidemiological studies to measure the exposure as a continuous variable, and for the outcome to be a dichotomous disease state. The commonly used measure of association is the *odds ratio*, i.e. the odds of disease at one level of exposure relative to the odds of disease at another (usually lower) level of exposure; it is an estimate of the rate ratio.

Studies of dichotomous outcomes, whether they are case–control or cohort designs, can be thought of as a comparison of two population groups, the diseased and non-diseased. Extending the measurement error model to the two groups, the exposure measure X_N in the non-diseased group differs from the true exposure T_N by

$$X_{iN} = T_{iN} + b_N + E_{iN}$$

and similarly for the diseased group,

$$X_{iD} = T_{iD} + b_D + E_{iD}.$$

Differential exposure measurement error occurs when b_N, the bias in the exposure measure in the non-diseased group, differs from b_D, the bias in the diseased group, or when the precision of X_N differs from that of X_D.

Figure 3.3 gives a graphical presentation of an example of differential measurement error, specifically differential bias between cases and controls. In the figure, the true mean exposure μ_{T_D} in the diseased group is greater than the true mean exposure μ_{T_N} in the non-diseased group. This leads to a positive slope in the true odds ratio curve (OR_T). (The odds ratio curve is shown as the odds ratio for disease among those with exposure level X or T versus an arbitrary reference point r.) In this example, exposure is overestimated in the non-diseased group (positive bias), so that the distribution of X_N is shifted to the right relative to T_N, and the exposure is underestimated among those with disease (negative bias) so that the distribution of X_D is shifted to the left relative to T_D. This leads the observable odds ratio curve (OR_O) to cross over the null value of 1: it indicates less disease risk with increasing exposure, rather than the true increasing disease risk.

The effect of differential measurement error in X on the odds ratio can be easily quantified when certain simplifying assumptions are made. Results can be derived for unmatched case–control studies under the following assumptions:

- X_N and X_D are modelled as above with $\rho_{TE} = 0$ for each group
- T_N and T_D are normally distributed with means μ_{T_N} and μ_{T_D}, respectively, and the same variance σ_T^2
- E_N and E_D are normally distributed with mean zero and common variance σ_E^2.

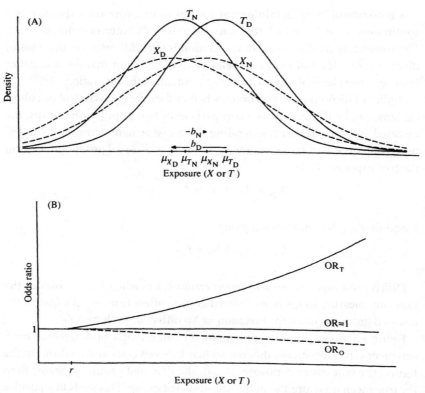

Figure 3.3 The effects of differential measurement error (differential bias) on (A) the distributions of exposure among the non-diseased and diseased groups, and (B) the odds ratio curve. T_N and T_D are the true exposures among the non-diseased group and the diseased group, respectively, X_N and X_D are the exposures measured with error among the non-diseased group and the diseased group, respectively, OR_T is the true odds ratio for exposure versus reference level r, and OR_O is the observable odds ratio for exposure versus reference level r.

The last assumption means that only differential bias, not differential precision, will be considered.

The above assumptions imply a logistic regression model for the probability of disease ($\Pr(d)$) as a function of true exposure T, with a true logistic regression coefficient β_T (Wu *et al.* 1986):

$$\log[\Pr(d) / (1 - \Pr(d))] = \alpha_T + \beta_T T$$

where $\beta_T = (\mu_{T_D} - \mu_{T_N}) / \sigma_T^2$. The true odds ratio for any u unit increase in T is $OR_T = \exp(\beta_T u)$.

With measurement error in the exposure variable X, the assumptions also lead to a logistic model (Armstrong *et al.* 1989):

$$\log[\Pr(d) / (1 - \Pr(d))] = \alpha_O + \beta_O X$$

where

$$\beta_O = [(\mu_{T_D} - \mu_{T_N}) + (b_D - b_N)] / (\sigma_T^2 + \sigma_E^2).$$

The observable logistic regression coefficient β_O differs from β_T because of the measurement error in X. β_O can be expressed in terms of β_T (if $\beta_T \neq 0$) as follows:

$$\beta_O = \left(1 + \frac{b_D - b_N}{\mu_{T_D} - \mu_{T_N}}\right) \rho_{TX}^2 \beta_T.$$

Therefore the observable odds ratio OR_O for a u unit increase in X can be expressed in terms of OR_T (if $\mu_{T_D} \neq \mu_{T_N}$) as follows:

$$\left.\begin{array}{l} OR_O = OR_T^{C\rho_{TX}^2} \\[2mm] \text{where } C = \left(1 + \dfrac{b_D - b_N}{\mu_{T_D} - \mu_{T_N}}\right). \end{array}\right\} \qquad [3.3]$$

OR_O differs from OR_T by two exponential factors. The effect of ρ_{TX}^2 is more predictable because it can only range from zero to one. However, the factor C can be any magnitude and either positive or negative. Thus the observable odds ratio could be closer to the null value of 1, further from the null value, or cross over the null value in comparison with the true odds ratio.

Example. Suppose that the study of weight and hip fracture had a case–control design and that the true average weight among cases was 2 kg less than the weight among controls. If the bias of the weight measure among controls (b_N) was 1 kg, but cases had gained an additional 2 kg ($b_D = 3$ kg) between their hip fracture and their participation in the study because of their immobility, then (assuming non-differential precision) by Equation 3.3:

$$C = \left(1 + \frac{3 - 1}{-2}\right) = 0$$

and

$$OR_O = 1.$$

> This shows that a differential bias between cases and controls of 2 kg would completely obscure a true difference of -2 kg, leading to no observable association between weight and hip fracture in the study.

The section on measurement and interpretation of differential bias in Chapter 4 provides further explanation of assessment of differential bias, as does the article by White (2003).

The above equations and Figure 3.3 were based on the assumption of equal precision for the diseased and non-diseased groups, but differential measurement error will also occur if precision differs between groups. If the biases were equal but if σ_E^2 differed (and σ_T^2 were equal for the two groups), the shape of the odds ratio function could change. For example, the observable curve could be U-shaped when, in reality, disease frequency increases consistently with increasing exposure (Gregorio *et al.* 1985). These effects of differential precision are generally less of a problem in interpretation of the exposure–disease association than the effects of differential bias described above. Therefore, the assessment of differential bias is of greater concern.

Effects of non-differential measurement error on the odds ratio

When the assumptions made in the previous section hold, there is *non-differential exposure measurement error* if there is equal bias and equal error variance (or equivalently equal ρ_{TX}) between the diseased and non-diseased groups. Figure 3.4 illustrates the effects of non-differential measurement error. Under non-differential measurement error, the two distributions may shift, but they are not shifted with respect to each other because there is equal bias for the two groups. Thus, based on the model presented, the observable difference in the mean values of X between cases and controls $(\mu_{X_D} - \mu_{X_N})$ is equal to the true difference $(\mu_{T_D} - \mu_{T_N})$. However, the lack of precision in X widens each distribution and leads to more overlap and less distinction between the distributions of X_N and X_D compared with the true distributions. The odds ratio curve is flattened towards the horizontal line of odds ratio equal to 1 for all X.

When there is non-differential measurement error, and the assumptions of the last section hold, we obtain (Whittemore and Grosser 1986; Wu *et al.* 1986)

$$\beta_O = \rho_{TX}^2 \beta_T. \tag{3.4}$$

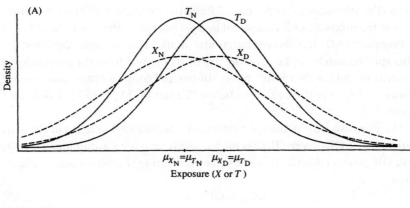

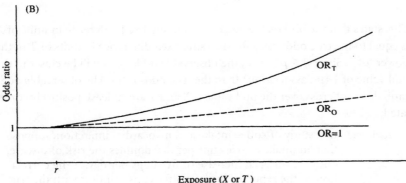

Figure 3.4 The effects of non-differential measurement error on (A) the exposure distributions of the non-diseased and diseased groups, and (B) the odds ratio curve. T_N and T_D are the true exposures among the non-diseased group and the diseased group respectively, X_N and X_D are the exposures measured with error among the non-diseased group and diseased group respectively, OR_T is the true odds ratio for exposure versus reference level r, OR_O is the observable odds ratio for exposure versus reference level r.

This states that the observable logistic regression coefficient β_O from analyses with X measured with non-differential error is closer to the null value of zero the true β_T by the factor ρ_{TX}^2. Equation 3.4 is referred to as an *attenuation equation*, because it shows that the observable association is attenuated towards the null hypothesis of no association.

While the difference in bias of X between cases and controls ($b_D - b_N$) can play a major role in the bias in the odds ratio under differential measurement error (Equation 3.3), Equation 3.4 shows that the bias in the odds ratio (the attenuation) under non-differential measurement error is a function of the precision of X (measured by ρ_{TX}) but not of the bias in X.

Prentice (1982) has shown that, under similar assumptions, Equation 3.4 also approximately applies to estimates of β obtained from the proportional hazards model for data from cohort studies and from matched case–control studies. Therefore the equations below (Equations [3.5]–[3.7]) would also apply.

There are two ways to interpret attenuation formula 3.4 in terms of the odds ratio. First, if $OR_T = \exp(\beta_T u)$ is the true odds ratio for a u-unit increase in T, and $OR_O = \exp(\beta_O u)$ is the observable odds ratio for a u-unit increase in X, then

$$OR_O = OR_T^{\rho_{TX}^2}. \tag{3.5}$$

This states that the observable odds ratio for any fixed difference in units of X is equal to the true odds ratio for the same fixed difference in units of T to the power ρ_{TX}^2. Since $0 \leq \rho_{TX}^2 \leq 1$, the observable odds ratio will be closer to the null value of 1 (no association) than the true odds ratio. The observable odds ratio does not cross over the null value if X and T are, at least, positively correlated.

> *Example.* In a study of coffee intake and myocardial infarction, suppose that an intake of five cups per day doubles the risk of disease: $OR_T = 2$ for each increase of five cups per day. If the correlation of the reported 'usual' coffee consumption with the true intake is 0.7, then the observable odds ratio for a five-cup intake is $2^{0.49} = 1.4$ (from Equation 3.5). Thus even when the association between X and T is moderately strong, the resulting attenuation in the odds ratio can be large.

The attenuation formula can also be looked at in another important way. Since one effect of measurement error is to increase the variance of X compared with T (Equation 3.2), there would be a greater spread of misclassified exposures than true exposures within the groups of cases and controls (as in Figure 3.4). Rather than comparing OR_T with OR_O based on some fixed difference in *units* of T or X, one might compare OR_T for a difference in terms of the standard deviation of T ($OR_T = \exp(\beta_T s \sigma_T)$) with OR_O for the same difference in terms of the standard deviation of X ($OR_O = \exp(\beta_O s \sigma_X)$). Then the observable odds ratio of disease for an increase in X of s standard deviations of X is (de Klerk *et al.* 1989)

$$OR_O = OR_T^{\rho_{TX}}. \tag{3.6}$$

This states that the observable odds ratio for a difference of s standard deviations of X is equal to the true odds ratio for a difference of s standard deviations of T to the power ρ_{TX}. Comparing Equation 3.6 with Equation 3.5, it is apparent that the attenuation is less when the observable odds ratio is *interpreted* in terms of the standard deviation (or, more generally, the distribution) of X, rather than interpreting the odds ratio in actual units of X.

> *Example.* Using the coffee consumption and myocardial infarction example again, suppose that the true standard deviation of coffee intake per day is 2.5 cups and the true odds ratio OR_T for an increase of two standard deviations of T (five cups) is 2. If $\rho_{TX} = 0.7$, the standard deviation of X is 3.57 (2.5/0.7 from Equation 3.2). Then, from Equation 3.6, the observable odds ratio for an increase of two standard deviations of X is $2^{0.7} = 1.6$. The interpretation of the observable odds ratio of 1.6 as the odds ratio for a difference of two standard deviations in exposure is more accurate than interpreting the observable odds ratio of 1.4 (from the previous example) as a measure of the odds ratio for a five-cup difference in exposure.

Further examples of the effects of non-differential measurement error on the odds ratio, based on Equations 3.5 and 3.6, are given in Table 3.3 (columns 3 and 4). The table shows that exposures with a validity coefficient ρ_{TX} near 0.5 would obscure all but the strongest associations, while measures so accurate as to have $\rho_{TX} = 0.9$ still lead to appreciable attenuation.

Effects of non-differential measurement error on power and sample size

Measurement error in X also affects the power of a study, or the sample size needed. For example, unmatched case–control studies often employ a sample size calculation based on the normality assumption for the exposure variable as follows:

$$n = 2\left[(Z_{\alpha/2} + Z_\beta)^2 \sigma^2\right] / d^2$$

where $Z_{\alpha/2}$ denotes the upper $100\,(1-\alpha/2)$ centile of the standard normal distribution, d is the magnitude of the difference to be detected between the mean exposure of the cases and controls, σ^2 is the common variance of the exposure in each group, α is the significance level for a two-sided test of the hypothesis, β is 1 minus the required power, and n is the sample size needed in each group (Kelsey *et al.* 1996).

Table 3.3 Effect of non-differential measurement error in a normally distributed exposure X on the observable odds ratio (OR_O)

$\rho_{TX}{}^a$	$OR_T{}^b$	u-unit difference in X OR_O	$s\sigma_X$ difference in X OR_O	Upper versus lower quarter of X OR_O
0.5	1.5	1.11	1.22	1.19
0.7	1.5	1.22	1.33	1.29
0.9	1.5	1.39	1.44	1.39
0.5	2.0	1.19	1.41	1.35
0.7	2.0	1.40	1.62	1.54
0.9	2.0	1.75	1.87	1.76
0.5	4.0	1.41	2.00	1.81
0.7	4.0	1.97	2.64	2.35
0.9	4.0	3.07	3.48	3.11

[a] ρ_{TX} is the validity coefficient of X.

[b] OR_T represents the true odds ratio for a u-unit difference in T for comparison with OR_O for a u-unit difference in X, OR_T represents the true odds ratio for an $s\sigma_T$ difference in T for comparison with OR_O for an $s\sigma_X$ difference in X, and OR_T represents the true odds ratio for the upper versus lower quarter of T for comparison with OR_O for the upper versus lower quarter of X.

The effect of non-differential measurement error under the model used in this chapter is to increase the variance of X such that $\sigma_X^2 = \sigma_T^2 / \rho_{TX}^2$, while d would remain the same. Then the sample size n_X needed to detect a difference of d in a study with non-differential measurement error with reference to the sample size n_T needed in a study in which the exposure is measured without error is (Fleiss 1986)

$$n_X = n_T / \rho_{TX}^2. \qquad [3.7]$$

This formula may be of theoretical interest only, since an empirical estimate of σ_X^2 is usually available for the calculation of sample size. However, it can be used to show the potentially dramatic effects of poor exposure measurement on the sample size required. For example, if the correlation between T and X is 0.7 ($\rho_{TX}^2 = 0.49$), the sample size required when the imperfect measure is used is twice that required if a perfect measure were available.

Measurement error can also have adverse effects on the power of a study. The power of a case–control study involving a normally distributed exposure with common standard deviation σ and mean difference d can be derived from the following equation (Kelsey *et al.* 1996):

$$\text{power} = 1 - \Phi\left(\frac{d}{\sigma}\sqrt{\frac{1}{2}n} - Z_{\alpha/2}\right)$$

where $\Phi(z)$ is the probability that a standard normal variable is above z. As noted above, the effect of non-differential measurement error is to increase the standard deviation in the formula, such that $\sigma_X = \sigma_T/\rho_{TX}$. If an empirical estimate of σ_X is not available during the planning of a study, and if the sample size is miscalculated based on the variance of a more precise measure of exposure (as may be the case for measurements in a small-scale well-controlled pilot study), the power of the study will be less than predicted.

> *Example.* Suppose that a sample size for a study is calculated to be able to detect a difference between cases and controls of 10 months in the mean exposure to a certain drug. An estimated standard deviation of 40 months for duration of exposure was based on medical record reviews. Then the sample size for a two-sided α of 5 per cent and 80 per cent power would be
>
> $$n = 2\left[(1.96 + 0.84)^2\, 40^2\right] / (10)^2$$
> $$= 251 \text{ per group.}$$
>
> Suppose that the record review gave nearly perfect measurements of the exposure, but the study exposure will actually be measured by self-report which has a non-differential error such that $\rho_{TX} = 0.7$. Then the standard deviation of the study measure would be σ_T/ρ_{TX} or 57 months, and the study power would not be the calculated 80 per cent but instead only 50 per cent:
>
> $$\text{power} = 1 - \Phi\left(\frac{10}{57}\sqrt{\frac{251}{2}} - 1.96\right)$$
> $$= 50\%.$$

Effects of measurement error on measures of association between a continuous exposure and a continuous outcome

The effect of measurement error on the relationship of a continuous exposure with a continuous outcome also deserves mention. Suppose that the relationship between a continuous exposure X and a continuous outcome Y is to be studied, and their association is to be assessed by correlation and regression. Suppose that the measurement error in X is given by the model described on

p. 68, and Y is measured without error. There is a non-differential measurement error in X with respect to the outcome Y when E is uncorrelated with Y. The observable correlation coefficient of X with Y in these circumstances is given by (Allen and Yen 1979)

$$\rho_{XY} = \rho_{TY}\rho_{TX}. \qquad [3.8]$$

This equation states that the observable correlation ρ_{XY} is weaker than the true correlation ρ_{TY} by a factor equal to the validity coefficient of X.

> *Example.* Suppose that the true correlation of physical activity over the preceding 5 years and current body mass index (ρ_{TY}) is 0.5. Assume that body mass index (weight/height^2) is measured without error, but the correlation ρ_{TX} of true activity level with physical activity as ascertained by a self-administered questionnaire in the study population is 0.6. Also assume that the error in the assessment of physical activity is not correlated with body mass index. Then the observable correlation coefficient ρ_{XY} in the study is (by Equation 3.8) $0.5 \times 0.6 = 0.3$, a considerable attenuation from the true association of 0.5.

If β_T is the true regression coefficient from the regression equation

$$Y = \alpha_T + \beta_T T,$$

then the observable regression coefficient β_O from the regression equation

$$Y = \alpha_O + \beta_O X$$

is (Allen and Yen 1979)

$$\beta_O = \rho_{TX}^2 \beta_T. \qquad [3.9]$$

Note that Equation 3.9 is identical to Equation 3.4. Also note that the attenuation formulae 3.8 and 3.9 are functions of ρ_{TX} but not of the bias in X. This is because adding a constant to a variable does not change its coefficient of correlation with another variable, or its regression coefficient.

Differential measurement error can have any effect on the correlation or regression coefficients. Depending on the nature of the relationship between E and Y, the association between X and Y could be stronger or weaker than the true association, or even have the opposite sign.

Violations of the assumptions

In this chapter, several simplifying assumptions have been made. First, the model states that X is a measure of T with a simple additive error E, and that ρ_{TE} is 0. In other words, large positive errors are not more (or less) common for large values of T. However, it is likely that in some situations the size of the error would depend on T. For example, if X were a measure of the lifetime number of X-ray procedures, the under-ascertainment might become greater with increasing true lifetime numbers of procedures. A related violation may come about if X is a measure of T, but on a different scale of measurement. These violations are examples of a model in which X is a linear function of T (or, equivalently, part of the error is proportional to T) as follows:

$$X_i = cT_i + b + E_i.$$

Only Equations 3.6, 3.7, and 3.8 still hold under this model. These equations do not change under linear transformations of X.

Several other assumptions have been made, including the normality of T and E in equations expressing the effect of measurement error on logistic regression, and the assumptions of no sampling error, no confounding, and no error in ascertainment of disease. The purpose of the equations presented above is to permit estimation of the effects of varying degrees of measurement error in a simplified situation, to aid in the interpretation of the effects of measurement error. In actual studies of a continuous exposure, the distribution of the true exposure among cases and controls and the distribution of errors can take on almost any form. Unlike the simple model presented, the shape of the odds ratio curve could change under non-differential measurement error, and for some levels of exposure the odds ratio could be biased away from the null or cross over the null value of 1 (Dosemeci *et al.* 1990). Further discussion of these limitations, as well as references to results derived under less restrictive assumptions, are given in Chapter 5 in the section on adjustment of study results for the effects of measurement error.

Categorical Exposure Measures

Measurement error in categorical variables is usually referred to as misclassification. Categorical variables, including dichotomous, nominal categorical, or ordered categorical variables, are subject to all the sources of measurement error outlined in Table 3.1.

Measures of misclassification in categorical variables

Misclassification of exposure implies that a certain proportion of subjects who truly fall into a specific exposure category will be correctly classified, but the remainder will be misclassified into other categories. For all types of categorical variables, the measurement error for a population can be described in a *misclassification matrix.* This is a matrix of the proportions C_{ij} of those with true exposure category j who will be classified into category i. This matrix can be represented as follows:

$$
\begin{array}{cc}
& \text{True exposure } j \\
\end{array}
$$

$$
\begin{array}{ccccc}
& & 1 & 2 & . & . & k \\
\text{Classified} & 1 & \\
& 2 & \left[\begin{array}{ccccc} C_{11} & C_{12} & . & . & C_{1k} \\ C_{21} & C_{22} & . & . & C_{2k} \\ . & . & . & . & . \\ . & . & . & . & . \\ C_{k1} & C_{k2} & . & . & C_{kk} \end{array}\right] \\
\text{exposure } i & \\
& k & \\
\text{Total} & & 1 & 1 & . & . & 1
\end{array}
$$

where k is the number of categories. Note that the C_{ij} sum down each column to 1 (the sum over true exposure j). The diagonal elements quantify the proportions correctly classified; a measure is perfect when the diagonal elements are all 1. As noted for measures of measurement error in continuous variables, the misclassification matrix depends on the instrument, the operational procedures, and the population to which the instrument is applied, and can differ by disease status.

For a dichotomous exposure ($k = 2$), only two classification probabilities are needed: the sensitivity and the specificity of the exposure measure. (The terms sensitivity and specificity are more commonly used to define the accuracy of a diagnostic test for disease, but they apply equally to accuracy of a dichotomous exposure measurement.) The *sensitivity* of the exposure measure is the proportion of those who truly have the exposure who will be correctly classified as exposed, and the *specificity* is the proportion of those who are truly unexposed who will be classified as unexposed. If category 1 is 'exposed' and 2 is 'unexposed' the misclassification matrix would be

$$
\begin{bmatrix} \text{sensitivity} & 1 - \text{specificity} \\ 1 - \text{sensitivity} & \text{specificity} \end{bmatrix}.
$$

The probability of misclassifying a truly exposed person as unexposed is (1 − sensitivity) and the probability of misclassifying a truly unexposed person is (1 − specificity).

Even though both sensitivity and specificity can range from 0 to 1, it is assumed that

$$
\text{sensitivity} + \text{specificity} \geqslant 1.
$$

In other words, for the instrument to be considered a measure of the exposure, it should classify a truly exposed person as exposed with greater (or at least equal) probability than it classifies a truly unexposed person as exposed, i.e.

$$\text{sensitivity} \geq 1 - \text{specificity}.$$

Effects of misclassification on the observable distribution of exposure in a population

The misclassification matrix relates the true distribution of exposure in a population to the misclassified distribution. For a population whose true distribution into the k categories of exposure (expressed as proportions) is $[P_1, P_2, ..., P_k]$, the observable (misclassified) distribution would be $[p_1, p_2, ..., p_k]$ according to the matrix equation

$$\begin{bmatrix} C_{11} & . & . & C_{1k} \\ . & . & . & . \\ . & . & . & . \\ . & . & . & . \\ C_{k1} & . & . & C_{kk} \end{bmatrix} \times \begin{bmatrix} P_1 \\ . \\ . \\ . \\ P_k \end{bmatrix} = \begin{bmatrix} p_1 \\ . \\ . \\ . \\ p_k \end{bmatrix} \qquad [3.10]$$

or, in non-matrix form,

$$p_i = \sum_j C_{ij} P_j.$$

This equation shows that some proportion of people in each of the true categories may fall into each of the observable categories. Applying it to a dichotomous exposure, the observable proportion p of the population who are exposed is composed of a proportion (sensitivity) of those truly exposed (P) plus a proportion (1 - specificity) of those unexposed (1 - P):

$$p = \text{sensitivity} \times P + (1 - \text{specificity}) \times (1 - P). \qquad [3.11]$$

Effects of differential misclassification of a dichotomous exposure on the odds ratio

While the above equations express the effect of misclassification within one population, a more common situation in epidemiology is the comparison of exposure between two populations: those with the disease of interest and those without. The effects of misclassification of categorical exposure measures are straightforward for two types of studies: studies of the association between a dichotomous exposure and a dichotomous disease outcome (Bross 1954; Newell 1962; Gullen *et al.* 1968; Goldberg 1975; Copeland *et al.* 1977; Barron 1977; Fleiss 1981; Kleinbaum *et al.* 1982) and, under certain assumptions, studies of an ordered categorical exposure and a dichotomous disease outcome (Walker and Blettner 1985; de Klerk *et al.* 1989).

In an unmatched case–control study of a dichotomous exposure, under the assumption that the disease is measured without error, the effect of misclassification of exposure is to rearrange individuals in the true 2×2 table into an observable 2×2 table. Individuals remain in the correct disease group but may be misclassified as to exposure status, as shown in Figure 3.5. P_D and P_N are the true proportions exposed in the diseased and non-diseased groups, respectively, and similarly p_D and p_N refer to the observable proportions exposed in the two groups.

There is *differential misclassification* when the sensitivity of the exposure measure for the diseased group (sens_D) differs from that for the non-diseased group (sens_N), or the specificity of exposure for the diseased group (spec_D) differs from that for the non-diseased group (spec_N), or both. The observable odds ratio can be calculated by applying Equation 3.11 separately to the diseased and non-diseased groups (Goldberg 1975):

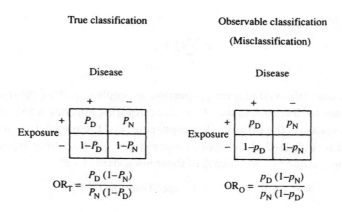

Figure 3.5 The effects of misclassification of a dichotomous exposure on the distribution of exposure and the odds ratio. (P_D and P_N are the true proportions exposed in the diseased and non-diseased groups respectively, p_D and p_N are the observable proportions in each group, OR_T is the true odds ratio and OR_O is the observable odds ratio).

$$p_D = \text{sens}_D P_D + (1 - \text{spec}_D)(1 - P_D)$$
$$p_N = \text{sens}_N P_N + (1 - \text{spec}_N)(1 - P_N) \quad [3.12]$$
$$OR_O = \left[p_D(1 - p_N) \right] / \left[p_N(1 - p_D) \right].$$

As with continuous exposures, differential misclassification can have any kind of effect on the odds ratio; in comparison with the true odds ratio, the observable odds ratio can be closer to the null hypothesis of OR = 1, be further from the null, or cross over the null.

Example. In a case–control study of the relationship between maternal use of illegal drugs during pregnancy and infant birth defects, suppose that all the exposed mothers of the children with birth defects felt committed to accurately disclose any illegal drug use ($\text{sens}_D = 1.0$), while only half of exposed mothers of control children were inclined to admit drug use ($\text{sens}_N = 0.5$). Similarly, suppose that some (10 per cent) unexposed mothers of cases reported using illegal drugs during pregnancy ($\text{spec}_D = 0.9$) out of concern about the effects of use before pregnancy, while the unexposed control mothers accurately reported no use ($\text{spec}_N = 1.0$). Then if the true classification is as shown, the observable classification and observable odds ratio would be as follows (from Equations 3.12):

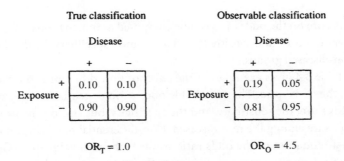

Thus, a true odds ratio of 1.0, i.e. no association between the disease and exposure, could appear as a strong association because of differential misclassification.

Effects of non-differential misclassification of a dichotomous exposure on the odds ratio

Non-differential misclassification occurs when the sensitivity and specificity of the exposure measurement for the diseased group are equal to those for the non-diseased group. The effect of non-differential misclassification of

Table 3.4 Effect of non-differential misclassification of a dichotomous exposure on the observable odds ratio (OR_O)

			True odds ratio		
			$OR_T = 1.5$	$OR_T = 2.0$	$OR_T = 4.0$
Exposure sensitivity	Exposure specificity	P_N^a	OR_O	OR_O	OR_O
0.6	0.9	0.1	1.17	1.34	1.93
0.6	0.9	0.5	1.24	1.42	1.86
0.6	0.99	0.1	1.40	1.79	3.20
0.6	0.99	0.5	1.30	1.54	2.12
0.9	0.9	0.1	1.24	1.48	2.41
0.9	0.9	0.5	1.38	1.73	2.85
0.9	0.99	0.1	1.45	1.89	3.61
0.9	0.99	0.5	1.43	1.82	3.11

[a] P_N is the true proportion exposed in the non-diseased group. The true proportion P_D exposed in the diseased group is, by definition,

$$P_N = P_N \, OR_T \, / \, (1 + P_N \, (OR_T - 1)).$$

exposure on the odds ratio can be computed as in Equations 3.12, except that there is a common sensitivity and a common specificity for the diseased and non-diseased groups.

Table 3.4 gives examples of the effect of non-differential misclassification on the odds ratio. The observable odds ratio depends not only on the true odds ratio, the sensitivity, and the specificity, but also on the probability of exposure among the non-diseased. Non-differential misclassification leads to an attenuation of the odds ratio towards the null value of 1 (Gullen *et al.* 1968). As can be seen from Table 3.4, the attenuation can be appreciable even with a high sensitivity and specificity. For example, a true odds ratio of 4 is attenuated to 2.85 when sensitivity is 0.9, specificity is 0.9, and P_N is 0.5. The observable odds ratio does not cross over the null value of 1 if, at least, the measurement classifies a truly exposed person as exposed with the same or greater probability as it classifies a truly unexposed person as exposed (i.e. sensitivity + specificity ≥ 1).

The results of Equations 3.12 for differential and non-differential misclassification of exposure in case–control studies also apply to cohort studies. However, for cohort studies in which exposed persons are over-sampled in comparison with unexposed persons, the sensitivity and specificity of the exposure measurement change after the sampling. In such cohort studies, the true 2 × 2 table can be considered to represent the entire population (before sampling), stratified by future disease status. Before one can sample by exposure, the population must be 'measured' as to exposure, leading to the misclassified 2 × 2 table and the resulting observable (future) odds ratio. The cohort sampling is based on the *misclassified* population, and that sampling does not change the observable odds ratio. However, *within* the cohort study after sampling, the sensitivity of the exposure measure is greater than the population sensitivity because exposed individuals who were correctly classified are more likely to enter the study than exposed individuals who were incorrectly classified as unexposed. The specificity also changes, as do the probabilities of exposure in the diseased and non-diseased groups.

Effects of non-differential misclassification of a dichotomous exposure on sample size and power

Non-differential misclassification leads to an increase in the sample size required for a study, because the observable odds ratio is attenuated. Sample size calculations for case–control studies usually depend on the hypothesized odds ratio and the proportion of the non-diseased group exposed. For cohort studies they depend on the odds ratio and the probability of disease among the non-exposed group. In planning a study, the sample size calculations should be based on estimates of the observable study parameters rather than estimates based on studies in which the exposure is measured with greater accuracy. If the increased sample size requirement due to misclassification is not taken into consideration in planning the study, non-differential misclassification results in a fall in study power (Bross 1954; Mote and Anderson 1965; Quade *et al.* 1980).

> *Example.* Suppose that animal experiments suggest that breast cancer risk is dependent on selenium intake. A case–control study of this relationship may classify case and control women into two exposure categories: those above the control median of selenium intake, and those below. The results of animal studies, which could measure selenium intake accurately, are extrapolated to yield a study hypothesis that those in the upper half of intake will have 0.6 times the risk as those in the lower half (OR = 0.6). The sample size based on this hypothesized odds ratio, equal-sized study groups, $\alpha = 0.05$, and 80 per cent power is (Kelsey *et al.* 1986)

$$n = \frac{2(Z_{\alpha/2} + Z_\beta)^2 \, \overline{P}(1 - \overline{P})}{(P_D - P_N)^2} = 247 \text{ per group}$$

where

$$P_D = \frac{P_N OR}{1 + P_N(OR - 1)} = 0.375$$

is the probability of exposure in the diseased group, P_N is the probability of exposure in the control group (0.5 in this example), and $\bar{P}$ is the mean exposure of the two groups. Suppose that selenium intake over the aetiologically relevant time period is difficult to measure in the study population, such that the sensitivity of the measure is 0.7 and the specificity is 0.7 for both cases and controls. Then the observable odds ratio would equal 0.8 (by Equations 3.12). If the sample size of 247 for each group were used, the actual study power would only be 20 per cent.

Effects of non-differential misclassification in an ordered categorical exposure on the odds ratio

The effects of differential and non-differential misclassification can also be predicted for categorical exposure variables other than dichotomous variables. If the misclassification matrix for cases and controls were known and the true distribution of exposure among cases and non-cases were known, then Equation 3.10 could be applied separately to cases and controls. The resulting observable distribution of exposure among cases and controls could be used to calculate the observable odds ratios for a comparison of disease risk for each category of exposure versus the reference category.

For categorical exposures with more than two categories, general conclusions cannot be drawn about the effect of non-differential misclassification on the odds ratio for each category (Dosemeci *et al.* 1990). However, for ordered categorical exposures, if the risk of disease either monotonically increases or decreases with the true exposure, and the mean value of the measured exposure increases monotonically with the true exposure, then, as with continuous variables, non-differential misclassification attenuates the odds ratios toward the null value of 1 (Weinberg *et al.* 1994).

One special case of interest is non-differential misclassification of an ordered categorical exposure variable when, as is common in epidemiology, the exposure variable is derived by dividing a continuous variable X into discrete categories. X is assumed to be measured with error as in the measurement error model presented for continuous variables, with X, T, and E normally distributed. Under these assumptions, the joint distribution of X and T is bivariate normal with correlation coefficient ρ_{TX}. This joint distribution can be used to quantify the misclassification matrix for an ordered categorical variable in which X is divided into categories (e.g. quarters or fifths) based on quantiles of X in the non-diseased group (Walker and Blettner 1985; de Klerk *et al.* 1989).

The last column of Table 3.3 gives examples of the attenuation of the odds ratio for those in the upper quarter of exposure versus the lowest quarter for several values of ρ_{TX} and OR_T, the true odds ratio for those in the upper quarter versus the lowest quarter. The attenuation appears to be somewhat *more* (by about 10 per cent of OR_T) than that which would be predicted based on the attenuation formula for the odds ratio in the logistic model interpreted in terms of the distribution of the measured exposure (last column versus fourth column of Table 3.3) (de Klerk *et al.* 1989).

This indicates that classifying a continuous exposure into a small number of categories does not reduce the effects of measurement error. Classifying subjects into broad categories of exposure may appear to lessen the chance of measurement error in comparison with attempting to classify subjects more finely (e.g. a 'continuous' measure), because small errors may not be sufficient to misclassify a subject. However, this apparent protection from error is lost as a consequence of the fact that when a subject does move from one broad category to another the error is larger than when a finer categorization is used.

However, categorizing a continuous variable does have an advantage. It generally leads to an interpretation of the odds ratio in terms of the distribution of exposure, an approach which lessens the consequences of measurement error in comparison with interpreting the odds ratio in terms of units of exposure (last column compared with third column of Table 3.3).

Effect of Measurement Error in the Presence of Covariates

In analysing the relationship between an exposure and an outcome, it is usually necessary to adjust for confounding factors. These factors, often exposures of interest themselves, are also subject to the sources of measurement error discussed in this chapter. For example, in a study with body weight as a primary exposure, it may be necessary to adjust for the potentially confounding effects of dietary intake of energy, an exposure which would be more difficult to assess accurately than the primary exposure.

The effects of measurement error in the primary exposure and covariates are not easy to quantify unless the exposure error is independent of the confounder and the confounder error, and vice versa. In this case, the effects of non-differential measurement error in an exposure and/or a confounder are predictable, and the same results apply for studies in which the primary exposure and confounder are continuous bivariate normal variables (Armstrong *et al.* 1989), or the exposure and confounder are dichotomous

(Greenland 1980). When the confounding factor is measured with non-differential error, but the exposure is measured perfectly, residual confounding can remain after adjustment for the confounding factor. Therefore the adjusted observed disease-exposure association could appear stronger (or weaker) than the true adjusted association. Adjustment by use of a poor measure of the confounder may be equivalent to no control of the confounder at all. When the exposure is measured with non-differential error and the covariate is measured perfectly, the attenuation toward the null of the adjusted disease–exposure association can be even greater than the attenuation of the crude association. When both the exposure and the confounder are measured with error, either of these effects can dominate so that the adjusted measure of association could be stronger or weaker than the true association.

Measurement error can also induce spurious effect modification. As noted earlier, the effect of measurement error on the odds ratio is dependent on the distribution of exposure (σ_T^2 for continuous variables and the true proportion exposed for dichotomous variables). Therefore when comparing, for example, the odds ratios across two or more groups categorized by the potential effect modifier, the observable odds ratios may differ even if the true odds ratios are identical because of the differential effect of measurement error in these groups.

Summary

Validity is not an inherent property of an instrument; it is a property of an instrument applied to a particular population using a specific protocol. For a continuous exposure X, the validity or measurement error in X can be represented by the bias ($\mu_X - \mu_T$) and by the validity coefficient ρ_{TX}, the correlation of the true exposure T with the measured exposure X in the population. For categorical variables, the measurement error is quantified by the misclassification matrix or, equivalently, by the sensitivity and the specificity for a dichotomous exposure measure. For studies comparing diseased and non-diseased groups, these measures should be assessed separately in the two groups.

Differential measurement error occurs when exposure measurement error varies by outcome status (e.g. diseased or non-diseased). It can cause the observed association between the measured exposure and the outcome to appear stronger or weaker than the true association, or can lead to an association in the opposite direction, thus completely invalidating the results of the study. For continuous exposures, differential bias is the major concern because it can lead to more untoward effects than differential precision.

Non-differential exposure measurement error can lead (although not invariably) to attenuation towards the null value of no association in the measure of association between the exposure and the outcome. For continuous variables, the attenuation is a function of ρ_{TX} only. The degree of attenuation is larger than commonly appreciated. For example, an exposure measured so well as to correlate with the true exposure with $\rho_{TX} = 0.7$ would lead to a true odds ratio of 4 being attenuated to an observed odds ratio of 2. This attenuation calls for a larger study sample size or, for a fixed sample size, leads to less power to detect an association.

There are some important conclusions regarding the effects of non-differential measurement error.

- The magnitude of the bias in the odds ratio or in a correlation coefficient does not depend on the sample size, so that increasing the sample size does not reduce the bias. However, increasing the sample size would increase the power to detect the attenuated association as significantly different from the null hypothesis.

- Interpreting the observed odds ratio in terms of the observed distribution of the exposure (e.g. the odds ratio for a one standard deviation increase in exposure, or for the upper quarter versus the lower quarter of exposure), rather than in terms of measured units of the exposure, provides a more accurate view of the odds ratio.

- A continuous exposure measurement that is 'good on average' (bias equal to zero for both diseased and non-diseased) does not eliminate the effects of measurement error from the results of an analytical study. When there is non-differential measurement error in a continuous exposure measure X, it is not the bias in the measure but rather the degree of precision of X (measured by ρ_{TX}) which leads to bias in the measure of association between X and the outcome.

- Classifying individuals into ordered categories generally does not lessen the attenuation of the odds ratio due to measurement error.

The effects of measurement error on measures of association between exposure and disease can be estimated from simple equations (Equations 3.3, 3.5, 3.6, 3.8, 3.12) under certain assumptions. These effects can be substantial and justify concern about the accuracy of exposure measurement in epidemiological studies. Elimination of differential measurement errors should be the highest priority and reduction of non-differential errors should be a major concern in the design and conduct of studies.

References

Allen, M. J. and Yen, W. M. (1979). *Introduction to Measurement Theory*, pp. 1–117. Brooks/Cole, Monterey, CA.

Armstrong, B. G., Whittemore, A. S., and Howe, G. R. (1989). Analysis of case–control data with covariate measurement error: application to diet and colon cancer. *Statistics in Medicine*, **8**, 1151–63.

Barron, B. A. (1977). The effects of misclassification on the estimation of relative risk. *Biometrics*, **33**, 414–8.

Bohrnstedt, G. W. (1983). Measurement. In *Handbook of Survey Research* (ed. P. H. Rossi, J. D. Wright, and A. B. Anderson), pp. 70–121. Academic Press, Orlando, FL.

Bross, I. (1954). Misclassification in 2 × 2 tables. *Biometrics*, **10**, 478–86.

Cochran, W. G. (1968). Errors of measurement in statistics. *Technometrics*, **10**, 637–66.

Copeland, K. T., Checkoway, H., McMichael, A. J., and Holbrook, R. H. (1977). Bias due to misclassification in the estimation of relative risk. *American Journal of Epidemiology*, **105**, 488–95.

de Klerk, N. H., English, D. R., and Armstrong, B. K. (1989). A review of the effects of random measurement error on relative risk estimates in epidemiological studies. *International Journal of Epidemiology*, **18**, 705–12.

Dosemeci, M., Wacholder, S., and Lubin, J. H. (1990). Does nondifferential misclassification of the exposure always bias a true effect toward the null value? *American Journal of Epidemiology*, **132**, 746–8.

Fleiss, J. L. (1981). *Statistical Methods for Rates and Proportions* (2nd edn), pp. 188–211. J. Wiley, New York.

Fleiss, J. L. (1986). *The Design and Analysis of Clinical Experiments*, pp. 1, 5. Wiley, New York.

Fuller, W. A. (1987). *Measurement Error Models*. Wiley, New York.

Goldberg, J. D. (1975). The effects of misclassification on the bias in the difference between two proportions and the relative odds in the fourfold table. *Journal of the American Statistical Association*, **70**, 561–7.

Greenland, S. (1980). The effect of misclassification in the presence of covariates. *American Journal of Epidemiology*, **112**, 564–9.

Gregorio, D. I., Marshall, J. R., and Zielenzny, M. (1985). Fluctuations in odds ratios due to variance differences in case–control studies. *American Journal of Epidemiology*, **121**, 767–74.

Gullen, W. H., Bearman, J. E., and Johnson, E. A. (1968). Effects of misclassification in epidemiologic studies. *Public Health Reports*, **83**, 914–8.

Hansen, M. H., Hurwitz, W. N., and Bershad, M. (1961). Measurement errors in censuses and surveys. *Bulletin of the International Statistical Institute*, **38**, 359–74.

Kelsey, J. L., Whittemore, A. S., Evans, D.S., and Thompson, W. D. (1996). *Methods in Observational Epidemiology*. (2nd edn), pp. 327–34. Oxford University Press, New York.

Kleinbaum, D. G., Kupper, L. L., and Morgenstern, H. (1982). *Epidemiologic Research*, pp. 183–93, 220–41. Lifetime Learning Publications, Belmont, CA.

Lord, F. M. and Novick, M. R. (1968). *Statistical Theories of Mental Test Scores*. Addison-Wesley, Reading, MA.

Mote, V. L. and Anderson, R. L. (1965). An investigation of the effect of misclassification on the properties of χ^2-tests in the analysis of categorical data. *Biometrika*, **62**, 95–109.

Newell, D. J. (1962). Errors in the interpretation of errors in epidemiology. *American Journal of Public Health*, **52**, 1925–8.

Nunnally, J. C. (1978). *Psychometric Theory* (2nd edn), pp. 190–225. McGraw-Hill, New York.

Prentice, R. L. (1982). Covariate measurement errors and parameter estimation in a failure time regression model. *Biometrika*, **69**, 331–42.

Quade, D., Lachenbruch, P. A., Whaley, F. S., McClish, D. K., and Haley, R. W. (1980). Effects of misclassification on statistical inferences in epidemiology. *American Journal of Epidemiology*, **111**, 503–15.

Thürigen, D., Spiegelman, D., Blettner, M., Carsten, H., and Brenner, H. (2000). Measurement error correction using validation data: a review of methods and their applicability in case–control studies. *Statistical Methods in Medical Research*, **9**, 447–74.

Walker, A. M. and Blettner, M. (1985). Comparing imperfect measures of exposure. *American Journal of Epidemiology*, **121**, 783–90.

Weinberg, C.R., Umbach, D.M., and Greenland, S. (1994). When will nondifferential misclassification of an exposure preserve the direction of a trend? *American Journal of Epidemiology*, **140**, 565–71.

White, E. (2003). Design and interpretation of studies of differential exposure measurement error (Review and Commentary). *American Journal of Epidemiology*, **15**, 380–7.

Whittemore, A. S. and Grosser, S. (1986). Regression methods for data with incomplete covariates. In *Modern Statistical Methods in Chronic Disease* (ed. S. H. Moolgavkar and R. L. Prentice), pp. 19–34. Wiley, New York.

Wu, M. L., Whittemore, A. S., and Jung, D. L. (1986). Errors in reported dietary intakes. I Short-term recall. *American Journal of Epidemiology*, **124**, 826–35.

4

Validity and reliability studies

One must go seek more facts, paying less attention to
techniques of handling the data and far more to the
development and perfection of the methods of
obtaining them.
(*Hill 1953*)

Introduction

The serious adverse effects of the use of invalid exposure measurements have
been described in Chapter 3. Selecting or developing an accurate measurement instrument is obviously a critical step in designing an epidemiological
study. First, the available literature on the validity and reliability of instruments which measure the exposure of interest should be reviewed. Then, if a
new instrument is to be developed which differs substantially from other
methods, its reliability or, preferably, its validity should be assessed.

The term *reliability* is generally used to refer to the reproducibility of a
measure, i.e. how consistently a measurement can be repeated on the same
subjects. Reliability can be assessed in a number of ways. *Intramethod reliability* is a measure of the reproducibility of an instrument, either applied in the
same manner to the same subjects at two or more points in time (*test–retest
reliability*) or applied by two or more data collectors to the same subjects
(*inter-rater reliability*). For example, a comparison could be made of exposure
information from two data abstractors who extracted information from the
medical records of the same group of subjects. *Intermethod reliability* is a
measure of the ability of two different instruments which measure the same
underlying exposure to yield similar results on the same subjects. Generally an
intermethod reliability study compares a measurement method to be used in
an epidemiological study with a more accurate but more burdensome method.
For example, a questionnaire might be compared with an exposure diary for a
group of subjects. Intermethod reliability studies of this type are sometimes
called *validity studies* or *validation studies*. Technically, however, a perfectly
accurate measure of exposure (criterion measure or 'gold standard') is needed

to measure validity directly, and so the term intermethod reliability is preferable. Intermethod reliability studies have also been called *method comparison studies* and studies of the *relative validity* of one measure in comparison to another. In most fields of study, the term reliability refers to intramethod reliability, and less work has been done on the design and interpretation of intermethod reliability studies. Intermethod reliability studies are dealt with in detail in this chapter because of their potential importance in epidemiology.

The first topic to be covered in this chapter is the relationship of measures of reliability to measures of validity. Measures of reliability are primarily important for what they reveal about the validity of a measurement because, as shown in Chapter 3, the bias in an epidemiological study is a function of the validity of the exposure measure. The second section covers additional issues in the design of reliability and validity studies, and the third covers the statistical analysis of reliability and validity studies.

Many of the examples in this chapter are based on real data and most are focused on dietary measurements. Part of this focus is a reflection of the difficulties in assessing diet. Additionally, by focusing on a few exposures, the reader can observe how measures of reliability are a function of the design of the reliability study as well as of the accuracy of the instrument itself.

Another type of reliability, *internal consistency reliability*, is not covered in this chapter, but is covered in Chapter 5 in the section on use of scores or averages based on multiple measures of exposure. Internal consistency reliability can be assessed when the exposure measure for each individual in the parent epidemiological study is a sum or average of two or more individual items. Examples are a disability scale calculated as the sum of multiple questions or the average serum beta carotene for each subject, averaged over three blood draws. For these types of exposure measures, a measure of reliability can be calculated based on the correlation between the individual items that were summed or averaged. The reliability statistic used is Cronbach's α (Carmines and Zeller 1979), which is discussed in Chapter 5.

The Interpretation of Measures of Reliability

This section covers the interpretation of measures of reliability in terms of measures of validity, and is meant to provide some general concepts for the interpretation of reliability studies. The concepts presented are important when evaluating the results of reliability studies conducted by others and in designing a reliability or validity study.

The results of this section are limited to continuous exposure measures, and assume that measures are obtained from an infinite population, i.e. issues of sampling error are ignored. In actual practice, validity and reliability studies are conducted on a small sample of subjects, and the results of the validity/reliability study are used to interpret the effects of exposure measurement error on the results from the larger parent epidemiological study.

A model of reliability and measures of reliability

Suppose that each person in a population of interest is measured twice, either with one instrument or two instruments that purport to measure the same exposure. If two instruments are used, X_1 will denote the measure of interest, i.e. the one to be used in the epidemiological study, and X_2 the comparison measure. For a given subject i, two (continuous) exposure measurements, X_{i1} and X_{i2}, are obtained. A simple model that could apply to intermethod or intramethod reliability studies is

$$X_{i1} = T_i + b_1 + E_{i1}$$
$$X_{i2} = T_i + b_2 + E_{i2}$$

where $\mu_{E_1} = \mu_{E_2} = 0$. The model can also be written

$$X_{ij} = T_i + b_j + E_{ij}$$

where X_{ij} is the observation on subject i of measure X_j.

This model states that subject i's first measure, X_{i1}, is equal to the true value of exposure T_i for subject i plus the constant bias b_1 of the first instrument in the population plus the error E_{i1} for subject i on measure 1. The second measure, X_{i2}, is equal to the same true value T_i plus the bias b_2 of the second instrument plus a second error E_{i2}.

In the population, $X_1, X_2, T, E_1,$ and E_2 are random variables with distributions. The population mean of X_1 is denoted by μ_{X_1}, the variance by $\sigma^2_{X_1}$, etc. Because the bias of X_1 in the population is expressed as a constant b_1 and the bias of X_2 as b_2, it follows that the population means of the subject error terms E_1 and E_2 are zero.

In a reliability study, information is available on X_1 and X_2 for each subject, but not on T. A reliability study can yield estimates of μ_{X_1}, μ_{X_2}, and the correlation $\rho_{X_1 X_2}$ between the two measures, termed the *reliability coefficient*.

In Chapter 3, two measures of the validity of a continuous exposure measure were shown to be important in assessing the impact of measurement error: the bias and the validity coefficient. The primary question is: If X_1 is the measure of interest, what can the estimates of μ_{X_1}, μ_{X_2} and $\rho_{X_1 X_2}$ from a reliability study tell us about the bias b_1 in X_1 and its validity coefficient ρ_{TX_1}?

The measurement of the bias in a measure and differential bias

Reliability studies often cannot provide information on the bias in X_1 or X_2. In a reliability study based on the above model, only the *difference* between the biases of X_1 and X_2 can be observed:

$$(b_1 - b_2) = \mu_{X_1} - \mu_{X_2}. \qquad [4.1]$$

This equation states that the difference between the population means of the two measures is equal to the difference between their biases. This difference is often not very informative. If a similar degree of bias is present in both measures—for example, if the same miscalibrated scale is used to weigh each subject twice—the difference between the means of the two measures can be close to zero even when there is considerable bias in both measures. However, if X_2 is an unbiased measure of T $(b_2 = 0)$, then

$$b_1 = \mu_{X_1} - \mu_{X_2}. \qquad [4.2]$$

Thus, only when the comparison measure X_2 is a perfect measure or when X_2 can be assumed to be unbiased (e.g. a well-calibrated scale) can a reliability study yield information about the bias in X_1.

As discussed in Chapter 3, differential bias in the exposure measure between cases and controls is a major concern because it can lead to invalid results in an epidemiological study. (Differential precision may also be a concern, but is not discussed in this chapter.) To assess differential bias, a reliability study would need to measure X_1 and X_2 in a population of cases and a population of controls to yield estimates of the means of X_1 and X_2 among those with disease $(\mu_{X_{1D}}, \mu_{X_{2D}})$ and among the non-diseased group $(\mu_{X_{1N}}, \mu_{X_{2N}})$. The difference between the bias in X_1 between cases and controls $(b_{1D} - b_{1N})$ can be measured *only* if the comparison measure X_2 is perfect or is unbiased, or if there is non-differential bias in $X_2 (b_{2D} = b_{2N})$. Then, if the simple additive model given above holds for both cases and controls,

$$(b_{1D} - b_{1N}) = (\mu_{X_{1D}} - \mu_{X_{2D}}) - (\mu_{X_{1N}} - \mu_{X_{2N}}). \qquad [4.3]$$

Example. To assess differential bias between breast cancer cases and controls in a retrospective food frequency estimate of dietary fibre intake (X_1), a reliability study was conducted within an existing cohort study (Giovannucci *et al.* 1993). X_1 was compared with the prospective (pre-diagnostic) food frequency estimate of fibre intake (X_2)

from the cohort study. Cases reported 19.5 grams of fibre prospectively and 20.0 grams retrospectively. Controls reported 20.5 grams of fibre prospectively and 20.2 grams retrospectively. Since there is reasonable certainty that any bias in X_2 is equal for cases and controls, the differential bias in X_1 can be estimated from Equation 4.3 as

$$b_{1D} - b_{1N} = (20.0 - 19.5) - (20.2 - 20.5)$$
$$= 0.8 \text{ grams.}$$

Interpretation of differential bias

Differential bias should be interpreted in terms of its effect on the odds ratio (OR). Equation 3.3 gives the effect of differential measurement error on the OR when the normality assumptions given in that section hold; otherwise that equation can be used as an approximation of the effect. The factor C in that equation requires an estimate of $(\mu_{T_D} - \mu_{T_N})$ as well as $(b_D - b_N)$. When X_2 is unbiased or has non-differential bias,

$$\mu_{T_D} - \mu_{T_N} = \mu_{X_{2D}} - \mu_{X_{2N}}.$$

Therefore a reliability study with an unbiased comparison measure X_2, or with X_2 with non-differential bias, can be used to estimate $\mu_{T_D} - \mu_{T_N}$ by $\bar{X}_{2D} - \bar{X}_{2N}$. However, if the parent epidemiological study has been completed, it may be more accurate to estimate $\mu_{T_D} - \mu_{T_N}$ using the mean of X_1 in the disease group $(\bar{X}'_{1D})$ and the non-disease group $(\bar{X}'_{1N})$ from the parent study and the bias from the validity or reliability study. Then

$$\mu_{T_D} - \mu_{T_N} = (\bar{X}'_{1D} - \bar{X}'_{1N}) - (b_{1D} - b_{1N}).$$

Example. Continuing the example from above, the exponential factor C in Equation 3.3 can be estimated as

$$C = \left(1 + \frac{b_D - b_N}{\mu_{T_D} - \mu_{T_N}}\right) = 1 + \frac{0.8}{19.5 - 20.5} = 0.2.$$

Suppose that the true odds ratio for dietary fibre and breast cancer was 0.25 for a 10 gram increase in fibre intake and the validity coefficient of dietary fibre intake from the food frequency questionnaire (ρ_{TX_1}) was 0.6 (for both cases and controls for the retrospective questionnaire). Then the bias in the odds ratio from both the differential bias (factor C) and the lack of precision would lead the observable OR for a 10 gram increase in fibre intake to be 0.91 (from Equation 3.3). This could be compared with the attenuation of the odds ratio due to non-differential measurement error in the prospective study, which would lead to an observed odds ratio of 0.61 (from Equation 3.5 if $\rho_{TX_2} = 0.6$ for the prospective food frequency questionnaire). Thus, in this example, a strong relationship of fibre with risk of breast cancer (75 per cent reduction in risk) would be attenuated to an observed 39 per cent reduction in risk in the cohort study, but the relationship would be almost completely obscured because of the differential measurement error in the retrospective study.

Relationship of reliability to validity under the parallel test model

The inability of many reliability study designs to yield information on bias or differential bias is a major limitation. However, it should be recalled, that under non-differential measurement error (and certain other assumptions), the attenuation equations depend only on the validity coefficient and not on the bias. Thus measures of reliability may be used to estimate at least some of the effects of measurement error in the absence of a measure of bias. When non-differential measurement error can be assumed, reliability can be assessed in a single population representative of the population in which the epidemiological study is to be conducted.

When certain assumptions are met, reliability studies can yield information about the validity coefficient. One such set of assumptions is the *model of parallel tests* (Lord and Novick 1968; Nunnally 1978; Allen and Yen 1979; Carmines and Zeller 1979; Bohrnstedt 1983). The model is the same as the general model above, but with some additional assumptions:

$$\rho_{TE_1} = \rho_{TE_2} = 0$$
$$\sigma_{E_1}^2 = \sigma_{E_2}^2 = \sigma_E^2$$
$$\rho_{E_1 E_2} = 0.$$

The first assumption of the parallel test model is that the error variables E_1 and E_2 are not correlated with the true value T. It is further assumed that E_1 and E_2 have equal variance σ_E^2. This also implies that X_1 and X_2 have equal variance and that X_1 and X_2 are equally precise ($\rho_{TX_1} = \rho_{TX_2}$) (see Equation 3.2). This is usually a reasonable assumption in intramethod studies, since X_1 and X_2 are measurements from the same instrument. Finally, it is assumed that E_1 is not correlated with E_2. This important (and often violated) assumption implies, for example, that an individual who has a positive error E_1 on the first measurement is equally likely to have a positive or a negative error E_2 on the second measurement. These assumptions are often summarized by saying that two measures are parallel measures of T if they have equal and uncorrelated errors. (The parallel test model generally includes the assumption that $b_1 = b_2 = 0$, but this assumption is not needed for the results in this chapter.)

Often a test–retest reliability study of an objective measure (e.g. a physical or biochemical test) can be assumed to meet the parallel test model if separate measures are taken over the aetiological time period of interest. For example, two measures of serum cholesterol measured from two blood draws over the time period of interest (e.g. over one year) could be assumed to have equal and uncorrelated errors. The two measures would have equal error variance, assuming the methods for blood drawing, handling, and laboratory analysis were identical. Uncorrelated error between the two measures is likely because if a subject's serum cholesterol were higher than his true one-year average at the first measure (e.g. because he had eaten a larger amount of saturated fat than usual the previous month or because of laboratory error), there is no reason to expect that his second measure from blood drawn at a different time would also be higher than his true one-year average. Thus those subjects with a positive error on the first measure are equally likely to have a positive or negative error on the second.

Under the assumptions of parallel tests it can be shown that (Allen and Yen 1979)

$$
\rho_{X_1 X_2} = \frac{\sigma_T^2}{\sigma_{X_1}^2} = 1 - \frac{\sigma_E^2}{\sigma_{X_1}^2} = \rho_{TX_1}^2
$$

[4.4]

or equivalently

$$
\rho_{TX_1} = \sqrt{\rho_{X_1 X_2}}.
$$

These equations state that the reliability coefficient $\rho_{X_1 X_2}$ is equal to the square of the validity coefficient for X_1 (or X_2). This result is important, because it shows that, if the assumptions are correct, the reliability coefficient, which is a measure of the correlation between two imperfect measures, can be used to estimate the correlation between T and X_1 *without* having a perfect measure of T. The correlation of X_1 with X_2 is less than the correlation of X_1, with T, because of the error in X_2.

Example. In a reliability study of fatty acid composition in serum phospholipids, fatty acids were measured from repeat blood draws over a two-year period for each subject (Zeleniuch-Jacquotte *et al.* 2000). The reliability coefficient for total saturated fat was 0.31. Suppose that the 'true measure' of interest was each subject's average measure over the two-year period. The assumptions of the parallel test model are likely to be appropriate, as discussed above. Therefore the correlation of X_1 with T can be estimated from Equation 4.4:

$$\rho_{TX_1} = \sqrt{0.31} = 0.56.$$

The definition of the reliability coefficient of X_1 as the correlation between X_1 and X_2, two parallel measures of T, is one definition of reliability. Based on Equation 4.4, the results in the last chapter on the attenuation of exposure – disease associations which were expressed in terms of ρ_{TX}^2 could have been (and often are) expressed in terms of $\rho_{X_1X_2}$. These expressions apply only when the reliability coefficient is restricted to the correlation between parallel measures of T. However, we use the term reliability coefficient to refer to the correlation $\rho_{X_1X_2}$ between measures of the same exposure even when the assumptions of parallel tests do not hold. This means that, for a given instrument X_1 applied to a given population, the reliability coefficient will vary with the choice of X_2.

In real reliability studies, the assumptions of parallel tests are often incorrect. Two common violations will be discussed: unequal variances of E_1 and E_2, and correlated errors. Even when these assumptions are violated, the correlation between X_1 and X_2 can still provide some information about the validity coefficient of X_1.

Relationship of reliability to validity under unequal variances of E_1 and E_2

In the model of parallel tests, the variances of E_1 and E_2 are assumed to be equal, which implies that X_1 and X_2 are equally precise ($\rho_{TX_1} = \rho_{TX_2}$). This assumption is incorrect for certain reliability studies, particularly for many intermethod reliability studies. First, consider a true validity study where X_1, the exposure measure of interest, is compared with a perfect measure of exposure, termed X_2 ($X_2 = T$). Then, by definition,

$$\rho_{X_1X_2} = \rho_{TX_1}. \qquad [4.5]$$

However, a perfect measure is often not available, and so the exposure measure of interest X_1 is often compared with an imperfect but more precise measure, X_2. This implies that $\rho_{TX_2} > \rho_{TX_1}$. If the other assumptions of the parallel tests model hold, including the assumption of uncorrected errors, then

$$\rho_{X_1 X_2} < \rho_{TX_1} < \sqrt{\rho_{X_1 X_2}}.$$ [4.6]

This equation states that when X_2 is more precise than X_1 and the errors in X_1 and X_2 are not correlated, the reliability coefficient $\rho_{X_1 X_2}$ can be used to yield an upper and a lower bound for the validity coefficient of X_1. The lower bound for the validity coefficient of X_1 is the interpretation as if X_2 were a perfect measure (Equation 4.5), and the upper bound is the interpretation as if X_2 had equal error variance (Equation 4.4). The more accurate X_2 is, the closer the *lower* bound is to ρ_{TX_1}.

Example. Willett *et al.* (1985) conducted an intermethod reliability study to evaluate a food frequency questionnaire estimate of average daily fat intake over the preceding year (X_1). The comparison measure was an estimate of average daily fat intake from four 1-week diet diaries spread over the year (X_2). The observed correlation between the food frequency estimate and the diary estimate (energy adjusted) among 173 subjects was $\rho_{X_1 X_2} = 0.5$.

One might argue that the errors in the estimate of fat from a diet diary are not correlated with those on the food frequency questionnaire. The primary source of error on a food frequency questionnaire may be poor recall, while on the diet diaries it may be whether 4 weeks are fully representative of yearly intake. It was assumed that the four diaries yielded a more accurate measure of fat and, in fact, the variance from the diary estimate appeared to be smaller than the variance from the food frequency estimate. Then Equation 4.6 might apply:

$$0.5 < \hat{\rho}_{TX_1} < 0.7$$

which suggests that the validity coefficient for X_1 would be between 0.5 and 0.7. Willett et al. argued that the use of four 1-week diaries is a near-perfect criterion (e.g. there was little increase in $\rho_{X_1 X_2}$ when X_2 was based on four diaries rather than two). This suggests that ρ_{TX_1} is near the lower limit 0.5.

In an effort to find a comparison measure X_2 with an error uncorrelated with the error in X_1, the comparison measure may be less accurate than X_1 ($\rho_{TX_2} < \rho_{TX_1}$). More specifically, X_2 may be a less accurate measure of T, the true exposure that X_1 is attempting to measure, than X_1. If X_2 is a less precise measure of T or if it is not known whether X_1 or X_2 is more accurate, it can still be assumed that (Allen and Yen 1979)

$$\rho_{TX_1} > \rho_{X_1 X_2}.$$ [4.7]

In other words, the correlation of X_1 with even a poor measure X_2 with uncorrelated errors gives a lower limit for the correlation of X_1 with the true measure. For example, suppose that a food frequency measure of fat intake (X_1) was compared with serum cholesterol (X_2). While serum cholesterol may be an accurate measure of cholesterol level, it is a poor measure of fat intake (T). If $\rho_{X_1 X_2}$ is found to be 0.2, and assuming that there are no sources of correlated error between X_1 and X_2, Equation 4.7 shows that the lower limit for ρ_{TX_1} would be 0.2.

A model of reliability allowing for correlated errors

One assumption of the model of parallel tests that is often violated is the assumption of uncorrelated errors. Often the errors in X_1 and X_2 are positively correlated. For example, physical activity may be over-reported by some subjects on a self-administered questionnaire, and those same subjects may be most likely to over-report their activity on an in-person interview used as a comparison measure. Since the same subjects with large positive errors on the first measure tend to have positive errors on the second measure, the errors are correlated. The correlated error can be due to the subject (e.g. social desirability bias may affect some subjects consistently across measures) or the instrument (e.g. a physical activity questionnaire which omitted swimming will repeatedly underestimate the total activity level for those subjects who are swimmers). Positive *correlated errors* occur when those subjects with positive error E_1, i.e. those for whom X_1 overestimates their true exposure (beyond the constant b_1 which affects everyone), are also more likely to have a positive error E_2, i.e. X_2 also overestimates their true exposure (beyond the constant b_2 which affects all subjects). (Note that if X_1 and X_2 have a similar bias (b_1 and b_2), this does *not* lead to correlated error because bias adds a constant error to *all* subjects.)

A model for reliability that makes the correlated errors explicit is

$$X_{ij} = T_i + b_j + E_{ij}$$

where $E_{ij} = B_i + F_{ij}$. The error terms E_{i1} and E_{i2} for a given subject are the sum of two parts: a part B_i which repeats itself on each measure of subject i, termed the *within-subject bias*, and a part F_{ij} which varies between measures (around a mean of zero for subject i), termed the *random error* (see Figure 4.1). E_1 and E_2 are correlated because they both include the within-subject bias.

To simplify the reliability coefficient under this model, let S_i be that part of X_1 and X_2 that is consistently measured for subject i on both instruments.

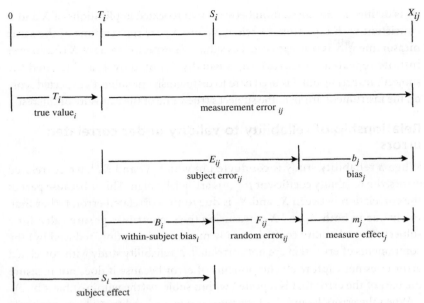

Figure 4.1 Measurement error in X_{ij}, the jth measure on subject i.

S_i would be the sum of T_i plus B_i (plus the average bias across measures). Then the model of reliability can be rewritten as

$$X_{ij} = S_i + m_j + F_{ij}$$

where S_i represents the effect of subject i and m_j represents the effect of measure j on X_{ij} (the m_j are the b_j minus the average bias across measures, such that $\Sigma m_j = 0$). If X_1 and X_2 are equally precise (and $\rho_{TF_1} = \rho_{TF_2} = 0$), then the reliability coefficient under this model is the proportion of the variance of X_1 explained by S, the part that is common to the repeated measures, i.e. (Allen and Yen 1979)

$$\rho_{X_1 X_2} = \frac{\sigma_S^2}{\sigma_{X_1}^2} = 1 - \frac{\sigma_F^2}{\sigma_{X_1}^2}. \qquad [4.8]$$

The right-hand side of this equation shows that when there are correlated errors, the reliability coefficient only measures (i.e. is only reduced by) the random component of error in X_1.

Equation 4.8 is essentially identical to the classical definition of the *reliability* of a measure X (Allen and Yen 1979; Dunn 1989):

$$\rho_X = \frac{\sigma_S^2}{\sigma_X^2}. \qquad [4.9]$$

ρ_X is defined as the correlation between two repeated applications of X and is consistent with Equation 4.8 when X_1 and X_2 are replications of the same measurement. S_i is conceptualized as subject i's expected value of X (mean over infinite repeated measures). (S_i is usually denoted by T_i and termed the subject's *true score*, but S is used here to distinguish 'the subject's expected score on the instrument' from T, 'the subject's true value of the exposure of interest').

Relationship of reliability to validity under correlated errors

When a reliability study is conducted in which X_1 and X_2 have correlated errors, the reliability coefficient $\rho_{X_1 X_2}$ is artificially high. This is because part of the correlation between X_1 and X_2 is due to the correlated error, rather than solely due to both X_1 and X_2 measuring the same true exposure value for a subject. The reliability coefficient only measures (i.e. is only reduced by) the components of error that are not correlated. A reliability study with correlated error does not capture all components of error because it does not measure the part of the error that is repeated within subjects (the within-subject bias).

When the errors E_1 and E_2 of the measures in a reliability study are positively correlated, the reliability study can only yield an *upper limit* for the validity coefficient. Specifically, when X_1 and X_2 are equally precise (or X_2 is more precise than X_1) and the assumptions of the above model hold, the validity coefficient is less than the square root of the reliability coefficient (Walker and Blettner 1985):

$$\rho_{TX_1} < \sqrt{\rho_{X_1 X_2}}. \qquad [4.10]$$

Thus a measure can be reliable (repeatable) even if it has poor validity. While a low reliability coefficient implies poor validity, a high reliability does not necessarily imply a high validity coefficient. The high reliability may be due instead to the correlated error.

To interpret a reliability study, one should evaluate whether there are potential sources of correlated errors between the two measures. As outlined in Table 3.1, there is a wide range of sources of measurement error, and most of these could be sources of correlated errors.

Example. A test–retest reliability study was also conducted in the study by Willett *et al.* (1985) presented in the previous example. The observed correlation between the estimates of average daily fat intake from two administrations of the food frequency questionnaire, 1 year apart, was 0.6.

Sources of correlated errors between two administrations of a food frequency questionnaire include the following.

(a) Some subjects may consistently tend to report their 'best' diet rather than their usual diet.

(b) Certain high-fat foods eaten frequently by a few subjects may have been omitted from the questionnaire. Those subjects would have their fat intake consistently underestimated.

(c) The nutrient database used to convert foods to grams of fat may be incorrect for certain subjects. For example, those subjects who reduce the fat content of standard recipes, such as stews, lasagna, etc., would have the fat content of their diet consistently overestimated.

(d) The time period assessed by the instrument (diet in last year) may differ from the true time period of interest (e.g. diet over the last 5 years). Then those who have lowered the fat in their diet in recent years will have their fat intake underestimated on both administrations of the instrument compared with their true 5-year average fat intake.

Under this strong likelihood of correlated errors, Equation 4.10 would apply in interpreting this reliability study:

$$\rho_{TX_1} < 0.77$$

and so only an upper limit on the validity coefficient of the measurement can be estimated. This outcome clearly provides less information about the validity of the food frequency measure of fat than did the outcome of the intermethod reliability study described in the last example.

Correlated errors commonly occur in intramethod studies, but they could occur in intermethod studies as well. In the example of an intermethod study of a food frequency estimate of fat intake compared with a diet diary estimate, it was argued that the errors on the two instruments were unlikely to be significantly correlated. However, of the four sources of correlated errors noted in the above example, at least two could lead to correlated errors between a food frequency measure and a diet diary measure (the tendency of some subjects to report their best diet, and the issue relating to the time period of measurement). Therefore the study used in that example might only provide an upper limit of the validity coefficient.

Table 4.1 summarizes the results presented in this chapter on the interpretation of the reliability coefficient ($\rho_{X_1 X_2}$) in terms of the validity coefficient of $X_1 (\rho_{TX_1})$. Further discussion about how to use these results to design and interpret reliability studies is given in the section on choice of comparison measures later in this chapter.

Table 4.1 Interpretation of reliability studies of X_1 and X_2: What does $\rho_{X_1X_2}$ (reliability coefficient) reveal about ρ_{TX_1} (validity coefficient of X_1)?

Error correlated between X_1 and X_2?	X_2 more or less precise than X_1?[a]	ρ_{TX_1} in terms of $\rho_{X_1X_2}$	Equation
No error in X_2 Validity study	X_2 perfect	$\rho_{TX_1} = \rho_{X_1X_2}$	[4.5]
No Parallel test model	Equally precise	$\rho_{TX_1} = \sqrt{\rho_{X_1X_2}}$	[4.4]
No	X_2 more precise	$\rho_{X_1X_2} < \rho_{TX_1} < \sqrt{\rho_{X_1X_2}}$	[4.6]
No	X_2 less precise or don't know	$\rho_{TX_1} > \rho_{X_1X_2}$	[4.7]
Yes	Equally precise or X_2 more precise	$\rho_{TX_1} < \sqrt{\rho_{X_1X_2}}$	[4.10]
Yes	X_2 less precise or don't know	One learns nothing	

[a] Is X_2 a more or less precise measure of T, the true exposure that X_1 is meant to measure?

Interpretation of the value of the reliability coefficient

Some authors have provided guidance on whether to consider the reliability of a measure poor, fair, or good from the value of the reliability coefficient. However, it is more appropriate first to consider what information the reliability study yields about the validity of the measure, as discussed above. Then consideration could be given to the effect of the estimated measurement error in the exposure on the epidemiological study which will use the measure, based on the tables and equations in the last chapter.

For example, suppose that a reliability study which complied with the parallel test model yielded $\rho_{X_1X_2} = 0.64$, leading to an estimate of the validity coefficient of $\hat{\rho}_{TX} = 0.8$. If the true odds ratio were 2.0, and if the assumptions of non-differential measurement error and the other assumptions of Equation 3.6 were reasonable, then the estimated observable odds ratio would be

$$\hat{OR}_O = OR_T^{\hat{\rho}_{TX}} = 2^{0.8} = 1.7.$$

This might be considered to be acceptable attenuation. On the other hand, if a reliability study of a different instrument produced the same reliability coefficient (0.64) but, because of correlated errors between the measures, only an upper bound for ρ_{TX} of 0.8 could be estimated, then applying Equation 3.6 would yield

$$\mathrm{OR}_o < 1.7.$$

This estimate of the attenuated odds ratio includes only the attenuation due to the random error in X, and the actual attenuation would be greater. This instrument might not be acceptable despite the same value of the reliability coefficient.

Other violations of the assumptions of the model

In some situations the assumption of the basic model, which states that both X_1 and X_2 measure T with additive errors E_1 and E_2, is incorrect. One alternative to this model is that X_1 or X_2, or both, may be a linear function of T:

$$X_{ij} = c_j T_j + b_j + E_{ij}.$$

This model states that only some fixed proportion of T is measured by X (i.e. there is systematic proportional error) or that X uses a different unit scale from T. (In intramethod studies it is assumed that c_1 and c_2 are equal, i.e. X_1 and X_2 have the same scale.) Reliability studies such as these can still yield information about the validity coefficient, but not about bias. The results presented so far in this chapter for interpreting the reliability coefficient $\rho_{X_1 X_2}$ in terms of the validity coefficient ρ_{TX_1} would also apply to the above model because $\rho_{X_1 X_2}$ is not affected by linear transformations of X_1 or X_2. For example, a food frequency questionnaire measure of beta-carotene (X_1) could be compared with serum beta-carotene (X_2) and interpreted by Equation 4.7 (if there were no sources of correlated errors) even though serum beta-carotene is not measured in the same units as beta-carotene intake.

Further violations of the assumption that T and E are uncorrelated are beyond the scope of this book, but several practical points should be noted. First, a transformation of X, such as the logarithmic transformation, may reduce the dependence of E on T (Altman and Bland 1983). Secondly, when T and E are negatively correlated, the measure X will have a variance less than $\sigma_T^2 + \sigma_E^2$, possibly even a smaller variance than T, therefore the variances of two measures should not be compared to determine which is more precise.

Finally, the equations given so far have assumed a population of infinite size. In practice, there will be sampling error in the estimate of $\rho_{X_1 X_2}$. The confidence interval around estimates of $\rho_{X_1 X_2}$ should be taken into consideration when using the equations in this section to interpret reliability in terms of validity.

Interpretation of reliability studies of categorical variables

Most of the concepts presented for continuous variables apply in a qualitative way to interpretation of reliability studies of categorical variables. For example, when two imperfect categorical measures of exposure are being compared, part of the agreement between them could be due to repeated error. Mathematical relationships between measures of reliability and measures of validity for categorical variables are not straightforward. However, some reliability study designs can yield estimates of the sensitivity and specificity of each measure or can be used to estimate the bias in the odds ratio that would result from the misclassification (Hui and Walter 1980; Walter 1984; Clayton 1985; Kaldor and Clayton 1985; Walter and Irwig 1988; Dunn 1989; Tavaré et al.1995).

Issues in the Design of Validity and Reliability Studies

Several issues need to be considered in the design of validity and reliability studies (Fleiss and Shrout 1977; Carmines and Zeller 1979; Dunn 1989, 1992; Willett 1998; Wong 1999a). Most of these issues are also important in interpreting reliability studies carried out by others.

Purpose and timing of the reliability study

When a new instrument is to be developed for an epidemiological study, or when an existing one is to be applied to a substantially different population, a validity or reliability study of the instrument should be carried out first. Estimates of the validity or reliability coefficient and, when possible, the bias of the instrument can then be used to decide whether it is necessary to develop a more accurate instrument. If the measure is shown to be reasonably reliable, and by inference reasonably valid, this will increase confidence in the outcome of the epidemiological study.

Reliability studies conducted before the main epidemiological study, or early in its course, can be used not only to evaluate but also to improve the instrument. For example, an inter-rater reliability study could identify interviewers, abstractors, or laboratory personnel who need more training or should be dropped from the study. Such a study could be done by comparing three or more raters who collect data on the same subset of subjects. Computation of reliability coefficients for each pair of raters may reveal an individual rater who compares poorly with the others. In addition, the researcher should investigate the situations in which discrepancies between the repeated measurements have occurred. This can often lead to improvement of the instrument or the protocol for its use. For example, if disagreements on the variable marital status of subjects usually involved divorced subjects being erroneously classified as 'single', the category 'single' might be clarified by the label 'never married'.

An additional use of reliability studies is to estimate the impact of exposure measurement error on the results of a study after the parent epidemiological study has been completed. Information from a reliability study conducted on a subset of subjects concurrently with the epidemiological study can yield information about the validity of the exposure measure. This information can be used to adjust the observed odds ratio for the effects of measurement error. Adjustment procedures are discussed in Chapter 5.

Choice of comparison measures

Many types of comparison measures have been used in reliability studies. An instrument can be compared with a re-administration of the same instrument at a different time, by a different rater, or with variation of some other condition of interest, for example proxy respondent versus index subject. For inter-method studies, questionnaire data have been compared with more detailed interviews (Hunter *et al.* 1997), medical records (Hunter *et al.* 1997; Fowles *et al.* 1998), physical or biochemical measures of exposure (Chasan-Tabar *et al.* 1996; McKeown *et al.* 2001), interviews by experts such as nutritionists, industrial hygienists, or physicians (Stewart *et al.* 2002), exposure diaries (Chasan-Tabar *et al.* 1996; Stewart *et al.* 2002), and direct observation (Stange *et al.* 1998). Information from medical records and vital records has been compared with subject interviews, physician interviews and direct observation (Stange *et al.* 1998). Diaries have been compared with biochemical measures (McKeown *et al.* 2001) and direct observation (Karvetti and Knuts 1992).

How is an appropriate comparison method selected? The issues discussed in the section on interpretation of measures of reliability (pp. 98–112) and summarized in Table 4.1 should provide some guidance in selecting a comparison measure. Ideally, measurements from the instrument whose accuracy is to be determined are compared with those provided by a perfect, or near-perfect, measure of exposure. This type of study, known as a *validity study*, allows one to estimate both dimensions of measurement error – the bias and the validity coefficient (Equations 4.2 and 4.5).

If a validity study is not possible, then one should consider comparing the instrument of interest with a measure of exposure with uncorrelated errors. A good choice is a comparison measure X_2 which is more precise than the measure of interest X_1 and has an error unlikely to be correlated with X_1. Intermethod studies comparing questionnaire measures which records (e.g. comparing a questionnaire on oral contraceptive use with complete medical or pharmacy records) or with multi-week diaries (e.g. comparing a questionnaire on leisure physical activity over the last year with six 1-week diaries) often meet these criteria. Equations 4.1 and 4.6 can aid in interpreting such studies. If a comparison measure can be selected with equal error as well as error uncorrelated with the instrument of interest, this can yield good information on the validity coefficient of the instrument (Equation 4.4). Test-retest studies of biochemical measures can often be assumed to have equal and uncorrelated errors if the replicates are sampled over the entire time period to which the exposure measure is intended to relate. Often questionnaire measures of behaviours can be compared with relevant physical or biochemical measures under the assumption of uncorrelated errors (e.g. a questionnaire on physical activity can be compared with a treadmill test), but such comparisons are often limited because the physical or biochemical measure may be a poor measure of the behaviour. Equation 4.7 can be useful in interpreting such studies. However, if both the questionnaire and the biochemical test reflect recent exposure, and the instrument is intended to represent exposure over a longer period of time, the errors could be correlated.

When a comparison measure with uncorrelated error is not available, then only part of the measurement error can be assessed in the reliability study. The part of the error that is repeated cannot be measured. The researcher can attempt to select the comparison measure X_2 so that the main sources of error in the measure of interest X_1 are not repeated in X_2. For example, in assessing a questionnaire covering diet 10 years in the past, long-term recall might be the greatest concern. One reliability study of this issue selected subjects who had answered a diet questionnaire years earlier and compared their measurements from the questionnaire of interest with those on the earlier version (Wu *et al.* 1988). This design would permit assessment of the main sources of error, that due to poor recall and that due to random variation, even though some sources of error (e.g. omission of certain foods on both questionnaires) could be repeated on both questionnaires. By careful selection of X_2, correlated errors between X_1 and X_2 can be minimized and the reliability study may then yield more information about the validity of X_1.

Finally, a simple test–retest reliability study is often quick and inexpensive to undertake. If there are sources of correlated error, the study will yield only an upper limit for validity (Equation 4.10). Nonetheless, if the reliability coefficient proves to be *low*, the instrument should probably be abandoned or extensively revised.

In reviewing reliability studies by others, the same issues should be considered. The key questions are as follows.

- Was the comparison method used close to perfect, a more precise measure of the true exposure than X_1, or a less precise measure than X_1?
- Are there sources of correlated error between X_1 and X_2?
- If two or more measures with correlated errors were used, were the errors likely to be strongly or weakly correlated?

The answers to these questions will guide the interpretation of the reliability study.

Separate studies on diseased and non-diseased groups

The researcher must decide whether or not to attempt to measure differential error. To assess differential measurement error, the reliability study needs to be conducted on a sample of cases and a sample of controls, and the comparison measure needs to be carefully selected.

Differential *bias* is a particular concern (Chapter 3). Therefore a comparison of the bias in the measure of interest X_1 between cases and controls would be of major interest. For reliability studies to assess differential bias in X_1, a comparison measure X_2 needs to be selected which is unbiased or can be assumed to have non-differential bias. Then the differential bias in X_1 can be estimated by Equation 4.3. For example, comparison of recall of a specific medication (X_1) with an abstract of medical records (X_2) among cases versus a similar comparison among controls may be a good way to assess differential bias; any bias in records is unlikely to be related to the disease under study, provided that a sufficient period prior to diagnosis is excluded. On the other hand, a test–retest reliability of recall of medications (assessed separately on cases and controls) would not reveal any differential bias between cases and controls, because the bias would occur in both measures.

Selection of subjects for reliability studies

Ideally, subjects in a reliability study should be a random sample of those in the population in which the epidemiological study will be carried out. This is because there are problems in generalizing reliability studies conducted on one population to another. These problems include the following.

- Reliability or validity studies which use self-selected volunteers might find the instrument to be more valid than it would be in the intended population, because of the higher level of motivation among the volunteers.
- Differences between populations in education, age, sex, and other factors could influence the validity and reliability of the instrument.

◆ Differences in the *distribution* of the true exposure between populations can influence the validity and reliability coefficients. Recall that ρ_{TX}^2 (also $\rho_{X_1 X_2}$ under parallel tests) is equal to

$$\frac{\sigma_T^2}{\sigma_X^2} = \frac{\sigma_T^2}{\sigma_T^2 + \sigma_E^2} = \frac{1}{1 + \sigma_E^2 / \sigma_T^2}. \qquad [4.11]$$

Thus even if the same instrument had the same error variance, σ_E^2, in two populations, the validity coefficient (or reliability coefficient) would be smaller in the population with least variation in true exposure, σ_T^2. For this reason, the use of the validity coefficient (and the reliability coefficient) to express measurement error has been criticized (Altman and Bland 1983). However, these *are* appropriate statistics in that they can be used to estimate the effect of measurement error on the bias in the observed odds ratio in the population of interest, which depends on the ratio σ_T^2 / σ_X^2. A validity or reliability coefficient assessed in one population may not apply to another with a different distribution of exposure.

Timing and order of measures

Correlated errors between measures in a reliability study may occur when subjects recall at the second or later testing the responses they gave on earlier tests. This recall can be minimized by separating the measures over time, usually by a month at least. However, when the two periods of testing are well separated, the two measures of exposure may refer to different time periods. Thus some lack of correlation between them may be due to true change in exposure over time. For example, a test–retest reliability study of a food frequency questionnaire estimate of fat intake over the last year, with the two administrations separated by a year, would not yield a perfect correlation even if the instrument was perfect, because of the one-year shift in the time period covered. However, this issue may not be a problem; depending on the true exposure of interest, it may be appropriate to include the variation in a measure over time as a source of measurement error.

In intermethod reliability studies, the instrument to be evaluated is generally given first because the comparison measure is usually less prone to error and therefore may be less affected by recall of the prior measurement. Knowledge that a measure is to be validated can influence subjects' responses (e.g. self-report of weight may be influenced by knowledge that they will be weighed), and so the invitation to subjects to participate in the second measure should be given after the first measurement has been completed. In intramethod reliability studies, the order of measures (e.g. raters) should be randomized (although X_1 would always be the measure by rater 1, X_2 by rater 2, etc.).

Review of studies using the instrument

There is an additional approach to assessing the validity of an instrument, which is similar to the concept of *predictive validity* from psychology (Nunnally 1978; Carmines and Zeller 1979). If an exposure measure has been shown to be associated with a disease or other outcome in several epidemiological studies, this provides some evidence that it is a valid measure. Specifically, it can be seen from Equation 3.8 that $\rho_{TX} > \rho_{XY}$, i.e. the correlation between a continuous exposure variable X and a continuous outcome Y is a lower limit for the validity coefficient of X. The assumption is that the errors in the outcome Y and exposure X are uncorrected. This approach of reviewing other epidemiological studies can also be applied in a qualitative way to studies with dichotomous disease outcomes. For example, if an estimate of vitamin A from a dietary questionnaire was significantly associated with disease in several studies, in agreement with prior hypotheses, this provides some evidence for the validity of the instrument.

Analysis of Validity and Reliability Studies

Selecting the appropriate measures of validity or reliability

This section covers some common approaches to the statistical analysis of validity and reliability studies. These are the statistics which one would present in the results section of a paper that described a validity or reliability study. (The concepts presented in this chapter on the *interpretation* of measures of reliability, including the interpretation of κ presented at the end of this section, would be appropriate for the discussion section of a paper.)

The selection of the appropriate analysis depends on certain aspects of the design of the study (Fleiss 1981, 1986; Maclure and Willett 1987; Dunn 1989, 1992; Kelsey *et al.* 1996). First, is the exposure measure a continuous variable, a nominal (including dichotomous) categorical variable, or an ordered categorical variable? All the statistical techniques to be discussed are for reliability and validity studies in which the two or more measures of exposure to be compared are on the same type of scale.

Secondly, is the study an intermethod reliability/validity study or an intramethod reliability study? In an intermethod reliability study or a validity study, the instruments usually differ, the variances of the measures may not be equal, and even the units of measure may not be the same (e.g. a measure of beta-carotene intake may be compared with serum beta-carotene concentration). Further, our discussion of intermethod reliability is limited to the comparison of only two measures at one time. In the intramethod type of study the instruments used are essentially the same, possibly with some difference in administration (e.g, two interviewers). Intramethod reliability studies can be performed using more than two measures per subject. One assumption of the analytical methods for intramethod studies is that the variances of the measures $X_1, X_2, ..., X_k$ are equal for continuous measures, or that the measures are 'equally precise' (Fleiss 1986) for categorical exposures.

The issue of correlated errors does not influence the choice of analytical method for reliability studies, only the interpretation of the results.

Table 4.2 gives an overview of methods for the analysis of validity and reliability studies. The upper half gives methods for intermethod studies, and the lower half gives approaches for intramethod studies. These techniques will be described in this section, with emphasis on intramethod reliability. It is assumed that the reader is already familiar with the assumptions and computations of the Pearson product-moment correlation coefficient, the one-and two-sample t-test, and the analysis of variance (ANOVA) (Armitage and Berry 1987).

The emphasis in the analysis of reliability and validity studies is on parameter estimation (e.g, estimation of $\rho_{X_1 X_2}$). Confidence intervals also add useful information. Statistical tests are less important, for it should almost be a 'given' that X_1 and X_2 are not related by chance.

Except for the evaluation of differential bias between cases and controls, the statistical techniques given in this section are for a single population. Many could be extended to the comparison of cases and controls, but these extensions are beyond the scope of this book.

Validity and intermethod reliability studies of continuous measures

Intermethod reliability studies and validity studies can be analysed using common statistical techniques.

For the analysis of continuous exposure variables, one would report $\bar{X}_1$, $\bar{X}_2$, and $\rho_{X_1 X_2}$ estimated by the Pearson correlation coefficient. Under the model of additive independent errors, the difference between the biases of the two measures can be estimated as the difference between the sample means of X_1 and X_2 (from Equation 4.1):

$$(b_1 - b_2) = \bar{X}_1 - \bar{X}_2.$$

Table 4.2 Analysis of validity and reliability studies

Type of exposure measures	Statistical measure of reliability or validity[a]	Condition under which statistic equals 1
Intermethod reliability and validity studies		
Continuous	Pearson correlation coefficient $(\rho_{X_1 X_2}), \bar{X}_1, \bar{X}_2,$ and $\bar{X}_1 - \bar{X}_2$	$X_{i1} = cX_{i2} + d$
Dichotomous	Sensitivity and specificity	(Not a summary measure)
Nominal	Misclassification matrix	(Not a summary measure)
Ordered categorical	Misclassification matrix or	(Not a summary measure)
	Spearman correlation coefficient	Ranking by X_1 same as ranking by X_2
Intramethod reliability studies		
Continuous: $X_1, ..., X_k$ are essentially the same measure	Intraclass correlation coefficient: one-way (R_1)	$X_{i1} = X_{i2} = ... = X_{ik}$
Continuous: $X_1, ..., X_k$ are the k measures (e.g. raters) to be used in the epidemiological study	Intraclass correlation coefficient: two-way fixed effects (R_2)	$X_{i1} = X_{i2} = ... = X_{ik}$
Continuous: $X_1, ..., X_k$ represent k of many measures (e.g. raters) that will be used in the study	Intraclass correlation coefficient: two-way random effects (R_3)	$X_{i1} = X_{i2} = ... = X_{ik}$
Continuous: same as two-way fixed effects except difference between means of measures not a source of error in parent study	Intraclass correlation coefficient with difference in means excluded in variance of X (R_4)	$X_{i1} = X_{i2} + d_2 = ... = X_{ik} + d_k$
Nominal or dichotomous	Cohen's κ	$X_{i1} = X_{i2}$
Ordered categorical	Weighted κ	$X_{i1} = X_{i2}$

[a] Statistical analysis would include an estimation of the statistical measure and its confidence interval.

For a validity or reliability study in which X_2 is unbiased, $\bar{X}_1 - \bar{X}_2$ is an estimate of b_1, the bias in X_1. The value of t calculated through a one-sample t-test on the variable $(X_{i1} - X_{i2})$ performed for each subject can be used to compute a confidence interval.

For reliability studies in which cases are compared with controls, if X_2 has non-differential bias then the difference in bias in X_1 between cases and controls can be estimated as (from Equation 4.3)

$$(b_{1D} - b_{1N}) = (\bar{X}_{1D} - \bar{X}_{2D}) - (\bar{X}_{1N} - \bar{X}_{2N}).$$

The value of t from a two-sample t-test on the variable $(X_{i1} - X_{i2})$ can be used to compute a confidence interval for the difference in b_1 between the two groups.

The Pearson product-moment correlation and its confidence interval can be used to estimate $\rho_{X_1 X_2}$ for intermethod or validity studies. If X_1 and X_2 are, at least, positively associated, then the Pearson correlation coefficient would range from zero to 1. The correlation is equal to 1 when X_1 is a perfect linear transformation of X_2 for all subjects:

$$X_{i1} = cX_{i2} + d.$$

For example, if subjects in an epidemiological study were to be weighed on a portable scale which was validated against a highly accurate scale, a Pearson correlation coefficient close to 1 would suggest that the portable scale was highly precise. If there was a consistent difference between the two measures (e.g. if the portable scale was miscalibrated 2 kg too heavy, or even if the portable scale weighed in pounds and the comparison scale was a kilogram scale), this would not reduce the correlation $\rho_{X_1 X_2}$.

Example. In an intermethod reliability study on 110 women, an estimate of percentage of energy intake from fat (X_1) from a food frequency questionnaire was compared with a 4-day diet record (X_2). The results of the study were as follows.

	Mean (% energy)	Standard deviation
X_1	39.1	6.6
X_2	37.5	6.0

Pearson correlation coefficient = 0.45

An estimate of the difference in the biases of X_1 and X_2 is

$$(b_1 - b_2) = 39.1 - 37.5 = 1.6\% \text{ dietary energy}$$

i.e. the food frequency questionnaire overestimates percentage dietary energy from fat by 1.6 per cent compared with a food record. The estimated reliability coefficient is based on the Pearson correlation coefficient $\rho_{X_1 X_2} = 0.45$.

In assessing the relationship between X_1 and X_2, one might also consider adjustment for potentially confounding factors which may explain the association of X_1 and X_2 other than by way of their relationship with T (Pearson partial corrrelation coefficient.)

Analysis of validity and intermethod studies of categorical measures

Several methods can be used to analyse validity or intermethod reliability studies of categorical exposure variables. For a nominal categorical variable the validity or intermethod reliability can be described by the misclassification matrix as described in Chapter 3. For a dichotomous exposure variable, the sensitivity and specificity are commonly used. (Alternatively, Marshall (1994) describes the parameters of sensitivity and specificity adjusted for chance agreement.)

The misclassification matrix is also appropriate for ordered categorical variables. Depending on the distribution of the ordered categorical variable, the Spearman rank correlation coefficient might be used. Recall from Chapter 3 that the effect of measurement error in an ordered categorical variable can also be described (under certain assumptions) in terms of the validity coefficient of the underlying continuous variable from which the categorical variable was created. This means that the difference in means and the correlation between the two underlying continuous variables could be appropriate.

Because the misclassification matrix is not a summary measure, κ (described below) is often used to analyse intermethod reliability studies of categorical variables. However, these methods were developed under assumptions more appropriate to intramethod reliability studies.

Analysis of intramethod reliability studies: the concept of interchangeable measures

The primary distinction we have made between intermethod and intramethod reliability studies is that intermethod studies use two instruments and intramethod studies involve repeated applications of one instrument. However, the most important distinction in terms of selecting an analytical method is that in intermethod studies only one measure, X_1, is to be used in the full epidemiological study, so one is interested in the reliability of X_1. In intramethod studies, the two or more measures compared are to be used interchangeably as a single exposure measurement in the epidemiological study. For example, in an intramethod reliability study, X_1 may refer to a measure by one interviewer and X_2 to one by a second interviewer, but in the parent epidemiological study each subject will be questioned by one or other of the two interviewers. In intramethod studies, we are interested not in the reliability of X_1 or X_2 but in the reliability of the interchangeable measure 'X', the measure to be used in the epidemiological study.

There is a key difference between intermethod and intramethod reliability. In intermethod reliability, any systematic difference between X_1 and X_2 reflects a consistent bias which affects all subjects in the parent study, and thus does not affect the precision of X_1. In intramethod reliability, on the other hand, a systematic difference between measures contributes to a lack of precision in X because it affects some subjects but not others. For example, if one interviewer weighs subjects on a correctly calibrated scale and a second rater's scale is miscalibrated 2 kg too heavy, this source of error will affect only the subjects measured by the second rater. Thus any consistent difference between study interviewers would increase the variance of the exposure measure (σ_X^2) in the full study and decrease the reliability compared with the use of only one inter-viewer. The Pearson product-moment correlation is not appropriate for intramethod studies, because systematic differences (in bias or scale) between X_1 and the comparison measure X_2 are not reflected in the Pearson correlation.

Special analytical methods have been developed for intramethod reliability studies, particularly in the context of inter-rater reliability studies. For contin-uous variables, the reliability ρ_X of X is estimated by a version of the intraclass correlation coefficient R. The *intraclass correlation coefficient* is an estimate of ρ_X as defined in Equation 4.9, i.e.

$$\hat{\rho}_X = R = \frac{\hat{\sigma}_S^2}{\hat{\sigma}_X^2}.$$

The variance σ_X^2 of X in the full epidemiological study is estimated under the assumption that in the full study each subject will be *randomly* assigned one measure (e.g. one interviewer). The intraclass correlation is diminished by the error in X due to systematic differences between measures $X_1, \ldots, X_k$ as well as that due to random error. Thus the intraclass correlation (except for R_4

discussed below) is equal to 1 only when there is *exact* agreement between measures, i.e. when $X_{i1} = X_{i2} = \ldots X_{ik}$ for each subject.

The intraclass correlation coefficient can be interpreted by Equation 4.4 or Equation 4.10, depending on whether or not there are correlated errors between X_1 and X_2. The bias in X cannot be estimated in an intramethod study. The mean difference $(\bar{X}_1 - \bar{X}_2)$ between measures can be used to reflect the systematic difference between measures, but any consistent difference between X_1 and X_2 beyond chance also contributes to a lower estimate of ρ_X the intraclass correlation coefficient.

Four versions of the intraclass correlation coefficient are discussed here. This discussion is followed by a presentation of an analogous statistic κ for intramethod reliability studies of categorical variables. Books by Fleiss (1981, 1986) and Dunn (1989) contain excellent discussions of the intraclass correlation coefficient and κ.

Intraclass correlation for a simple replication study

Intramethod reliability studies of continuous exposure measures are analysed by analysis of variance (ANOVA) techniques. The selection of the appropriate version of the intraclass correlation coefficient depends on the reliability study design, within the context of ANOVA models.

First, consider a simple replication reliability study in which there is no characteristic that distinguishes the first and second measures across all subjects. Examples of this type of design include a study in which blood from each subject is analysed three times in the laboratory, or a study in which medical records are abstracted twice for each subject by two randomly selected abstractors from a pool of three or more abstractors. In studies of this type, the order of the measures can be considered arbitrary. This study design is analysed by a one-way random effects model ANOVA.

Each of n subjects is measured k times, with X_{ij} being the jth measure on subject i, $\bar{X}_i$, the mean for subject i, and $\bar{X}$ the overall mean. The computations for a one-way ANOVA appear in Table 4.3. The model is $X_{ij} = S_i + F_{ij}$, where S is the subject effect and F the random error as described on pp. 106–8. The reliability coefficient of X can be estimated by the intraclass correlation coefficient from the one-way random effects model, termed R_1 here:

$$\hat{\rho}_X = R_1 = \frac{\hat{\sigma}_S^2}{\hat{\sigma}_X^2} = \frac{\text{BMS} - \text{WMS}}{\text{BMS} + (k-1)\text{WMS}}$$

where BMS is the between-subjects mean square and WMS the within-subjects mean square.

Table 4.3 One-way analysis of variance and two-way analysis of variance for the computation of intraclass correlation coefficients

Source of variance	Sum of squares (SS)	Degrees of freedom (df)	Mean square (MS = SS/df)	Expected mean square
One-way ANOVA				
Between subjects	$k\sum_i(\bar{X}_i - \bar{X})^2$	$n-1$	BMS	$\sigma_F^2 + k\sigma_S^2$
Within subjects (random error)	$\sum_i\sum_j(X_{ij} - \bar{X}_i)^2$	$n(k-1)$	WMS	σ_F^2
Total	$\sum_i\sum_j(X_{ij} - \bar{X})^2$	$nk-1$		
Two-way ANOVA				
Between subjects	$k\sum_i(\bar{X}_i - \bar{X})^2$	$n-1$	SMS	$\sigma_F^2 + k\sigma_S^2$
Between measures	$n\sum_j(\bar{X}_j - \bar{X})^2$	$k-1$	MMS	$\begin{cases}\sigma_F^2 + \frac{n}{k-1}\sum m_j^2\ (F)^a \\ \sigma_F^2 + n\sigma_M^2 \quad (R)^b\end{cases}$
Random error	by subtraction	$(n-1)(k-1)$	EMS	
Total	$\sum_i\sum_j(X_{ij} - \bar{X})^2$	$nk-1$		σ_F^2

[a] Fixed effects model
[b] Random effects model

Example. Table 4.4 presents a summary of the data and an analysis of variance for a test–retest study of a food frequency questionnaire measure of percentage energy from fat. The two measures were derived from two administrations of the questionnaire to 110 subjects 6 months apart. If this were considered to be a simple replication study, the reliability coefficient would be estimated as

$$\hat{\rho}_X = R_1 = \frac{64.37 - 15.81}{64.37 + 15.81} = 0.61.$$

Under the assumption of normality of X and the random error, a lower $100(1 - \alpha)$ per cent confidence interval for R_1 can be estimated, from

$$R_1 \geqslant \frac{\dfrac{\text{BMS}}{\text{WMS}} - f}{\dfrac{\text{BMS}}{\text{WMS}} + (k - 1)f}$$

Table 4.4 Example of an analysis of variance for a test-retest study of percentage energy from fat estimated from a food frequency questionnaire

Variable	*N*	Mean (% kcal)	Standard deviation
% energy at baseline (X_1)	110	37.5	5.96
% energy at 6 months (X_2)	110	35.5	6.53

Source of Variance	Sum of squares	Degrees of freedom	Mean square
One-way ANOVA			
Between subjects	7015.89	109	64.37
Within subjects (random error)	1739.52	110	15.81
Total	8755.41	219	39.98
Two-way ANOVA			
Between subjects	7015.89	109	64.37
Between measures	233.81	1	233.81
Random error	1505.71	109	13.81
Total	8755.41	219	39.98

where f denotes the $(1 - \alpha)$ centile from tables of the F distribution with $n - 1$ and $n(k - 1)$ degrees of freedom.

Fleiss (1986) gives a method for the analysis of reliability studies in which the number of measures k can vary across subjects.

Intraclass correlation for subjects by measures (two-way) design

The remaining designs to be considered are intramethod reliability studies in which the two or more measures may have different characteristics, i.e. the order of measures is not arbitrary. An example would be an inter-rater reliability study in which all subjects are interviewed by the same two interviewers, with X_1 being the measure by rater 1 and X_2 by rater 2. When the k raters in the reliability study are the same as the k raters who will participate in the epidemiological study, the intraclass correlation coefficient from the two-way fixed effects ANOVA model (R_2) is appropriate. When the k raters in the reliability study are a sample from a population of raters to be used in the epidemiological study, the intraclass correlation coefficient from the two-way random effects ANOVA model (R_3) applies. An example of this would be when two interviewers participate in the reliability study as representatives of the several interviewers who will participate in the full study.

The ANOVA table for this two-way (subjects by measures) design under the assumption of no interaction between subjects and measures is given in the lower half of Table 4.3. X_{ij} is the jth measure on subject i, $\overline{X}_i$ is the mean for subject i, and $\overline{X}_j$ is the mean for measure j. The computations of the mean squares given in Table 4.3 are the same for the fixed and random effects models, but the estimate of σ_X^2 and therefore of R differs. SMS, MMS, and EMS are the mean squares for subjects, measures, and error respectively.

The two-way fixed effects model, where m_j is the fixed effect of measure j, is

$$X_{ij} = S_i + m_j + F_{ij}.$$

Under this model, the intraclass correlation coefficient (R_2) is estimated by

$$R_2 = \frac{\hat{\sigma}_S^2}{\hat{\sigma}_X^2} = \frac{n(\text{SMS} - \text{EMS})}{n\text{SMS} + (k - 1)\text{MMS} + (n - 1)(k - 1)\text{EMS}}.$$

No simple method is available for a confidence interval.

Under the two-way random effects model $X_{ij} = S_i + M_j + F_{ij}$, where M_j, is the random effect of measure j, the intraclass correlation coefficient (R_3) is (Bartko 1966)

$$R_3 = \frac{\hat{\sigma}_S^2}{\hat{\sigma}_X^2} = \frac{n(\text{SMS} - \text{EMS})}{n\text{SMS} + k\text{MMS} + (nk - n - k)\text{EMS}}.$$

A lower $100(1 - \alpha)$ percentage confidence limit for R_3 has been derived by Fleiss and Shrout (1978) (see Fleiss 1986).

The estimates of the intraclass correlation for both fixed and random effects models include the variation between measures (e.g. between raters) as a source of variance in X. R_3 is generally less than R_2 when applied to the same data. This is because the error in X is estimated to be larger when the measures (e.g. raters) in the reliability study are only a sample of the measures to be used in the full study.

Example. Suppose that two interviewers administered a food frequency questionnaire to each subject in a reliability study, and the same two interviewers will be employed in the full study. Then the fixed effects model applies, and R_2 is an appropriate estimate of ρ_X. The computation is illustrated on the same data as in the previous example (Table 4.4). From the two-way ANOVA

$$R_2 = \frac{110\,(64.37 - 13.81)}{110\,(64.37) + 233.81 + 109\,(13.81)} = 0.63.$$

Intraclass correlation which excludes the mean differences between measures

For some reliability study designs, the systematic differences between the measures, the differences between the $\overline{X}_j$, do not need to be included as a source of variance in X. This is the case when it is intended to adjust for the systematic difference between measures in the epidemiological study. For example, if interviewers produced different mean estimates of exposure, one might adjust in the epidemiological study for interviewer effects. Under these circumstances the intraclass correlation coefficient R_4 is used. R_4 may also be appropriate for reliability studies in which the difference between X_1 and X_2 can be explained by a 'learning effect' or other factors that will not add error (variance) to the measure X in the full study.

When the measurement effects are to be excluded as a source of variance in X, the intraclass correlation coefficient for the fixed effects model is

$$R_4 = \frac{\text{SMS} - \text{EMS}}{\text{SMS} + (k - 1)\text{EMS}}.$$

It has a lower $100(1 - \alpha)$ confidence limit:

$$R_4 > \frac{\dfrac{\text{SMS}}{\text{EMS}} - f}{\dfrac{\text{SMS}}{\text{EMS}} + (k-1)f}$$

where f denotes the $(1 - \alpha)$ centile of the F distribution with $(n - 1)$ and $(n - 1)(k - 1)$ degrees of freedom.

R_4 will equal 1 when the measures are identical for each subject except for a constant difference between measures:

$$X_{i1} = X_{i2} + d_2 = \quad = X_{ik} + d_k.$$

(R_4 differs from the Pearson correlation coefficient, in that R_4 includes any differences in scale as a source of variance in X.)

When the k measures, $X_1,\ldots,X_k$, have identical distributions, all four versions of R are essentially the same and are equal to the Pearson product-moment correlation coefficient.

Cohen's κ for dichotomous or nominal variables

The intramethod reliability of nominal categorical variables, including dichotomous variables, is measured by Cohen's κ (Cohen 1960). This can be computed from a reliability study in which n subjects have each been measured twice where each measure is a nominal variable with k categories. (Note that k here refers to number of categories, not number of measures per subject.) It is assumed that the two measures are equally accurate. To compute κ the data are laid out as a $k \times k$ table as in Table 4.5. The p_{ij} are the proportions

Table 4.5 Layout of data for computation of Cohen's κ and weighted κ

		Measure 2					
		1	2	.	.	k	Total
	1	p_{11}	p_{12}	.	.	p_{1k}	r_1
	2	p_{21}	p_{22}	.	.	p_{2k}	r_2
Measure 1	.	.	.	.	.	.	.
	.	.	.	.	.	.	.
	.	.	.	.	.	.	.
	k	p_{k1}	p_{k2}	.	.	p_{kk}	r_k
	Total	s_1	s_2	.	.	s_k	1

of subjects who fall into the ith category in measure 1 and the jth category in measure 2. Note that the p_{ij} proportions in the table sum to 1 over the entire table. The r_i and s_i are the marginal proportions for the first and second measure, respectively.

An obvious measure of agreement between two measures is the proportion of subjects for whom there was agreement. The observed proportion of agreement P_o is the sum of the proportions on the diagonal:

$$P_o = \sum_{i=1}^{k} p_{ij}.$$

However, this simple measure is not appropriate, because it does not take into consideration the agreement that would be expected by chance. For example, if 10 per cent of people in the population had a high alcohol intake and one interviewer accurately classified subjects but the second interviewer randomly assigned 90 per cent to low intake and 10 per cent to high intake, then there would be 82 per cent agreement (i.e. of 100 people, 81 of the 90 low intake subjects would be in agreement by the two interviewers as would one of the 10 high alcohol intake subjects). This high percentage agreement obscures the fact that *all* of the agreement occurred by chance, not because the measurement was repeatable across interviewers.

κ is a measure of agreement which corrects for the agreement that would be expected by chance. The expected agreement (on the diagonal) P_e is:

$$P_e = \sum_{i=1}^{k} r_i s_j.$$

κ is estimated as the observed agreement beyond chance divided by the maximum possible agreement beyond chance:

$$\hat{\kappa} = \frac{P_o - P_e}{1 - P_e}.$$

$\hat{\kappa}$ is equal to 1 when there is exact agreement between the two measures for all subjects. It is greater than zero when agreement is greater than chance, but can be less than zero if agreement is less than expected by chance.

An approximate lower $100(1 - \alpha)$ per cent confidence bound for $\hat{\kappa}$ (if $\kappa \neq 0$) is (Fleiss *et al.* 1969; Fleiss 1981)

$$\hat{\kappa} - Z_\alpha \times \text{s.e.}(\hat{\kappa})$$

where Z_α is the value of the $(1 - \alpha)$ centile of the standard normal variable and s.e. $(\hat{\kappa})$ is the estimated standard error of $\hat{\kappa}$:

$$\text{s.e. } (\hat{\kappa}) = \sqrt{\frac{a + b - c}{(1 - P_e)^2 n}}$$

where

$$a = \sum_{i=1}^{k} P_{ii}[1 - (r_i + s_i)(1 - \hat{\kappa})]^2$$

$$b = (1 - \hat{\kappa})^2 \sum_{i=1}^{k} \sum_{\substack{j=1 \\ i \neq j}}^{k} P_{ij}(r_i + s_j)^2$$

$$c = [\hat{\kappa} - P_e(1 - \hat{\kappa})]^2.$$

Example. Consider the reliability study described above in the intraclass correlation examples, and suppose that subjects were to be divided into only two categories of fat intake: those above the median in percentage energy from fat and those below. Cross-classifying the 110 subjects by the two measures yields the following table, with the proportions in brackets:

		2nd measure		
		Upper half	Lower half	
1st measure	Upper half	40 (0.364)	15 (0.136)	55 (0.5)
	Lower half	15 (0.136)	40 (0.364)	55 (0.5)
		55 (0.5)	55 (0.5)	110 (1.0)

Then

$$P_o = 0.364 + 0.364 = 0.727$$
$$P_e = (0.5 \times 0.5) + (0.5 \times 0.5) = 0.50$$
$$\hat{\kappa} = \frac{0.727 - 0.5}{0.5} = 0.45.$$

When there are more than two categories, the source of unreliability may become clearer by computing a κ for each category compared with all other categories combined. When there are more than two measures per subject, another version of κ has been derived under the assumption that there is no order to the measures (Landis and Koch 1977; Fleiss 1986). The assumptions and resulting κ are similar to the one-way ANOVA intraclass correlation coefficient.

Weighted κ for ordered categorical variables

The κ presented above for nominal categories is a measure of exact agreement, with all disagreements considered to be equally serious. For example, if rater 1 categorizes a subject as falling into category 1 and rater 2 disagrees, κ will be the same whether the second rating is category 2, 3, 4, etc. When the measure of interest in an intramethod reliability study is an ordered categorical variable, the use of κ is not appropriate. Instead, κ_w, *weighted* κ (Cohen 1968) is used, as this measure yields a higher reliability when disagreements between raters are small than when they are large. In other words, weighted κ gives 'partial credit' for close but not exact agreement.

Weighted κ is estimated as follows:

$$\hat{\kappa}_w = \frac{P_o - P_e}{1 - P_e}$$

where P_o is the weighted observed proportion of agreement (across the entire table)

$$P_o = \sum_{i=1}^{k}\sum_{j=1}^{k} w_{ij} p_{ij},$$

P_e is the weighted expected proportion of agreement (across the entire table)

$$P_e = \sum_{i=1}^{k}\sum_{j=1}^{k} w_{ij} r_i s_j,$$

and p_{ij}, r_i, and s_j are the proportions shown in Table 4.5.

The usual weight applied for one measure yielding category i and the other category j is

$$w_{ij} = 1 - \frac{(i-j)^2}{(k-1)^2}.$$

This gives a weight of 1 for exact agreement and a weight of zero when one measure yields the lowest category and the other the highest (kth) category.

A confidence interval for $\hat{\kappa}_w$ can be computed based on the large-sample estimate of the standard error of $\hat{\kappa}_w$ (for $\kappa_w \neq 0$):

$$\text{s.e.} (\hat{\kappa}_w) = \sqrt{\frac{a - b}{(1 - P_e)^2 n}}$$

where

$$a = \sum_{i=1}^{k} \sum_{j=1}^{k} p_{ij} [w_{ij} - (\bar{w}_i + \bar{w}_j)(1 - \hat{k}_w)]^2$$

$$b = [\hat{\kappa}_w - P_e(1 - \hat{\kappa}_w)]^2$$

$$\bar{w}_i = \sum_{j=1}^{k} s_j w_{ij}$$

and

$$\bar{w}_j = \sum_{i=1}^{k} r_i w_{ij}.$$

For the reliability study used in the previous examples, if percentage calories from fat were divided into four equal ordered categories, κ_w would be 0.57.

Ordered categorical variables are often created by categorizing a continuous variable. In these situations, the intraclass correlation coefficient could also be computed on the underlying variable.

Interpretation and limitations of κ and weighted κ

Certain similarities allow κ and κ_w to be interpreted as reliability coefficients. κ for binary variables and κ_w are equal to the intraclass correlation coefficient based on the two-way random effects model (R_3), except for a term that goes to zero as n increases (Fleiss and Cohen 1973; Fleiss 1975; Dunn 1989), when the categories are numerically coded 1 for category 1, 2 for category 2, etc. κ_w is also equal to the Pearson product-moment correlation coefficient if the marginal distributions of the two measures are identical (Cohen 1968).

The value of κ for dichotomous measures or κ_w can be interpreted in terms of the attenuation of the odds ratio due to non-differential measurement error. When κ is derived from a study in which the two dichotomous measures compared have equal sensitivity, equal specificity, and independent error (similar to the parallel test model), it has been shown to be approximately related to the attenuation of the odds ratio by (Tavaré *et al.* 1995)

$$OR_O = OR_T^{\sqrt{\kappa}}.$$

This is equivalent to using $\sqrt{\kappa}$ to estimate ρ_{TX}, similar to Equation 4.4, and then substituting $\sqrt{\kappa}$ for ρ_{TX} in Equation 3.6 (the attenuation equation based on the distribution of X, not absolute units). In addition, since κ_w could be interpreted as an intraclass correlation coefficient, the above equation might crudely apply to κ_w if the ordered categorical measures that were compared in the reliability study met the assumptions of equal and uncorrelated errors. If these assumptions are not met, then κ_w could be used for $\rho_{X_1 X_2}$ in the other interpretations given for $\rho_{X_1 X_2}$ in terms of ρ_{TX_1} in this chapter (and subsequently in terms of the attenuation of the odds ratio given by Equation 3.6). For example, if the categorical measures in the reliability study had correlated errors, then the above equation only represents the attenuation of the odds ratio due to the random component of error, and the actual attenuation would be greater.

There are several limitations to the interpretation of κ and κ_w (Maclure and Willett 1987). The value of κ_w varies with the number of exposure categories. In the reliability study of percentage energy from fat used in the previous examples, κ was 0.45 when the measure was divided into two categories and κ_w was 0.57 when four categories were used. (The intraclass correlation was 0.61 when percentage energy from fat was treated as a continuous variable.)

In addition, the value of κ or κ_w depends on the distribution of exposure in the population. Thus κ cannot be used to compare the reliability of two instruments measuring the same underlying exposure if the two reliability studies were conducted in populations which may have different distributions of the true exposure. This is similar to the problem of comparing reliability coefficients across populations which differ in the variance of exposure. However, this dependence of κ on the prevalence of exposure may be a desirable property because, as noted in Chapter 3, the attenuation of the odds ratio depends on the exposure prevalence as well as the sensitivity and specificity of the measurement.

Neither κ nor weighted κ_w is sufficient to detect differential misclassification between cases and controls. κ is a single summary measure of the misclassification in the measure, while the assessment of differential misclassification requires estimates of sensitivity and specificity for cases and controls (or the misclassification matrices for $k > 2$). κ could be similar for cases and controls even when there is differential misclassification, i.e. when the underlying sensitivity and specificity of the exposure measurement differs substantially between the two groups. This is analogous to the problem that intramethod reliability studies of continuous variables can provide information only on precision but not on bias, and therefore cannot assess differential bias between cases and controls.

Other types of analysis of reliability studies

Some authors (Liu *et al.* 1978) present the reliability of a continuous measure X in terms other than the reliability coefficient ρ_X. The *ratio of the within-subject variance* σ_W^2 *to the between-subject variance* σ_S^2, where S is the subject effect and σ_W^2 is defined as $\sigma_X^2 - \sigma_S^2$, is sometimes used. This ratio is a simple transformation of ρ_X

$$\frac{\sigma_W^2}{\sigma_S^2} = \frac{1 - \rho_X}{\rho_X}$$

where ρ_X is based on the appropriate measure of the reliability coefficient. Because the ratio of within- to between-subject variance provides the same information as the reliability coefficient, the equations presented in Chapters 3, 4, and 5 as functions of ρ_X (or of ρ_{TX}^2 when ρ_X can be considered as an estimate of ρ_{TX}^2) could be presented in terms of σ_W^2 / σ_S^2 by substituting

$$\rho_X = 1 / [(\sigma_W^2 / \sigma_S^2) + 1].$$

One additional analytical technique for reliability studies of continuous measures deserves mention: the *coefficient of variation* (Garber and Carey 1984). For laboratory measures, reliability is often assessed by repeated analysis of a single reference material with known true measurement t. For example, a fluid with a known concentration of retinol might be repeatedly analysed to yield measures of X, the measured retinol concentration. (This type of study only assesses the laboratory error, of course, and excludes errors due to storage and handling of specimens, and error due to the variation in the measure over time within individuals.) In such studies, the mean and variance of X can be used to assess the reliability of X. The bias of the measure can be estimated as

$$b = \bar{X} - t.$$

Because t is a constant, the variance of X in the reliability study is equal to the variance of the random error F:

$$\hat{\sigma}_F^2 = \hat{\sigma}_X^2.$$

A reliability coefficient cannot be estimated because the comparison measure is constant (t) for each measurement of X. Instead, a coefficient of variation CV, defined as the estimated standard deviation divided by the mean of $X \times 100$, is often used:

$$CV\% = \frac{\hat{\sigma}_X}{\bar{X}} \times 100.$$

A small CV is considered to indicate a reliable measure. However, it may be more informative to relate the variance of the random error $\hat{\sigma}_F^2$ to the expected variance of X in the population of interest (see right-hand side of Equation 4.8) to yield information closer to the reliability coefficient of X in the population of interest.

Reliability study designs may be more complex than those covered in this chapter, in order to yield more information about the measurement error. For example, an intramethod reliability study of a laboratory measure could use blood drawn at two points in time for each subject and have each sample tested by two laboratory technicians. This design could separately assess the errors due to variation over time within subjects and those due to variation between technicians. Or, an intermethod reliability study could have two comparison measures for X_1, one on the correct scale but with correlated errors and one with uncorrelated error but on a different scale from X_1. For example, a food frequency measure of beta-carotene could be simultaneously compared with a seven-day diet record and with serum beta-carotene. Approaches to the analysis of these more complex designs are given by Dunn (1989, 1992), Kaaks et al. (1994), and Wong et al. (1999a,b).

Finally, reliability studies of some instruments do not require a comparison measure. In the social sciences, the reliability of a total score on a test is often assessed by the reliability of parts of the test, for example by the correlation between test items (Carmines and Zeller 1979; Dunn 1989). This is termed *internal consistency reliability* and is discussed in Chapter 5 in the section on use of multiple measures of exposure. This approach may be useful for some applications in epidemiology. (One note of caution: in some packaged programs, SPSS in particular, the term reliability is often used to refer to the reliability of the sum of the measures. If you are interested in the reliability of the individual measures X_1, X_2, etc., the reliability coefficient that is reported by the program may not be the statistic you require.)

Sample size for reliability studies

The computation of the required sample size depends on the design and aim of the reliability study. For an intermethod reliability study conducted to assess differential bias between cases and controls, the required sample size could be based on the standard sample size formula for a two-sample comparison of means (Kelsey *et al.* 1996), where the variable of interest is $(X_{i1} - X_{i2})$.

For a validity or intermethod reliability study conducted to estimate $\rho_{X_1 X_2}$, the sample size would be that needed to estimate the Pearson correlation coefficient between two variables. Note that the null hypothesis to be tested would not be $\rho_{X_1 X_2} = 0$, for it should be assumed that X_1 and X_2 are at least positively correlated. Rather, the study should have sufficient power to detect whether $\rho_{X_1 X_2}$ is greater than some minimum value r_L. Based on the transformation of $\rho_{X_1 X_2}$ to a standardized normal distribution (Snedecor and Cochran 1971), the required sample size n is

$$n = 3 + \frac{4\left(Z_\alpha + Z_\beta\right)^2}{\left(\ln C\right)^2}$$

where

$$C = \frac{\left(1 - r\right)\left(1 + r_L\right)}{\left(1 + r\right)\left(1 - r_L\right)},$$

and where r is the hypothesized (expected) value of the correlation coefficient, r_L is the minimally acceptable correlation, Z_α is the $(100 - \alpha)$ centile of the standard normal distribution, α is the significance level for a one-sided test (or significance level for a lower bound for a confidence interval), and β is 1 minus the required power. $Z_{\alpha/2}$ would be substituted for Z_α for a two-sided confidence interval. For example, for an expected $r = 0.6$, a lower bound $r_L = 0.4$, 80 per cent power ($Z_\beta = 0.84$) and a two-sided 95 per cent confidence interval ($Z_{\alpha/2} = 1.96$), the required sample size is 111 subjects.

For intramethod reliability studies, Walter *et al.* (1998) give a simple approximation formula for the required number n of subjects needed to estimate an intraclass correlation coefficient based on one-way ANOVA:

$$n = 1 + \frac{2\left(Z_\alpha + Z_\beta\right)^2 k}{\left(\ln C\right)^2 \left(k - 1\right)}$$

where

$$C = \frac{\left(1 - R\right)\left[1 + \left(k - 1\right)R_L\right]}{\left[1 + \left(k - 1\right)R\right]\left(1 - R_L\right)}.$$

Z_α and Z_β are as above, k is the number of replicates per person, R is the hypothesized (expected) value of the intraclass correlation coefficient, and R_L is the lower limit of acceptable reliability. For $k = 2$, the first term should be 3/2 rather than 1. Walter *et al.* (1998) state that the above formula can also be used for approximate sample size guidelines for two-way ANOVA, especially if the rater effects are small.

In the above equation, the number of replicates per person is assumed to be fixed, because it is often based on practical constraints such as respondent burden. However, one could vary k to see which value of k minimizes the total number *(nk)* of measures in the reliability study. For R in the range 0.5–0.8 and $(R - R_L) = 0.2$, the optimal number of replicates to minimize the total number of measures is 3.

Jannarone *et al.* (1987) give an approach for selecting the number of subjects and number of measures per subject for studies which estimate κ.

Summary

Reliability studies can be designed to provide information about the validity of a measure if the comparison measure is carefully selected. If a comparison measure without differential bias between cases and controls is chosen, then a reliability study can yield estimates of differential bias in the measure of interest. Useful information about the validity coefficient can be obtained from a comparison of the measure of interest with an equally accurate or more accurate measure when the errors between the two measures are uncorrelated. When the measures in a reliability study have correlated errors, the reliability coefficient can provide only an upper limit to the validity coefficient.

The choice of an analytical technique for a validity or reliability study depends on whether the exposure is measured as a continuous variable, a nominal categorical (or dichotomous variable), or an ordered categorical variable. The choice also depends on whether the two or more measures in the reliability study will be used interchangeably in the full epidemiological study or only one will be used, and on other design issues. For example, for a reliability study in which a continuous exposure measure from proxy respondents was compared with the same measure from the subjects themselves, the Pearson correlation coefficient might be appropriate for the analysis if all interviews in the full study were to be from proxy respondents, a version of the intraclass correlation coefficient (R_2) might be used if both proxies and index cases were to be included in the full study, and another version (R_4) might be used if both were included but a factor indicating whether the interview was by index or proxy respondent was to be adjusted for in the full study. Versions of Cohen's κ are most commonly used to summarize the information obtained in reliability studies involving nominal or ordered categorical variables.

References

Allen, M.J. and Yen, W.M. (1979). *Introduction to Measurement Theory*, pp. 1–117. Brooks/Cole, Monterey, CA.

Altman, D.G. and Bland, J.M. (1983). Measurement in medicine: the analysis of method comparison studies. *Statistician*, **32**, 307–17.

Armitage, P. and Berry, G. (1987). *Statistical Methods in Medical Research* (2nd edn). Blackwell Scientific, Oxford.

Bartko, J.J. (1966). The intraclass correlation coefficient as a measure of reliability. *Psychological Reports*, **19**, 3–11.

Bohrnstedt, G.W. (1983). Measurement. In *Handbook of Survey Research* (ed. P. Rossi, J. Wright, and A. Anderson), pp. 70–121. Academic Press, Orlando, FL.

Carmines, E.G. and Zeller, R.A. (1979). *Reliability and Validity Assessment*. Sage, Beverly Hills, CA.

Chasan-Taber, S., Rimm, E.B., Stampfer, M.J., *et al.* (1996). Reproducibility and validity of a self-administered physical activity questionnaire for male health professionals. *Epidemiology*, **7**, 81–6.

Clayton, D. (1985). Using test–retest reliability data to improve estimates of relative risk: an application of latent class analysis. *Statistics in Medicine*, **4**, 445–55.

Cohen, J. (1960). A coefficient of agreement for nominal scales. *Educational and Psychological Measurement*, **20**, 37–46.

Cohen, J. (1968). Weighted kappa: nominal scale agreement with provision for scaled disagreement or partial credit. *Psychological Bulletin*, **70**, 213–20.

Dunn, G. (1989). *Design and Analysis of Reliability Studies*. Edward Arnold, London, and Oxford University Press, New York.

Dunn, G. (1992). Design and analysis of reliability studies. *Statistical Methods in Medical Research*, **1**, 123–57.

Fleiss, J.L. (1975). Measuring agreement between two judges on the presence or absence of a trait. *Biometrics*, **31**, 651–9.

Fleiss, J.L. (1981). *Statistical Methods for Rates and Proportions* (2nd edn), pp. 188–236. Wiley, New York.

Fleiss, J.L. (1986). *The Design and Analysis of Clinical Experiments*, pp. 1–32. Wiley, New York.

Fleiss, J.L. and Cohen, J. (1973). The equivalence of weighted kappa and the intraclass correlation coefficient as measures of reliability. *Educational and Psychological Measurement*, **33**, 613–19.

Fleiss, J.L. and Shrout, P.E. (1977). The effects of measurement errors on some multivariate procedures. *American Journal of Public Health*, **67**, 1188–91.

Fleiss, J.L. and Shrout, P.E. (1978). Approximate interval estimation for a certain intraclass correlation coefficient. *Psychometrika*, **43**, 259–62.

Fleiss, J.L., Cohen, J., and Everitt, B.S. (1969). Large sample standard errors of kappa and weighted kappa. *Psychological Bulletin*, **72**, 323–7.

Fowles, J.B., Fowler, E.J., and Craft, C. (1998). Validation of claims diagnoses and self-reported conditions compared with medical records for selected chronic diseases. *Journal of Ambulatory Care Management*, **21**, 24–34.

Garber, C.C. and Carey, R.N. (1984). Laboratory statistics. In *Clinical Chemistry: Theory, Analysis, and Correlation* (ed. L. Kaplan and A. Pesce), pp. 290–2. Mosby, St. Louis, MO.

Giovannucci, E., Stampfer, M.J., Colditz, G.A., *et al.* (1993). A comparison of prospective and retrospective assessments of diet in the study of breast cancer. *American Journal of Epidemiology*, **137**, 502–11.

Hill, A.B. (1953). Observation and experiment. *New England Journal of Medicine*, **248**, 995–1001.

Hui, S.L. and Walter, S.D. (1980). Estimating the error rates of diagnostic tests. *Biometrics*, **36**, 167–71.

Hunter, D.J., Manson, J.E., Colditz, G.A., *et al.* (1997). Reproducibility of oral contraceptive histories and validity of hormone composition reported in a cohort of US women. *Contraception*, **56**, 373–8.

Jannarone, R.J., Macera, C.A., and Garrison, C.Z. (1987). Evaluating inter-rater agreement through 'case–control' sampling. *Biometrics*, **43**, 433–7.

Kaaks, R., Riboli, E., Estève, J., van Kappel, A.L., and van Staveren, W.A. (1994). Estimating the accuracy of dietary questionnaire assessments: validation in terms of structural equation models. *Statistics in Medicine*, **13**, 127–42.

Kaldor, J. and Clayton, D. (1985). Latent class analysis in chronic disease epidemiology. *Statistics in Medicine*, **4**, 327–35.

Karvetti, R.L. and Knuts, L.R. (1992). Validity of the estimated food diary: comparison of 2-day recorded and observed food and nutrient intakes. *Journal of the American Dietetic Association*, **92**, 580–4.

Kelsey, J.L., Whittemore, A.S., Evans, A.S., and Thompson, W.D. (1996). *Methods in Observational Epidemiology* (2nd edn), pp. 327–34, 341–62. Oxford University Press, New York.

Landis, J.R. and Koch, G.G. (1977). The measurement of observer agreement for categorical data. *Biometrics*, **33**, 159–74.

Liu, K., Stamler, J., Dyer, A., McKeever, J., and McKeever, P. (1978). Statistical methods to assess and minimize the role of intra-individual variability in obscuring the relationship between dietary lipids and serum cholesterol. *Journal of Chronic Diseases*, **31**, 399–418.

Lord, F.M. and Novick, M.R. (1968). *Statistical Theories of Mental Test Scores*, pp. 13–278. Addison-Wesley, Reading, MA.

Maclure, M. and Willett, W.C. (1987). Misinterpretation and misuse of the kappa statistic. *American Journal of Epidemiology*, **126**, 161–9.

McKeown, N.M., Day, N.E., Welch, A.A., *et al.* (2001). Use of biological markers to validate self-reported dietary intake in a random sample of the European Prospective Investigation into Cancer United Kingdom Norfolk cohort. *American Journal of Clinical Nutrition*, **74**, 188–96.

Marshall, R.J. (1994). Misclassification of exposure in case–control studies: assessment by quality indices. *Epidemiology*, **5**, 309–14.

Nunnally, J.C. (1978). *Psychometric Theory*, pp. 190–255. McGraw-Hill, New York.

Snedecor, G.W. and Cochran, W.G. (1971). *Statistical Methods*. Iowa State University Press, Ames, IA.

Stange, K.C., Zyzanski, S.J., Smith, T.F., *et al.* (1998). How valid are medical records and patient questionnaires for physician profiling and health services research? A comparison with direct observation of patients visits. *Medical Care*, **36**, 851–67.

Stewart, W.F., Lipton, R.B., Dowson, A.J., and Sawyer, J. (2001). Development and testing of the Migraine Disability Assessment (MIDAS) questionnaire to assess headache-related disability. *Neurology*, **56**, S20–8.

Tavaré, C.J., Sobel, E.L., and Gilles, F.H. (1995). Misclassification of a prognostic dichotomous variable: sample size and parameter estimate adjustment. *Statistics in Medicine*, **14**, 1307–14.

Walker, A.M. and Blettner, M. (1985). Comparing imperfect measures of exposure. *American Journal of Epidemiology*, **121**, 783–90.

Walter, S.D. (1984). Commentary on 'Use of dual responses to increase validity of case–control studies.' *Journal of Chronic Diseases*, **37**, 137–9.

Walter, S.D. and Irwig, L.M. (1988). Estimation of test error rates, disease prevalence and relative risk from misclassified data: a review. *Journal of Clinical Epidemiology*, **41**, 923–37.

Walter, S.D., Eliasziw, M., and Donner, A. (1998). Sample size and optimal designs for reliability studies. *Statistics in Medicine*, **17**, 101–10.

Willett, W. (1998). *Nutritional Epidemiology* (2nd edn), pp. 33–147. Oxford University Press, New York.

Willett, W., C., Sampson, L., Stampfer, M.J., *et al.* (1985). Reproducibility and validity of a semiquantitative food frequency questionnaire. *American Journal of Epidemiology*, **122**, 51–65.

Wong, M.Y., Day, N.E., Bashir, S.A., and Duffy, S.W. (1999a). Measurement error in epidemiology: the design of validation studies. I: Univariate situation. *Statistics in Medicine*, **18**, 2815–29.

Wong, M.Y., Day, N.E., and Wareham, N.J. (1999b). Measurement error in epidemiology: the design of validation studies. II: Bivariate situation. *Statistics in Medicine*, **18**, 2831–45.

Wu, M.L., Whittemore, A.S., and Jung, D.L. (1988). Errors in reported dietary intakes. II: Long-term recall. *American Journal of Epidemiology*, **128**, 1137–45.

Zeleniuch-Jacquotte, A., Chajès, V., Van Kappel, A.L., Riboli, E., and Toniolo, P. (2000). Reliability of fatty acid composition in human serum phospholipids. *European Journal of Clinical Nutrition*, **54**, 367–72.

5

Reducing measurement error and its effects

In most statistical approaches to observer variability, ...
no efforts have been made to detect and remove
sources of inconsistency. After noting the
disagreements and quantifying them with kappa scores
or other indices of concordance, investigators write the
paper and depart from the analytic scene.
(Feinstein 1983)

Introduction

In Chapters 3 and 4 we described the effects of exposure measurement error and how the degree of measurement error can be assessed. However, the primary focus on exposure measurement error should not be on its assessment but on the reduction of measurement error and its effects.

Several approaches to the reduction of measurement error and its effects are discussed in this chapter. First, adjustment procedures are briefly covered; these are methods of 'correcting' study results for the effect of measurement error by using information from a validity or reliability study. Next is the use of multiple measures of exposure, an important method of reducing measurement error. Then several other methods to reduce measurement error, which can be considered in design of an epidemiological study or during data analysis, are covered. Finally, minimization of error by way of quality control procedures is discussed. These procedures include a wide range of methods of reducing measurement error during instrument development, data collection, and creation of the dataset for analysis. Quality control procedures for specific methods of exposure measurement are also discussed in Chapters 6–10.

Adjustment of study results for the effects of measurement error

Adjustment using information from a validity study

One approach to accounting for the effect of measurement error is to estimate its impact on the results of the epidemiological study results after it has been conducted. By use of estimates of the exposure measurement error from a validity study, it is possible to adjust the observed exposure–disease association from the epidemiological study to yield an estimate of the true association.

Table 5.1 Equations for the true measure of association as a function of the observable measure of association and the exposure measurement error. (See Chapter 3 for the notation, the assumptions used in derivation of the equations, and the interpretation of equations.)

Equation	From equation	Differential or non-differential
Continuous exposure, dichotomous outcome		
$OR_T = OR_O^{C'/\rho_{TX}^2}$	[3.3]	
where $C' = \left(1 - \dfrac{b_D - b_N}{\mu_{X_D} - \mu_{X_N}}\right)$		differential
$\beta_T = \beta_O / \rho_{TX}^2$	[3.4]	non-differential
$OR_T = OR_O^{1/\rho_{TX}^2}$	[3.5]	non-differential
$OR_T = OR_O^{1/\rho_{TX}}$	[3.6]	non-differential
Continuous exposure, continuous outcome		
$\rho_{TY} = \rho_{XY} / \rho_{TX}$	[3.8]	non-differential
$\beta_T = \beta_O / \rho_{TX}^2$	[3.9]	non-differential
Dichotomuous exposure, dichotomous outcome		
$OR_T = \dfrac{P_D(1 - P_N)}{P_N(1 - P_D)}$	[3.12]	differential or non-differential
where $P_D = (p_D - 1 + spec_D) / (sens_D + spec_D - 1)$		
and $P_N = (p_N - 1 + spec_N) / (sens_N + spec_N - 1)$		

The equations presented in Chapter 3 which give the observable measure of association as a function of the true association and the measurement error can be used to derive equations that yield estimates of the true measure of association, given the observed measure of association and estimates of the measurement error. These *correction* or *de-attenuationd equations* are given in Table 5.1. The reader is referred to Chapter 3 for the notation and assumptions used in the derivation of the equations. Also, as noted in Chapter 3, the equations for the odds ratio from case–control studies would also apply to the hazard ratio from cohort studies.

Example. Suppose that a case–control study of years of occupational exposure to rubber, assessed by interview, in relation to bladder cancer yielded an odds ratio of 1.3 for 10 years of reported exposure. Suppose also that a validity study among a subset of the subjects yielded an estimate of 0.6 for the validity coefficient ρ_{TX} between self-report of years of exposure and industrial records of exposure (assumed here to be a near-perfect measure). Information from these two studies can then be used to adjust the observed odds ratio to yield an estimate of the true odds ratio (based on the equation in Table 5.1 derived from Equation 3.5, provided that the assumptions hold):

$$\widehat{OR}_T = \left(1.3\right)^{1/0.6^2} = 2.1.$$

This suggests that poor exposure measurement may have led to the weak observed association between the exposure and disease, because the observed odds ratio is consistent with a true odds ratio of 2.1 for 10 years of exposure.

In Chapter 3 it is noted that, for a cohort study in which sampling is by exposure status, the degree of misclassification changes after sampling. Adjustment procedures for cohort studies should be based on the estimates of exposure measurement error within the cohort(s) after any sampling by exposure status.

Adjustment using information from a reliability study

Information from reliability studies can also be used in adjustment procedures, to the extent that the reliability study provides information about the validity of the exposure variable (see Chapter 4). If the reliability study were of two measures with equal and uncorrelated errors (parallel measures), $\sqrt{\rho_{X_1 X_2}}$ could be substituted for ρ_{TX} in the equations in Table 5.1. However, when there is correlated error in a reliability study, it may only yield an upper limit for the validity coefficient. In this case, substitution of $\sqrt{\rho_{X_1 X_2}}$ for ρ_{TX} in the equations in Table 5.1 would lead to a conservative estimate of the true odds ratio under non-differential measurement error. This is because the estimate of the true odds ratio would only be corrected for the uncorrelated components of the measurement error, and not the components that were correlated in the reliability study.

Example. Using the previous example, suppose that only a test–retest reliability study of the interview was conducted, yielding a correlation $\rho_{X_1 X_2}$ over the two administrations of 0.7. Because the test–retest reliability study is likely to have correlated error, $\rho_{TX} < \sqrt{\rho_{X_1 X_2}}$. Substituting this in the equation in Table 5.1 derived from Equation 3.5 would yield $OR_T > 1.3^{1/0.7} = 1.5$. This adjustment only leads to a lower limit for OR_T because it only partially corrects for the measurement error.

In other circumstances, a reliability study would lead to a lower bound (or both upper and lower bound) for ρ_{TX} (see Table 4.1). This information could then be used to estimate an upper bound (or both an upper and a lower bound) for the corrected odds ratio. Applying adjustment equations without paying attention to the type of information provided by the reliability study can lead to over-correction of the odds ratio (Wacholder *et al.* 1993).

For reliability studies of categorical variables, Chapter 4 gives interpretations of κ and weighted κ that can be used to approximate the true odds ratio from the observed odds ratio. If the parallel test model holds, $\sqrt{\kappa}$ for dichotomous variables (Tavaré *et al.* 1995) or $\sqrt{\kappa_W}$ for ordered catgorical variables can be substituted for ρ_{TX} in the equation in Table 5.1 derived from Equation 3.6 to yield a crude estimate of the true odds ratio:

$$OR_T = OR_O^{1/\sqrt{\kappa}} .$$

Limitations of these methods and more advanced statistical methods

While adjustment procedures may aid in understanding the results of a study, caution should be exercised in interpreting the results. First, the assumptions used in the derivation of the equations in Table 5.1 may not be appropriate. In particular, an assumption of non-differential measurement error could be incorrect, and so it is preferable if the exposure measurement error can be assessed separately for the diseased and non-diseased groups to account for differential misclassification. For continuous exposures, the assumptions of the simple measurement error model, normality of exposure and error, and the logistic model of the disease–exposure relationship often also fail to hold.

Secondly, both the observed measure of association between the disease and exposure (e.g. the odds ratio) and the estimated measurement error (e.g. ρ_{TX}) would have sampling errors; this needs to be considered in the estimation of the true association. Thirdly, the estimates of the measurement error should be from a validity or reliability study from the same population as the study to be corrected, but such estimates may not be available. Finally, as noted in Chapter 3, the presence of covariates modifies the effect of exposure measurement error. Information on the multivariate measurement error structure of the primary exposure and covariates is required in order to correct fully for measurement error. Therefore, unless these issues have been accounted for, the emphasis of the adjustment procedure should be on interpretation of the observed estimate of association, not on the corrected estimate.

A great deal of statistical work has been done on adjustment procedures for correction of the odds ratio or risk ratio for the effects of measurement error. These procedures incorporate information from a validity or reliability study of the exposure in the statistical analysis of the disease–exposure relationship. Many of these approaches take into consideration some of the issues discussed above; in particular, some make less restrictive assumptions about the error model, yield confidence intervals that incorporate sampling error from the validity/reliability study, and/or allow a multivariate (exposure and covariate) measurement error structure. Most adjustment procedures need information from a validity study of the exposure, which requires a near-perfect comparison measure, while some incorporate information from a reliability study which has a comparison measure with uncorrelated errors. Reviews of the large number of approaches for continuous and/or categorical exposures are given by Chen (1989), Thomas et al. (1993), Holford and Stack (1995), Bashir and Duffy (1997), Thürigen et al. (2000), and Carroll et al. (2006). One method, the regression calibration method, is straightforward to implement and can be applied when the researcher has conducted a validity substudy or an intra- or intermethod reliability study with uncorrelated errors between the measures (plus certain other assumptions) (Rosner et al. 1989, 1990; Spiegelman et al. 1997a,b). In addition, some of these statistical methods and others (Liu and Liang 1992; Kim and Zeleniuch-Jacquotte 1997) would be appropriate for the analysis of epidemiological studies which use multiple (parallel) measures of exposure on each subject in the parent study (see next section) rather than only on a subset of subjects.

In designing an epidemiological study which will use adjustment techniques to correct for measurement error, the researcher needs to consider how to allocate study resources between the costs of the parent epidemiological study versus the substudy. Methods to determine the number of subjects to be allocated to the parent study versus the validity/reliability substudy to minimize total costs have been developed, and can provide guidance in specific design situations (Greenland 1988; Buonaccorsi 1990; Spiegelman and Gray 1991; Duffy *et al*. 1992; Holford and Stack 1995; Rippin 2001). However, under some circumstances it might be most efficient to use the more accurate measure of exposure on all subjects in the parent epidemiological study rather than only in the substudy (because this would lead to a smaller required sample size and possibly lower total costs) or to include multiple (imperfect) measures of exposure on all subjects in the parent study. These topics are discussed below.

Use of scores or averages based on multiple measures of exposure

The use of the average or sum of two or more measures of the exposure for each subject in an epidemiological study can be an effective method of decreasing measurement error that is due to variations over time, laboratory error, and other sources, in comparison with the use of a single measurement. The concepts presented in this section apply to a wide range of measures, including the following:

- ◆ average of repeated administrations of the same instrument (e.g. serum cholesterol could be measured by use of an average of measurements from two samples collected over two years)

- ◆ average of measures from two different instruments for the same exposure (e.g. dietary fat could be assessed as an average of a food frequency measurement and a measurement from a seven-day diet diary)

- ◆ average or sum of information from multiple days of a diary (e.g. a physical activity diary covering seven days)

- ◆ average or sum of information from multiple days or weeks of environmental exposure sampling

- ◆ use of scores, scales, or indices which are the sum of multiple questionnaire items, such as a physical function scale.

The term *multiple measures* refers to repeated measurement of *all* subjects in an epidemiological study to *reduce* measurement error; this differs from a reliability study in which a *sample* of subjects would be repeatedly measured to *assess* measurement error. However, these two approaches are related, and many of the concepts introduced in the previous chapter are important in understanding the benefits of multiple measures.

The methods in this section can apply to multiple measures of the same exposure collected over a short time period or over a long time period in prospective studies when one assumes that the average measure over time is the best predictor of disease. (Other models for multiple measures of exposure over time, such as those that use the most recent measure to predict outcome or use the change in measure over time to predict outcome are different concepts and are not covered.)

The concepts and equations presented in this section apply to both the average of multiple measures and the sum. Although we focus on the average, the sum has the same validity and reliability as an average because it only differs from the average by a constant multiple $1/k$.

The material below covers ways to estimate the benefits of multiple measures of exposure, including the advantage in terms of increased accuracy of the measure, and hence less attenuation of the odds ratio and smaller required sample size (under non-differential measurement error). Methods to determine the number of measures per subject that are needed to increase exposure precision or to minimize study costs are also presented.

The use of multiple measures to increase validity under parallel tests

The improvement in the validity of a continuous exposure variable resulting from the combination of multiple measures is easily demonstrated when the errors in the two or more measures to be averaged are equal and uncorrelated (the parallel test model) (Carmines and Zeller 1979; Bohrnstedt 1983; Fleiss 1986; Dunn 1989).

Suppose that each individual in a population is measured k times, by use of parallel measures of the underlying true exposure T, yielding observations of variables $X_1, ..., X_k$. Recall from Chapter 4 that, under the model of parallel tests, the errors of the measures $(E_1, ..., E_k)$ are uncorrelated with each other and with T and the variances σ_E^2 of the errors are equal. This implies that the correlation ρ_{TX} of each X_j with T is identical. The average measure A_i for individual i is computed as follows:

$$A_i = \frac{X_{i1} + ... + X_{ik}}{k}$$

where X_{ij} represents the observation on subject i of variable X_j. Then the variable A has a validity coefficient

$$\rho_{TA} = \sqrt{\sigma_T^2 / (\sigma_T^2 + \sigma_E^2 / k)}. \qquad [5.1]$$

It can be seen from Equation 5.1 that, as k increases, the term σ_E^2/k goes to zero. This shows that the validity coefficient of A is greater than that of the individual measures, $X_1, ..., X_k$ (i.e. equation 5.1 is greater for $k = 2$ or more than $k = 1$), and that the validity coefficient of A approaches 1 as k increases.

Equation 5.1 can be rewritten as a function of the validity coefficient ρ_{TX} of the parallel measures:

$$\rho_{TA} = \sqrt{\frac{k\rho_{TX}^2}{1+(k-1)\rho_{TX}^2}} .$$ [5.2]

However, ρ_{TX} is not usually known; rather, it is estimated from a reliability study as $\sqrt{\rho_{X_1X_2}}$, where $\rho_{X_1X_2}$ represents the common correlation between any two of the k measures. $\rho_{X_1X_2}$ can be estimated from the average Pearson correlation coefficient of the pairs of measures (Carmines and Zeller 1979; Bohrnstedt 1983). When $\rho_{X_1X_2}$ is substituted for ρ_{TX}^2 in Equation 5.2, it yields the formula for the validity coefficient of the average A as a function of $\rho_{X_1X_2}$:

$$\rho_{TA} = \sqrt{\frac{k\rho_{X_1X_2}}{1+(k-1)\rho_{X_1X_2}}} .$$ [5.3]

This would then be compared with the validity coefficient of one measure alone, $\sqrt{\rho_{X_1X_2}}$.

Table 5.2 gives examples of the improvement in validity that can be achieved by using multiple parallel measures of T. For example, if the reliability coefficient

Table 5.2 Improvement in the validity of a measure by averaging k parallel measures[a] and the effect on the odds ratio[b]

Number of measures k	$\rho_{X_1X_2} = 0.25$		$\rho_{X_1X_2} = 0.4$		$\rho_{X_1X_2} = 0.5$	
	ρ_{TA}	OR_O	ρ_{TA}	OR_O	ρ_{TA}	OR_O
1	0.50	1.41	0.63	1.73	0.71	2.01
2	0.63	1.73	0.76	2.23	0.82	2.54
3	0.71	2.01	0.82	2.54	0.87	2.86
4	0.76	2.23	0.85	2.72	0.89	3.00
5	0.79	2.38	0.88	2.93	0.91	3.15
7	0.83	2.60	0.91	3.15	0.94	3.40
10	0.88	2.93	0.93	3.32	0.95	3.49

[a] $\rho_{X_1X_2}$ is the reliability coefficient between the parallel measures and ρ_{TA} is the validity coefficient of the average A of the parallel measures.

[b] OR_O is the observed (attenuated) odds ratio under non-differential measurement error, based on Equation 3.5, when the true odds ratio is 4.

between parallel measures were 0.25, this would mean that a single measure would have a validity coefficient of 0.50, but averaging five such measures would yield a new exposure measure with a validity coefficient of 0.79.

The reliability ρ_A of A as a function of the reliability of X is the square of the validity coefficient of A:

$$\rho_A = \frac{k\rho_{X_1X_2}}{1+(k-1)\rho_{X_1X_2}} \ . \tag{5.4}$$

The validity coefficient of A (Equation 5.3) can be interpreted as the correlation between the k-item measure (sum or average) and the true measure, and the reliability coefficient of A (Equation 5.4) can be interpreted as the estimated correlation between two k-item measures on the same person. When k is the actual number of items administered to the subjects (e.g. when A is a scale made up of 10 items and one wants to estimate the reliability of the 10-item score), ρ_A is referred to as *Cronbach's α*. It is discussed in more detail below in the sections on use of a score, scale, or index and on use of the sum or average when the individual items are categorical variables. When k is not the actual number of items measured on the subjects, but instead equation 5.4 is being used to predict the reliability of the sum or average of k measures, this equation is called the *Spearman–Brown prophesy formula*.

The advantage of using multiple parallel exposure measures for each subject in an epidemiological study, assuming non-differential misclassification, is that it would result in less attenuation of the observed odds ratio (or other measure of association) due to measurement error. Examples of this are given in Table 5.2. Less attenuation of the odds ratio also yields the benefit of a smaller required sample size for a given power. Specifically, in a case–control study with equal numbers of cases and controls, the sample size n_k required with k measures per subject relative to the sample size n_1 needed when only one measure per subject is used is given by (Fleiss 1986)

$$n_k = \frac{1+(k-1)\rho_{X_1X_2}}{k} n_1 \ . \tag{5.5}$$

Example. Suppose that a case–control study is to be conducted on the relationship between serum cholesterol and colon cancer in a large health maintenance organization where records of pre-diagnostic serum cholesterol levels are available. A test–retest reliability study of serum cholesterol levels over the time period of interest yields an estimate of the reliability coefficient $\hat{\rho}_{X_1X_2} = 0.60$. Under the assumptions of parallel measures, the validity coefficient can be estimated as

$\hat{\rho}_{XT} = \sqrt{0.60} = 0.77$ (from Equation 4.4). If three measures of serum cholesterol over the relevant time period were averaged per subject, the validity of the average would be (from Equation 5.3)

$$\hat{\rho}_{TA} = \sqrt{\frac{3 \times 0.60}{1 + 2 \times 0.60}} = 0.90.$$

To interpret the effect of the use of three replicate measures on the bias in the odds ratio of the study of interest, Equation 3.6 might be used. With three measures per subject, if the true odds ratio were 2, the observable odds ratio would be $2^{0.90} = 1.9$, rather than $2^{0.77} = 1.7$ if only one measure per subject were used. Moreover, the number of subjects needed would be (from Equation 5.5)

$$\hat{n}_3 = \frac{1 + (3 - 1) \times 0.6}{3} n_1 = 0.73 n_1$$

i.e. 27 per cent fewer subjects than would be required if one measure per subject were used.

Determining the number of measures under parallel tests

One method of determining k, the number of parallel measures per subject, is to select k so as to yield a desired level of the validity coefficient ρ_{TA} of A. The number of measures can be calculated from Equation 5.3 as follows:

$$k = \frac{\rho_{TA}^2 \left(1 - \rho_{X_1 X_2}\right)}{\rho_{X_1 X_2} \left(1 - \rho_{TA}^2\right)}.$$ [5.6]

Example. Continuing with the last example, suppose that a measure of serum cholesterol with validity coefficient of 0.85 was required. Then it would be necessary to average k independent measures per subject, where

$$\hat{k} = \frac{0.85^2 \left(1 - 0.60\right)}{0.60 \left(1 - 0.85^2\right)} = 1.7$$

or two measures per subject.

Of course, there are disadvantages to the use of multiple measures. One is the increased burden on respondents which may lead to a fall in the participation rate, particularly if more study visits are required. Another is the increase in cost per subject which, depending on the trade-off between this increase and the reduced sample size required, could increase the total cost of the study. The choice of the number of measures requires balancing the expected reduction in bias in the odds ratio against total study cost and respondent burden.

One approach is to select the number of measures per subject to minimize total study costs (Fleiss 1986). Costs are minimized by selecting k measures per subject, where

$$k = \sqrt{\frac{1 - \rho_{X_I X_2}}{c \rho_{X_I X_2}}}$$ [5.7]

and c is the ratio of the cost of one exposure measurement to all other data collection costs per subject (recruitment costs, costs of other data collection). (Fixed costs such as scientific oversight and data analysis costs that are constant independent of the number of subjects do not enter the equation because they are the same for all choices of k.) If k is not an integer, the total study cost t for the two integers around k can be estimated, and the lowest cost selected, using

$$t \quad \left(\frac{1 + (k - 1)\rho_{X_I X_2}}{k}\right)(1 + ck)$$

which states that total costs t are proportional to the number of subjects multiplied by the cost per subject. A single measure is optimal when $c > \left(1 - \rho_{X_I X_2}\right)/\rho_{X_I X_2}$.

Example. Suppose that in the preceding example the number of replicate measures were to be selected so as to minimize total study costs. If each cholesterol measure costs \$20 and all other data collection costs were \$80 per subject ($c = 0.25$), then

$$\hat{k} = \sqrt{\frac{1 - 0.6}{0.25 \times (0.6)}} = 1.6$$

which means that the optimal number of replicates is between 1 and 2. For two measures per subject:

$$\hat{t} \sim \left(\frac{1 + (2 - 1) \times 0.6}{2}\right)(1 + 0.25 \times 2) = 1.2 .$$

For one measure per subject:

$$t \sim (1)(1 + 0.25) = 1.25.$$

Therefore two measures would minimize study costs.

The use of multiple measures when there are unequal variances or correlated errors

The possibility of violation of the assumptions of the parallel test model must be considered when assessing the use of multiple measures. It may be that the two or more measures to be averaged do not have equal error variance. In this situation, averaging a precise measure with a less precise measure may result in a variable A which is less valid than the good measure alone. An obvious example would be the use of the average of a perfect measure of exposure and an imperfect measure.

When the two or more measures to be averaged have positively correlated errors, but the other assumptions of parallel tests hold, the improvement in the validity of the exposure measure will be less than that predicted by Equations 5.1–5.3. Only the uncorrelated part of the error will be reduced by averaging, not the within-person bias (Liu 1988). If the errors are perfectly correlated (i.e. the measure is perfectly repeatable even though it is not a perfect measure of exposure), the use of multiple measures will lead to no improvement in validity. When there are correlated errors, the reliability coefficient of A can be calculated as in Equation 5.4, but then the square root of the reliability coefficient will only yield an upper limit of the validity of A (i.e. $\rho_{TA} < \sqrt{\rho_A}$).

The use of a score, scale, or index

Often the sum of different questionnaire items is used to create a *score*, which is often called a *scale* or *index*. Examples include a scale for depressive symptoms or an index of degree of chronic pain, each based on multiple questions. Details about development of health measurement scales are given in Streiner and Norman (2003).

If each of the individual items to be summed is a measure of the same underlying true exposure T, the concepts and equations relating to multiple measures presented above apply. (As noted above, the sum has the same validity and reliability as an average, because the sum only differs from the average by a constant multiple $1/k$.) For example, a scale on pain could sum five questions, with each designed to elicit information on degree of pain. These five items would measure the same underlying true exposure and therefore would be positively correlated.

Cronbach's α is often used as the measure of the reliability of a scale (see Equation 5.4 and the associated assumptions above). This is termed *internal consistency reliability* because the reliability of the total score is assessed by the correlation between the items rather than by the correlation of two administrations of the instrument. Cronbach's α for a total score S, i.e. the sum of k items X_j, is usually computed from the formula

$$\alpha = \frac{k}{k-1}\left(1 - \frac{\sum_{j=1}^{k}\sigma^2_{X_j}}{\sigma^2_S}\right) \qquad [5.8]$$

where α is the internal consistency reliability of S, σ^2_S is the variance of the total score S, and the $\sigma^2_{X_j}$ are the variances of the X_j items.

However, for many scores or indices used in epidemiology, each item used in the score is a measure of only one component of the true exposure rather than a measure of the true (total) exposure. For example, a recreational physical activity score might sum for each subject the times per week of walking, running, use of exercise machines, etc. The sum would be a more accurate measure of recreational activity than any item alone. However, each item is a measure of a component of physical activity, not the entire physical activity construct. Therefore one would not expect the items to be positively correlated; for example, times per week of running and times per week of walking might even be negatively correlated, because those who run the most often might rarely walk for exercise. (The negative correlation would be due to negatively correlated errors between the items, as measures of the total true exposure.) In these situations, the reliability and validity of a sum or average of multiple items cannot be estimated from the correlation between items, and so none of the equations presented in this section hold.

Use of the sum or average when the individual items are categorical variables

The concept of internal consistency reliability and the use of Cronbach's α can also be applied to a total score S, that is the sum of k binary or ordinal items. Equation 5.8 can be used when the X_j to be summed are binary or ordinal, as well as continuous.

When the *true* exposure measure is a binary variable, i.e. each person is truly exposed or is not exposed, the use of the sum of multiple imperfect methods has a different meaning from a score. An example would be exposure to human papillomavirus, which might be assessed by k different laboratory tests, each of which has measurement error. The sum of these binary variables creates an exposure variable equal to the number of measures on which a subject was positive. If there are only two measures per subject, the summation would lead to an exposure variable with three categories: classified as exposed on both, exposed on one, or exposed on neither. The resulting exposure variable could be treated as an ordered categorical variable; however, it would not be a scale (since the subject was either exposed or not exposed) but rather an indicator of the measurement error in the exposure. There are statistical methods for replicate binary or categorical variables which incorporate information on the multiple measures of the underlying (latent) categorical exposure to yield an estimate of the true odds ratio (see discussion in previous section on adjustment procedures).

Further use of multiple measures to reduce measurement errors

There is another approach to the use of multiple measures to improve the validity of the exposure measure. In this approach, when the two or more measures are inconsistent beyond some tolerance level, further information is obtained to resolve the difference.

For example, in a study of the concentration of selenium in toenails, which may be technically difficult to measure, the specimen was divided into several samples (Hunter *et al.* 1990). If analysis of the first two did not yield consistent results, another analysis was performed and then three measures, rather than two, were averaged. The tolerance could be set by requiring $|X_{i1} - X_{i2}|$ or the standard deviation for each subject (or the coefficient of variation for each subject) to be within some limit. When this approach is possible, it could improve the validity of a measure more than could be done by simple averaging.

Other methods to reduce measurement error

Take measurement error into account in calculating the sample size

Non-differential measurement error attenuates the risk ratio and therefore reduces the power of a study. One method of taking this loss of power into consideration was discussed in Chapter 3. When designing an epidemiological study, the sample size calculations should be based on estimates of the observable parameters (the standard deviation of the exposure, the observable odds ratio, etc.) as they will be affected by measurement error and not based on estimates from more accurate measures which may be available from pilot work. This approach does not lead to a more accurate risk ratio; rather, it provides more power to detect the attenuated risk ratio as different from the null value of 1. However, if the attenuated association is quite weak, increasing the sample size so that a weak association can be detected may lead to results that are difficult to interpret. Weak associations are often spuriously produced in epidemiological studies through selection bias or inadequate control of confounding factors.

Use a more accurate exposure measure on fewer subjects

The most important approach to reducing the effects of exposure measurement error is, of course, to choose a more accurate method to measure the exposure. If one can select a more accurate measure, the observed risk ratio will be closer to the true risk ratio and therefore the required sample size will be smaller (under non-differential measurement error). However, more accurate measures generally cost more, and so there is a trade-off between the costs of better exposure measurement on fewer subjects versus recruiting more subjects and using the less expensive method. If one has the opportunity to choose between two methods which measure the same exposure, with X_1 denoting the less accurate measure and X_2 denoting the more accurate measure, one can evaluate which will result in the lower total study costs. The total data collection costs t_1 for a study which uses X_1 would be the data collection cost per subject c_1 (for recruitment and all data collection) multiplied by the number of subjects needed if the less accurate instrument were selected. The number of subjects needed is $n_T / \rho_{TX_1}^2$ (see Equation 3.7), where ρ_{TX_1} is the validity coefficient for measure X_1 and n_T is the number of subjects needed without measurement error. (Fixed costs that are independent of sample size do not enter the equation because they are the same for both choices of exposure method.) Similarly, for the same power to detect the same mean difference between the diseased and non-diseased groups, the study which uses X_2 would have total data collection costs t_2, which is the data collection cost c_2 per subject multiplied by the number of subjects needed when X_2 is used. Thus the ratio of t_2 to t_1 is

$$\frac{t_2}{t_1} = \frac{c_2 / \rho_{TX_2}^2}{c_1 / \rho_{TX_1}^2}. \qquad [5.9]$$

By examining this ratio, it can be seen that an investment in the increased precision of X_2 is cost efective if

$$\frac{\rho_{TX_2}^2}{\rho_{TX_1}^2} > \frac{c_2}{c_1},$$

i.e. if the ratio of the square of the validity coefficient of X_2 to the validity coefficient of X_1 is more than the ratio of the data collection costs per subject for use of X_2 versus X_1 (Armstrong 1995).

Example. Suppose that using a more accurate exposure measure (X_2) would increase the data collection costs per subject from $100 to $125, i.e. the ratio of participant costs for use of X_2 versus X_1 is 1.25. If the estimated validity coefficient of X_1 is 0.5 and the estimated validity coefficient of X_2 is 0.6, then the ratio of these validity coefficients squared is 1.44. Then, by Equation 5.9, $t_2/t_1 = 0.87$. One could then justify spending the $25 more per subject to use X_2 because it would lead to a total data collection cost savings of 13 per cent through reduced required sample size for the same study power.

This example shows that using more expensive and more accurate exposure measurement methods can easily lead to cost savings.

Select a study population with greater true exposure variance

In designing epidemiological studies, it is well known that studying a population with a small variability of exposure leads to an increase in the required sample size, even in the absence of measurement error. McKeown-Eyssen and Thomas (1985) have shown that by selecting a population with larger exposure variance (population 2) versus one with smaller variance (population 1), the study sample size can be reduced by a factor equal to the ratio of the smaller to the larger variance:

$$\frac{n_2}{n_1} = \frac{\sigma_{T_1}^2}{\sigma_{T_2}^2}, \qquad [5.10]$$

where n_1 is the sample size needed in population 1 and n_2 is the sample size needed in population 2. (Note that this result is not obvious from the common sample size equation because the mean difference in exposure between diseased and non-diseased groups is greater in the population with greater exposure variance for a fixed risk ratio (McKeown-Eyssen and Thomas 1985)).

This sample size benefit may be even greater when the exposure is measured with error. When there is measurement error, the sample size requirements are greatly increased (as shown in Equation 3.7). White *et al.* (1994) have shown that the proportional reduction in sample size from selecting a population with larger true exposure variance may be even greater when there is measurement error than when there is not. If the same instrument is used in both populations (and if the variance of the exposure measurement error is the same in both populations), the validity coefficient $\rho_{T_2 X_2}$ of the exposure measure in population 2 is greater than the validity coefficient $\rho_{T_1 X_1}$ in population 1. This follows because the validity coefficient of a measure is a function of the true exposure variance in a population (Equation 4.11). This provides the additional sample size benefit. Then the sample size n_2 needed for a study in the population with a greater true exposure variance ($\sigma^2_{T_2}$) relative to the sample size n_1 needed for the population with the smaller true exposure variance ($\sigma^2_{T_1}$) when there is measurement error is (White *et al.* 1994)

$$\frac{n_2}{n_1} = \left(\frac{\sigma^2_{T_1}}{\sigma^2_{T_2}} \right) \left(\frac{\rho^2_{T_1 X_1}}{\rho^2_{T_2 X_2}} \right) . \qquad [5.11]$$

Example. Suppose that one is designing a case–control study of beta-carotene intake and cataract surgery. The study could be conducted in one of two populations: a white population with the standard deviation of (true) beta-carotene of 1000 or an Asian population with the standard deviation of (true) exposure of 1300. If the exposure were perfectly measured in the study, n_2/n_1 would be $1000^2/1300^2 = 0.59$ (from Equation 5.10), i.e. a 41 per cent reduction in sample size if the Asian rather than the white population is studied. More likely, the exposure would be measured with error, for example with a validity coefficient of 0.6 in the white population. Then selecting the Asian population would lead to an expected validity coefficient of 0.70 in that population (see White *et al.* (1994) for the derivation). Then the saving in sample size would be (from Equation 5.11)

$$\frac{n_2}{n_1} = \left(\frac{1000^2}{1300^2} \right) \left(\frac{0.6^2}{0.7^2} \right) = 0.43 ,$$

i.e. 57 per cent less than if the the the study was conducted using the mismeasured exposure in whites. In terms of actual numbers, suppose that the sample size was 1000 for each of the case and control groups for the study in whites with use of a perfect exposure measure. Then studying the Asian population instead would reduce the sample size to 590 per group. Using an imperfect measure of beta-carotene with a validity coefficient of 0.6 in the white population would yield a required sample size of 2780 for each group (by Equation 3.7). However, using the same instrument (with the same error variance) in the Asian population would only require 1210 subjects per group (by Equation 5.11).

The assumption made above that the error variance σ_E^2 is the same in the two populations implies that the error is predominantly a function of the measuring instrument as applied to an individual, and does not depend on the range of exposures in a population. While this is a reasonable assumption, it may not hold in practice. However, in using Equation 5.11, one should have actual estimates of the validity coefficient of the instrument in each population, in which case this assumption is no longer needed.

Control for factors associated with measurement error

Another method for reducing the effects of measurement error was briefly mentioned in Chapter 4. In the analysis of an epidemiological study, statistical adjustment for a covariate that is related to the exposure measurement error may reduce the effect of the error on the measure of association between the exposure and disease. Examples include adjustment for interviewer effects if different interviewers (randomly assigned to subjects) yielded different mean exposure levels, or adjustment for the season in which a food frequency questionnaire was completed if season influenced the subjects' perception of, for example, their diet over the last year. While this is an established technique for studies of continuous outcomes (Fleiss 1986), its usefulness has not been fully evaluated for studies in which the outcome is a dichotomous variable, as is common in epidemiology (Greenland and Robins 1985). However, such control would reduce differential error due to say unequal assignment of interviewers to cases and controls.

Control of a factor related to measurement error can also be accomplished by matching cases and controls on the factor. For example, for laboratory measures of exposure, it is common to match cases and controls within a batch. This avoids case-control differences due to variation in the chemicals or instrument calibration between batches.

Quality control procedures

Quality control procedures implemented at each stage of an epidemiological study can play an important role in reducing measurement error. Many of the approaches to quality control in data collection come from randomized clinical trials, vital statistics and disease registries, and large government surveys of economic, social, and health factors (Hilsenbeck *et al.* 1985; Meinert 1986; Groves 1989; Lyberg *et al.* 1997; McFadden 1998). Some of these can be applied to data collection in epidemiology, as can some of the new approaches to quality improvement from the business world (Biemer and Caspar 1994).

Table 5.3 General quality control procedures for the collection of data in epidemiological studies

Design of the instrument

Design of forms

Include all items needed to compute dose, timing of exposure, etc.

Include adequate subject identifiers—at least an identification number and a check digit or alphabetic code on all forms

Use separate forms for each method of exposure measurement

Make instructions clear and data collection items unambiguous

Use different typefaces for instructions, data collection items, and responses

Provide mutually exclusive and exhaustive response categories for closed-ended items

Make forms self-coding for simple items (e.g. data collector circles a number corresponding to the appropriate response category)

Make response codes consistent within and across forms (e.g. 1 = no, 2 = yes)

Provide for coding without loss of information, i.e. do not design forms so that continuous data are categorized at the coding stage.

Do not require computation by data collectors; rather, enter the data items needed for later computer calculations

Design forms for ease of data capture into an electronic record

Study procedures manual

Always have a study procedures manual

Include at least the following in the study procedures manual:

- ◆ description of the study in general terms
- ◆ sample selection, recruitment, and tracking procedures
- ◆ informed consent and confidentiality procedures
- ◆ data forms
- ◆ general methods of data collection
- ◆ item by item clarification of questions and responses, including special cases
- ◆ editing procedures
- ◆ coding instructions for items not self-coded on form
- ◆ codebooks for raw and computed variables

Update manual and distribute updated pages whenever procedural changes are made

Preparing for data collection

Pre-testing instruments

Have instruments reviewed by other researchers

Pre-test instruments on samples of convenience

Pre-test instruments on samples similar to study subjects

Identify problems through feedback from pre-test subjects and data collectors and by monitoring data collection (e.g. observing interviews, re-abstracting records) and make appropriate changes as early as possible

Review frequencies of responses to identify items with little variation in responses or large percentages of 'don't know' or missing

Modify instrument

Training data collectors

Discuss importance of complete and accurate data

Review study manual

Table 5.3 (continued) General quality control procedures for the collection of data in epidemiological studies

Practice data collection
Monitor initial data collection by each data collector
Resolve problems

Quality control during data collection

Supervision of data collectors

Assign cases and controls in a case–control study (or exposed and unexposed subjects, where this is known in advance, in a cohort study) in the same proportions to each data collector

Maintain ignorance of data collectors to exposure and disease status of subjects as far as possible

Replicate some proportion of data collection (e.g. 10% of subjects) to identify fictitious data, items with poor reliability, data collectors with errors on certain items, etc.

Compare the distributions of study variables among data collectors

Compare distributions of study variables over time

Conduct staff meetings for maintaining motivation and for discussion of problems and their solutions

Editing and coding

Check for inadmissible codes, missing data, and inconsistencies among responses through computer-assisted interviewing or by data collector immediately after interview

Correct errors by querying subjects (or checkbacks to records)

Have data collectors or editor code open-ended questions and query those inadequately answered for coding

Have one staff member maintain an editors' log to ensure consistency of recording and coding of unanticipated responses, and to record comments and responses coded as 'other'

Quality control during data processing

Data capture and editing by computer

Enter data contemporaneously with data collection

Perform quality control procedures appropriate to the data capture method[a]

Edit data by computer by performing range and logic checks contemporaneously with data entry

Correct errors by querying subjects (or check-backs to records)

Data documentation and creation of new variables

Create a codebook with detailed descriptions of raw (original) variables, corrected raw variables, and derived (computed) variables created from two or more original variables, including the programming code used to create them

Check and recheck the programming code used to create new variables

Check the correctness of new variables by manual computation from the raw data for a few subjects

Review distributions of original and derived variables

[a] See text for methods

Because many quality control procedures are common to a number of methods of exposure measurement, it is useful to summarize them here (Table 5.3). These procedures relate particularly to collection of data via interviews and abstraction of records, and their subsequent processing to the point of carrying out an analysis by use of original or derived variables. Many of these quality control methods also apply to exposure assessment from questionnaires and diaries completed by the subject and from collecting and processing biological or environmental samples for laboratory-based measurements. Quality control for each method is dealt with more extensively in Chapters 6–10.

Design of the data collection instrument

Design of forms

In addition to questionnaires, data collection forms can include forms for abstraction of data from medical records, diaries to be kept by subjects, etc. In designing or reviewing the data collection forms to be used in a study, the first concern should be whether they include complete coverage of the items necessary to compute the analytical exposure variables of interest (dose, time of commencement of exposure, duration of exposure, etc.) and the necessary covariates.

Generally, there should be one form per subject per method of exposure measurement. Colour coding of forms may help in studies with multiple forms per subject. Each form should have the subject's identity coded in a way that a simple typographical error (e.g. in the identification number (ID)) does not lead to misidentification of the subject. A *check digit* on the subject ID, i.e. an arithmetic combination of the other numbers in the ID (Anderson *et al.* 1974), allows identification of incorrect ID numbers (e.g. errors due to transposing two numbers). The check digit is computed as part of the ID before ID numbers are assigned, and is then checked each time the ID is entered as part of computer editing of the data. An incorrect check digit implies an incorrect ID number. Alternatively, or in addition, an alphabetic code based on the subject's name, such as the first three letters of the last name, could be part of the subject ID. Check digits or an alphabetic code are particularly useful when merging data from several forms.

Data forms should be designed for both accuracy and ease of use during data collection, coding and editing, and data capture into electronic form. Coding, i.e. assigning numbers to responses that are words, is handled in one of two ways. For items with a small number of possible responses (e.g. marital status), the form should be pre-coded (e.g. 1 = married, ..., 5 = never married). Codes used in the form (and preferably across all forms used in a data collection unit) should be consistent. For example, no = 1, yes = 2 should be the same on all forms. Circling the code number simplifies data entry and is an unambiguous way of signifying the correct response. If a new code needs to be added as a response to a question once data collection has begun, it should be given a different code from those already in use. A new response code should not be added in the middle and old codes renumbered, even if the new code logically falls between two other codes. For items with a large number of possible responses (e.g. occupations), the responses should be recorded as words with space provided for coding at a later time.

The data collector or the subject should not perform calculations unless they are necessary for the data collection. Instead, information should be sought as simple 'raw' data items and calculations performed during data processing. Units of measurement should be specified on the form. Generally, numerical data should be recorded without losing information, i.e. continuous data should not be categorized at the time of data collection.

Other aspects of form design are listed in Table 5.3. A more detailed treatment of the formatting of questionnaires is given in Chapter 6, and additional information about record abstraction forms and diaries is given in Chapter 8.

Study procedures manual

A data collection instrument should include detailed instructions on its use. For forms being completed by study staff rather than study subjects, these instructions should form part of a study procedures manual and should include an explanation of every item and the interpretation of each response to the item. The editing and coding procedures should also be included in the manual. This manual serves initially as a training manual, then as a reference for data collectors, and finally as a detailed record of the data collection procedures. Table 5.3 lists the contents of a typical study procedures manual. An interviewer's manual, a particular kind of study procedures manual, is outlined in Chapter 7, Table 7.6. One staff member, usually the project director, should be responsible for any changes to the manual and for the distribution of those changes to other staff members.

Preparing for data collection

Pre-testing instruments

Before data collection can begin, the instrument must be pre-tested and the data collectors trained in the study procedures. Steps in pre-testing are listed in Table 5.3. More detailed accounts of pre-testing in relation to questionnaires and of pre-testing medical record abstraction are given in Chapter 6 and Chapter 8, respectively. In addition, as noted in Chapter 4, validity and reliability studies can be used during the pre-test phase to investigate sources of error.

Training of data collectors

The study procedures manual can serve as the major training tool. Training begins with an overview of the study and the importance of accurate data to the success of the study. Standardized execution of the protocol should be emphasized. To reduce differential bias introduced by the data collectors, the hypothesis should be presented in only general terms (e.g. 'We are looking at a range of lifestyle factors that may be associated with colon cancer'). After review of the procedures manual, the trainees practise the data collection tasks that they will perform and have their work both observed and reviewed by the instructor. For large-scale studies, there is often a formal examination, leading to *certification* of the data collectors in the data collection procedures. This promotes uniform training, which is particularly necessary for multi-site studies. The initial data collection from study subjects by each new data collector should also be monitored closely and any problems resolved.

The principal investigator of the study should be actively involved in this phase of the study and in the early data collection by observing pilot data collection and by discussing problems with data collectors. This often provides additional insights leading to improvements in the data collection instruments.

Quality control during data collection

Supervision of data collectors

Methods of quality control during data collection include assignment of equal proportions of cases and controls to each data collector in a case–control study (or of exposed and unexposed subjects in a cohort study, if exposure status is known) and keeping the data collectors in ignorance of the case–control status (or exposure status) of subjects if possible. These approaches reduce differential measurement error.

Quality control during data collection should also include:

♦ replication of some proportion of each data collector's work by another or a senior data collector

♦ comparison of the distribution of variables among data collectors

♦ an analysis of trends in the variables over time.

Replication of data collection (e.g. re-interview by telephone of a 10 per cent sample, covering a few key questions) detects, at least, the worst type of error—complete fabrication of the data by the data collector! The data collector should be told that data collection will be replicated on some subjects, records, or specimens, but should not be told which ones. Analyses of trends over time might uncover interviewer fatigue or drift in laboratory methods. For large studies, these analyses of key variables can yield periodic formal quality control reports.

Staff meetings can be useful for discussion of problems, continued training, and for maintaining the interest of the staff in the quality of the data. A new philosophy about staff meetings and staff organization comes from the total quality management or continuous quality improvement approaches. Although these approaches come from the manufacturing world, they have some application to quality control in data collection (Biemer and Caspar 1994). Some of the basic principles are as follows.

- It is better to do a process correctly the first time rather than inspect for quality.
- Having separate 'inspectors' takes the responsibility away from those conducting the work.
- Errors are often due to the system itself rather than to individual workers not doing their job.

Applying these approaches to data collection suggests that it is important to provide the data collectors with the motivation and responsibility to improve data quality. Staff should be encouraged to identify problems relating to specific questions or items, procedures, or post-data collection processing, and the staff should be involved in the solutions. Biemer and Caspar (1994) applied this approach to a large-scale project involving the coding of occupations by using teams of coders to identify reasons for inaccurate coding and to implement solutions. This reduced the error rate from 21 per cent to 5 per cent, while decreasing costs.

Editing and coding

Traditionally there were several steps of editing questionnaires after data collection. First, the data collectors would immediately review their work for missing or unclear data and check back with the subject (or medical record) to complete missing items or clarify uncertain items. Shortly after completion of the data collector's work on a subject or the return of self-administered questionnaires, the forms would be reviewed by an editor (the project director, a person designated as the editor, or another data collector) to check for missing items, illegible responses, inadmissible codes (range checks), and logical inconsistencies among responses (e.g. in an abstract of a hospital birth record, it would be inconsistent for the type of birth to be reported as 'vaginal birth' but anaesthesia to be coded as 'general'). The editor would also check for inadequate answers to questions requiring detailed coding (e.g. 'business owner' for occupation) and code these items. Finally, range and logic checks would also be performed by computer. For items that could not be resolved with the data collector, the subject would be telephoned or the medical record pulled to correct the data.

Currently, most data collection, except that by self-administered questionnaire, is computer assisted. This includes computer-assisted interviewing (CAI), either *computer-assisted personal interviewing (CAPI)* using a laptop computer in the subject's home or *computer-assisted telephone interviewing (CATI)*, as well as medical record abstraction using a computer. These computer-based systems can incorporate computerized editing concomitantly with the data collection process, and generally eliminate the need for a human editor, except to resolve problems (see editor's log below). Specifically these systems allow range checks to occur immediately after the answer is entered, and allow checks for inconsistencies to be made as soon as the relevant items are entered. These systems can then produce prompts to the interviewer or abstractor to correct the answers during the interview or record abstraction. Furthermore, because the skip patterns (routing to appropriate subquestions based on prior answers) can be programmed, the system can ensure that all required items have responses (Nicholls *et al.* 1997). Other advantages of CAI are discussed in Chapters 2 and 7. Unfortunately, improper programming of the CAI adds a new source of error from this technology. The program, especially the skip patterns, needs to be checked carefully before the study enters the field. Without adequate checking, a simple programming error can lead to a final data set with a key variable missing for all subjects!

Coding, i.e. assigning codes to responses to open-ended questions where the number of possible responses is too large to be included on a form, was traditionally done by the study editor or a specialized coder after data collection. With the increased use of computer-assisted coding systems and the total quality management approach of less specialization (discussed above), the interviewers now also do the coding in some survey groups. The advantages of this are that some simple computerized 'look-up' coding systems, or even more complex systems which provide automated potential matches, can sometimes be fast enough for the coding to occur during the interview or record abstraction. This allows the interviewer to probe the subject or medical record more deeply, when necessary, to select the correct code. However, coders need good training and experience, and so this suggests that specialized coders should be used. Several studies have shown that coding by specialized coders is more reliable than interviewer coding (Dodd 1985; Martin *et al.* 1995).

For coding of most exposures (e.g. drugs or occupations), completely automated coding is unlikely ever to be as accurate as human judgement. Computer-assisted systems, i.e. those that automatically code some responses and for others provide a list of choices from which a human coder selects, probably provide little gain in accuracy over human coding; however, they generally save time and reduce coding costs for very large surveys (Campanelli *et al.* 1997). Again, the computerized system must be carefully designed and checked, and should simulate manual coding by allowing synonyms, mis-spellings, and abbreviations in the text (Lyberg and Kasprzyk 1997).

A second coder should review all or a sample of records to check the coding. To be most accurate in identifying discrepancies, the second review should be independent (i.e. blind to the first assigned code), rather than a review of the text and assigned code.

Errors or problems identified by any of the quality control procedures during data collection should be resolved by checking back with the subject or the original records, by improving the study procedures, by additional training for some or all data collectors, or a combination of these strategies.

An additional quality control procedure is the keeping of an *editor's log*, a record of all problems in recording or coding answers, problems in specimen handling or analysis, and subject comments that could affect the analysis or interpretation of the data. The log generally includes the date of the problem, the subject ID, the item (e.g. question number or variable name), the problem, the date of resolution, the resolution, and by whom. The editor's log is kept by one person (e.g. the project director), which ensures uniform handling of problems. For example, a question on marital status may lead to unanticipated responses such as 'common law marriage' or 'married but husband has been in a nursing home for five years'. These responses should be coded consistently and, when appropriate, the question or responses should be clarified. The log may also include the verbatim responses that were coded as 'other'. For example, a family history of breast cancer in a half-sister may have been coded as 'other relative', but the researcher would be likely to choose to include this response along with other second-degree relatives (aunts, grandmothers) during data analysis. It will be much easier to do this by reference to an electronic editor's log which can be sorted by item rather than by having to refer back to the original records. This also allows the editor easier reference to previous problems with the same item, and allows the investigator to review all problems with a specific item during data collection or at the time of data analysis. Figure 5.1 shows a sample editor's log.

Quality control during data processing

Data capture and editing by computer

Errors can be introduced in almost any phase of a study (Table 3.1), including during data capture and during programming of the variables derived from the raw data. Methods for data capture include data entry during a computer-aided interview (CAI), key entry from hand-completed forms, optical scanning of mark sense ('bubble') forms, and computer character recognition of hand-written responses from forms that have been scanned (digitized).

Quality control varies by data capture method. For traditional post-survey key entry, the data can be entered twice using a verification program which signals disagreements. However, with the increased use of CAI, double entry is no longer possible, and the interviewers need to be accurate at key entry as well as skilled at interviewing. Optical scanning (mark recognition) methods are good for large studies using self-administered questionnaires, but all question-naire responses must be categorized (or this technique can be combined with key entry of some written text or numeric responses). Quality control usually consists of the review of all forms before scanning to white out (with tape) responses that were crossed out, and to re-mark forms completed in a way not readable by the scanner (e.g. by pen, red pen, or a light pencil, depending on the scanner). Optical scanner programs are good at selecting the darkest bubble if two or more are erroneously marked when only one is allowed. Therefore hand review of duplicate marks before scanning, or review of duplicate marks which the scanner could not distinguish after scanning, are probably not worthwhile (except to signal call-backs to subjects). Character

Question A.5—Present weight

Date	Subject ID	Question	Problem	Date	Resolution	By whom
15/10/06	10027	A.5	On steroid drugs, gained 21 lb	25/10/06	Change to missing to omit from analyses of weight	EW
27/01/07	10102	A.5	Had gallbladder problems, then surgery 3 weeks ago – lost 17 lb	20/02/07	Change to missing to omit from analyses of weight	EW
17/02/07	10142	A.5	On weight loss diet – lost 15 lb in 6 weeks	20/02/07	OK as recorded	EW

Figure 5.1 Example of an editor's log.

recognition software that 'reads' numbers and letters that were hand-written by subjects allows more detailed information to be ascertained (e.g. exact height and weight). There is substantial error in reading the handwriting of untrained subjects; however, the software can provide a percentage certainty for each character (e.g. 75 per cent certainty that the letter in the first box was an 'n'). For this reason, quality control procedures for this technology should include human verification of 100 per cent of the data (except for simple checked boxes) or verification of all items not read with high certainty. Verification programs allow an editor to correct the data by viewing the digitized facsimile of the response field along with the program interpretation of the characters.

If computer data editing for range and logic checks was not done as part of a computer-aided data collection method, then it should be done after data capture. Both the data capture and the computer editing should be done contemporaneously with data collection. This allows call-backs to subjects soon after an interview to clarify responses and allows the researcher to be alerted to data problems in a timely manner.

Data documentation and creation of new variables

Codebooks which describe three types of variables should be developed.

- The raw data variables as they were originally collected from participants. A sample codebook for raw data is shown in Figure 5.2. An alternative format is an annotated questionnaire with the variable names, codes used, and codes for missing values added.

- New variables that are corrected versions of raw variables. These 'corrected raw variables' include new versions of raw variables for which outliers are set to missing or for which a main question is changed (e.g. when it is missing) when answers to the sub-questions make the answer to the main question obvious. Computer-assisted data collection with programmed range and logic checks and automated skip patterns often obviates the need to correct raw data variables. In contrast, data collected from self-administered questionnaires will require numerous corrected raw variables based on corrections from range and logic checks.

- New variables derived or computed from more than one raw variable during the course of analysis. A sample codebook for documenting corrected and computed variables is shown in Figure 5.3. The programming code for all the computed variables should be in a single file and forms a second more detailed level of documentation for these variables. (Documentation of variables created only for analysis of a specific paper

		CODEBOOK – RAW DATA		
Variable name	**Item no.**	**Description**	**Codes or range**	**Question**
ID		ID number	As given	
SEX	1	Sex	1 = female 2 = male . = missing	
AGE	2	Age	20 – 70 . = missing	
SMOKE	3	Ever smoked	1 = no 2 = yes . = missing	Have you ever smoked cigarettes regularly (at least 1 cigarette a day) for at least a year?
CIGNO	3a	Cigarettes per day	1 – 100 . = N/A or missing	During the years you smoked, how many cigarettes did you usually smoke each day?
CIGYRS	3b	Years smoked	1 – 60 . = N/A or missing	How many years have you been (or were you) a regular smoker? *Do not count years you stayed off cigarettes.*
SMOKENOW	3c	Current smoker	1 = no 2 = yes . = N/A or missing	Do you smoke cigarettes now?

Figure 5.2 Example of a codebook for raw data as collected.

and not stored in the main study database can be kept on a separate file with the documentation of the analyses for the paper.)

Errors in programming the computed exposure variables (e.g. cumulative dose) are another source of error in exposure measurement. These errors can easily occur as a consequence of not considering all possible combinations of the responses to the items that are used in creating the new variable. In particular, missing values need to be handled carefully. For example, suppose that a variable for diabetes (yes, no, missing) was to be created based on self-administered questions on use of insulin and on use of 'pills for diabetes or to lower blood sugar' that were part of a longer list of medications taken in the last two weeks. If each medication question was coded as yes, no, or missing, there are nine possible response combinations for the two items. In many statistical packages, when one variable in a statement is missing, the computation using that variable is set to missing. Instead, the researcher should decide how missing data should be handled and override this standard handling of missing data by the statistical package. For example, diabetes could be computed from the two items as 'yes' if either medication was taken, 'no' if both items were 'no' or missing, and 'missing' only when the entire section (page) was left blank. This assumes that a missing item in a list means 'no' as long as some items on the page were completed. Figure 5.3 gives another example of how missing data are handled in a computed variable.

The programming for the computation of new variables should be checked by review of the programming code by a second person, by hand calculation in some cases, and, when possible, by cross-classifying subjects by the items used to create the new variable and the new variable itself. Finally, the researcher should always review the frequency distributions of all raw and computed variables; errors are sometimes identified during this review.

Summary

The design and interpretation of an epidemiological study should take into account the effects of exposure measurement error, i.e. that the observed odds ratio (or other measure of association) will be biased and, under non-differential measurement error, the power to detect an association will be reduced. For the study to have sufficient power, the sample size calculations should be based on parameters as they will be affected by measurement error. In addition, after a study has been completed, an estimate of the bias in the risk ratio can be calculated based on estimates of the magnitude of the measurement error obtained from validity or reliability studies.

CODEBOOK – CORRECTED AND COMPUTED VARIABLES			
Variable name	Description	Codes or range	Computation
SMOKEC	Ever smoked (corrected)	1 = no 2 = yes . = missing	SMOKEC = SMOKE but set to yes if either CIGNO or CIGYRS has values in allowable range
PACKYRS	Cigarette pack-years	0 – 600 . = missing	PACKYRS = CIGNO/20 × CIGYRS Set to missing if (CIGNO =. or CIGYRS = .) and (SMOKEC = 2 or SMOKEC = .). Set to zero for non-smokers (if SMOKEC = 1)

Figure 5.3 Example of a codebook for corrected and computed variables.

More importantly, the design and execution of a study should incorporate methods to reduce measurement error. One such method is the collection of multiple measures of certain exposure(s) for each subject in the study. If two or more measures of the same exposure have equal and uncorrelated errors, the average (or sum) of the measures will be a more precise measure of the exposure than only one of the measures on its own. Use of the average or sum will lead to less bias in the observed odds ratio (or other measure of the effect of the exposure) and a reduction in the required sample size. When the errors are not equal, or they are correlated, there may be less or even no reduction in measurement error. The use of multiple measures increases both the cost per subject and respondent burden, and these effects need to be taken into consideration when determining the number of measures to be used.

Systematic quality control procedures before, during, and after data collection are necessary to identify and correct measurement errors. Careful design of the data collection forms, complete documentation of study procedures, and pre-testing of the data collection instrument will eliminate some sources of error. The training and supervision of data collectors should emphasize uniform execution of the study protocol and collective responsibility to maintain and improve the data quality. Review of the completed data forms by an editor and/or automated editing for range and logic checks will uncover data items that need clarification or correction.

References

Anderson, L.K., Hendershot, R.A., and Schoolmaker, R.C. (1974). Self-checking digit concepts. *Journal of Systems Management*, **25**, 36–42.

Armstrong, B. (1995). Study design for exposure assessment in epidemiological studies. *Science of the Total Environment*, **168**, 187–94.

Bashir, S.A. and Duffy, S.W. (1997). The correction of risk estimates for measurement error. *Annals of Epidemiology*, **7**, 154–64.

Biemer, P. and Caspar, R. (1994). Continuous quality improvement for survey operations: some general principles and applications. *Journal of Official Statistics*, **10**, 307–26.

Bohrnstedt, G.W. (1983). Measurement. In *Handbook of Survey Research* (ed. P. Rossi, J. Wright, and A. Anderson), pp. 70–121. Academic Press, Orlando, FL.

Buonaccorsi, J.P. (1990). Double sampling for exact values in the normal discriminant model with application to binary regression. *Communications in Statistics: Theory and Methods*, **19**, 4569–86.

Campanelli, P., Thomson, K., Moon, N., and Staples, T. (1997). The quality of occupational coding in the United Kingdom. In *Survey Measurement and Process Quality* (ed. L. Lyberg, P. Biemer, M. Collins, *et al.*), pp. 437–53. Wiley, New York.

Carmines, E.G. and Zeller, R.A. (1979). *Reliability and Validity Assessment*. Sage, Beverly Hills, CA.

Carroll, R.J., Ruppert, D., Stefanski, L.A. and Crainiceanv, C.M. (2006). *Measurement Error in Nonlinear Models.: A Modern perspective.* Chapman & Hall CRC Press, London/Boca Radon, FL.

Chen, T.T. (1989). A review of methods for misclassified categorical data in epidemiology. *Statistics in Medicine,* **8,** 1095–1106.

Dodd, T. (1985). *An Assessment of the Efficiency of the Coding of Occupation and Industry by Interviewers. New Methodology Series NM 14.* Office of Population Censuses and Surveys, London.

Duffy, S.W., Maximovitch, D.M., and Day, N.E. (1992). External validation, repeat determination, and precision of risk estimation in misclassified exposure data in epidemiology. *Journal of Epidemiology and Community Health,* **46,** 620–4.

Dunn, G. (1989). *Design and Analysis of Reliability Studies.* Oxford University Press, New York.

Feinstein, A.R. (1983). An additional basic science for clinical medicine. IV: The development of clinimetrics. *Annals of Internal Medicine,* **99,** 843–8.

Fleiss, J.L. (1986). *The Design and Analysis of Clinical Experiments.* Wiley, New York.

Greenland, S. (1988). Statistical uncertainty due to misclassification: implications for validation substudies. *Journal of Clinical Epidemiology,* **41,** 1167–74.

Greenland, S. and Robins, J.M. (1985). Confounding and misclassication. *American Journal of Epidemiology,* **122,** 495–506.

Groves, R.M. (1989). *Survey Errors and Survey Costs.* Wiley, New York.

Hilsenbeck, S.G., Glaefke, G.S., Feigl, P., *et al.* (1985). *Quality Control for Cancer Registries.* US Department of Health and Human Services, Washington, DC.

Holford, T.R. and Stack, C. (1995). Study design for epidemiologic studies with measurement error. *Statistical Methods in Medical Research,* **4,** 339–58.

Hunter, D.J., Morris, J.S., Chute, C.G., *et al.* (1990). Predictors of selenium concentration in human toenails. *American Journal of Epidemiology,* **132,** 114–22.

Kim, M.Y. and Zeleniuch-Jacquotte, A. (1997). Correcting for measurement error in the analysis of case–control data with repeated measurements of exposure. *American Journal of Epidemiology,* **145,** 1003–10.

Liu, K. (1988). Measurement error and its impact on partial correlation and multiple linear regression analyses. *American Journal of Epidemiology,* **127,** 864–74.

Liu, X. and Liang, K.-Y. (1992). Efficacy of repeated measures in regression models with measurement error. *Biometrics,* **48,** 645–54.

Lyberg, L. and Kasprzyk, D. (1997). Some aspects of post-survey processing. In *Survey Measurement and Process Quality* (ed. L. Lyberg, P. Biemer, M. Collins *et al.*), pp. 353–70. Wiley, New York.

Lyberg, L., Biemer, P., Collins, M., *et al.* (eds) (1997). *Survey Measurement and Process Quality,* Wiley, New York.

McFadden, E. (1998). *Management of Data in Clinical Trials.* Wiley, New York.

McKeown-Eyssen, G.E. and Thomas, D.C. (1985). Sample size determination in case–control studies: the influence of the distribution of exposure. *Journal of Chronic Diseases,* **38,** 559–68.

Martin, J., Bushnell, D., Campanelli, P., and Thomas, R. (1995). A comparison of inter-viewer and office coding of occupations. In *Joint Proceedings of ASA/AAPOR: Section of Survey Research Methods*. American Statistical Association, Washington, DC.

Meinert, C.L. (1986). *Clinical Trials: Design, Conduct, and Analysis*. Oxford University Press, New York.

Nicholls, W.L., II, Baker, R.P., and Martin, J. (1997). The effect of new data collection technologies on survey data quality. In *Survey Measurement and Process Quality* (ed. L. Lyberg, P. Biemer, M. Collins *et al.*), pp. 221–48. Wiley, New York.

Rippin, G. (2001). Design issues and sample size when exposure measurement is inaccu-rate. *Methods of Information in Medicine*, **40**, 137–40.

Rosner, B., Willett, W.C., and Spiegelman, D. (1989). Correction of logistic regression relative risk estimates and confidence intervals for systematic within-person measure-ment error. *Statistics in Medicine*, **8**, 1051–69.

Rosner, B., Willett, W.C., and Spiegelman, D. (1990). Correction of logistic regression relative risk estimates and confidence intervals for measurement error: the case of multiple covariates measured with error. *American Journal of Epidemiology*, **132**, 734–45.

Spiegelman, D. and Gray, R. (1991). Cost-efficient study designs for binary response data with Gaussian covariate measurement error. *Biometrics*, **47**, 851–69.

Spiegelman, D., McDermott, A., and Rosner, B. (1997a). Regression calibration method for correcting measurement-error bias in nutritional epidemiology. *American Journal of Clinical Nutrition*, **65** (Suppl.), 11795–1865.

Spiegelman, D., Schneeweiss, S., and McDermott, A. (1997b). Measurement error correc-tion for logistic regression models with an 'alloyed gold standard'. *American Journal of Epidemiology*, **14**, 184–96.

Streiner, D.L. and Norman, G.R (2003). *Health Measurement Scales: A Practical Guide to Their Development and Use* (3rd edn). Oxford University Press.

Tavaré, C.J., Sobel, E.L., and Gilles, F.H. (1995). Misclassification of a prognostic dichoto-mous variable: sample size and parameter estimate adjustment. *Statistics in Medicine*, **14**, 1307–14.

Thomas, D., Stram, D., and Dwyer, J. (1993). Exposure measurement error: influence on exposure–disease relationships and methods of correction. *Annual Review of Public Health*, **14**, 69–93.

Thürigen, D., Spiegelman, D., Blettner, M., Carsten, H., and Brenner, H. (2000). Measurement error correction using validation data: a review of methods and their applicability in case–control studies. *Statistical Methods in Medical Research*, **9**, 447–74.

Wacholder, S., Armstrong, B.G. and Hartge, P. (1993). Validation studies using an alloyed gold standard. *American Journal of Epidemiology*, **137**, 1251–8.

White, E., Kushi, L.H., and Pepe, M.S. (1994). The effect of exposure variance and exposure measurement error on study sample size: implications for the design of epidemiologic studies. *Journal of Clinical Epidemiology*, **47**, 873–80.

6

The design of questionnaires

Words are the building blocks for all question structures,
but deciding which words to be used and in what order
is far from simple. The wrong choice of words can create
any number of problems, from excessive vagueness to
too much precision, from being misunderstood to not
being understood at all, and from being too
objectionable to being uninteresting and irrelevant.
(Dillman 2000, p. 50)

Introduction

For our purposes, a *questionnaire* can be defined as a tool designed to elicit
and record, or guide the elicitation and recording of, recalled exposures from
subjects of an epidemiological study. It contains questions to be put to the
subject, and may also include answers to those questions from which the
subject must choose those that are appropriate to him/her.

The objectives of questionnaire design are:

- to obtain measurements of exposure variables essential to the objectives of
  the study
- to minimize error in these measurements
- to create an instrument that is easy for the interviewer and subject to use,
  and for the investigator to process and analyse.

These objectives are potentially in conflict, and any questionnaire usually
represents a compromise among them. For example, it may be necessary to
trade off some ease in processing and analysis against ease in completion by the
interviewer or the subject. Similarly, the addition of some questions essential to
the objectives of the study, for example questions about sexual behaviour in a
study of the aetiology of cancer of the cervix, may make a questionnaire more
difficult for an interviewer to administer and more threatening to the respondent. Judgement must be exercised in making decisions about the content and

structure of questionnaires. Where compromise is necessary, the designer should favour decisions that maximize the usefulness of the questionnaire to the objectives of the study and minimize error in measurement.

In this chapter, we cover the major topics of importance in the design of questionnaires:

- choice of the items of data to be covered by the questionnaire
- the types of question that can be used
- the material covered by each question
- the wording of questions
- question order
- physical format and structure of questionnaires
- the problem of collecting information on behaviours that vary with time
- aids to recall
- pre-testing questionnaires.

More comprehensive accounts of the design of questionnaires can be found in Bennett and Ritchie (1975), Sudman and Bradburn (1983), Schwarz and Sudman (1996), Aday (1996), Dillman (2000), and Tourangeau *et al.* (2000). Decisions about choice of mode of administration of the questionnaire (i.e. telephone interview, in-person interview, self-administered questionnaire, or various types of computer-assisted interviews) are discussed in Chapter 2. Chapter 7 covers issues specific to administering questionnaires by in-person and telephone interviewing.

Choice of items to be covered

Questionnaire design usually begins with selection of the items of data that must be translated into questions. The ground to be covered is determined by two main factors: the objectives of the study, and the limitations imposed by the burden that can be placed on respondents, including the feasible length of the questionnaire.

Objectives of the study

'The content of a questionnaire is generally designed to investigate the minimum amount of an individual's total experience that will provide sufficient information concerning the problem under study' (Bennett and Ritchie 1975). Just as the objectives of the study determine the variables to be measured as a whole, they also determine the specific items to be covered in the questionnaire. If a question does not contribute to the achievement of the objectives, it has no place in the questionnaire.

Adequately detailed data should be sought for each essential exposure variable, as described in Chapter 1. For example, for exposure that happens frequently, it is usual to ask about the time exposure began, the time it ended, and the frequency and intensity of the exposure and their variation over time. A comprehensive list of potential confounders and effect modifiers should also be developed. A well thought out plan for data analysis, and a description of the algorithms that will be used to create exposure dose variables and covariate variables, is essential in determining the items and detail required. Developing the exposure and covariate algorithms that will be used at the end of the study *before* questionnaire development at the beginning of a study is important to avoid a surprising common problem—that at the time of data analysis, the researcher realizes that an item needed to compute an exposure dose variable had not been collected!

Length of the questionnaire

The topics to be covered in a questionnaire and the detail in which they are covered are limited first and foremost by the length of time that subjects are willing to spend on the questioning process. While there are inevitable exceptions, it may be taken as a general rule that the maximum time that can be spent administering a questionnaire is 1–2 hours by face-to-face interview and 30–40 minutes by telephone interview. Self-administered questionnaires are at an added disadvantage in that the subject can gain an impression of the size of the response task before deciding whether to embark on it. Response rates are reduced with longer mailed questionnaires (Edwards *et al.* 2002).

Other aspects of respondent burden

'Respondent burden concerns the level of demand placed on the respondent necessary to answer the survey instrument questions' (Sudman and Andersen 1977). Length of the questionnaire is one aspect of respondent burden. Additional contributors to respondent burden are:

- length and distance (from the present) of the period of time over which recall is requested
- salience (or impact) to the subject of the topic of questioning, including its sensitivity
- frequency of the event
- complexity or detail of the data sought.

In general, recall over a long period of time or from the distant past, topics of low salience or impact, questioning regarding frequent events (such as eating), and complex questions (e.g. a full occupational history with details of exposure to hazards in each occupation) will all add to respondent burden. Being a proxy respondent for someone else is generally a further burden.

Increased burden on the respondent has several consequences:

- risk increases for termination of the interview or non-completion of a self-administered questionnaire
- quality of data obtained is reduced
- response rate is threatened
- the population may become alienated from survey research and cooperation in future studies may be reduced (Sudman and Andersen 1977).

The last effect is a particular problem for longitudinal studies requiring recurrent surveys in one population.

There is often a conflict between collecting information considered to be necessary to the objectives of the study, keeping the questionnaire to an acceptable length, and minimizing other aspects of respondent burden. In resolving this conflict, it is important not only to collect the amount of information necessary to the objectives of the study, but also to ensure that questionnaire length and respondent burden are kept to levels that do not threaten subject participation or cause a material increase in measurement error.

Types of question

Questions are generally classified as either 'open-ended' or 'closed-ended'. *Open-ended questions* are questions to which no answers are provided by the investigator. Only the question is asked, and the respondent's answer is recorded verbatim. In an interview, extensive probing may be used to ensure that all relevant aspects of the topic are covered by the answer. *Closed-ended questions* are questions for which the range of possible answers is specified by the investigator and the respondent is asked to make a choice from among the answers provided.

Open-ended questions

Open-ended questions should be used in epidemiology for eliciting and recording *simple* facts to which there are a large number of possible answers, for example, age, occupation, country of birth, number of cigarettes smoked a day, amount of alcohol drunk in a particular period of time, etc. The use of closed-ended questions for these topics leads to loss of information and, when asking about a socially undesirable behaviour, a greater degree of error. For example, reporting of intake of beer was nearly 50 per cent less when a closed-ended rather than an open-ended question was used (Blair *et al.* 1977).

One advantage of open-ended questions is that subjects cannot be influenced by the response options, as they may be for closed-ended questions. Schwarz *et al.* (1985) found that when offered a range of categories from 'up to half an hour' to 'more than 2½ hours' for daily TV watching, 16.2 per cent of subjects estimated that they watched more than 2½ hours. When offered the range 'up to 2½ hours' to 'more than 4½ hours', 37.5 per cent estimated that they watched more than 2½ hours. It appears that the response categories offered are seen as normative by some respondents, and their responses are influenced away from the extremes, particularly if one or other extreme is viewed as socially undesirable.

The collection of data on income (used in epidemiology as a measure of socio-economic status) may be an exception to the rule that simple factual data are best sought through open-ended questions. While there is probably no particular tendency for subjects to over- or understate their income, they are sensitive about disclosing the exact amount. Thus a closed-ended question with income categories might be acceptable, where an open-ended question would not. It is also usual in self-administered questionnaires to ask questions with a limited range of categorical responses (such as 'What is your sex?' or 'What is your marital status?') as closed-ended questions to permit maximum use of self-coding responses.

When the likely answer to an open-ended question is neither simple nor factual, the use of such a question increases the burden on both respondent and interviewer and produces answers that are difficult both to code and to analyse.

Closed-ended questions

The use of closed-ended questions is comparatively uncommon in epidemiology for exposure measurement, and appropriately so for the reasons given above. Most data sought are both simple and factual, and are best dealt with by open-ended questions. However, closed-ended questions are needed more often on self-administered questionnaires than on interviews, for at least two reasons. First, self-administered questionnaires need to be simpler to complete than interviews. For example, an interview may ask an open-ended question on frequency of a behaviour, for which the interviewer records both the frequency and the period: for example, for a response of 'three times per week', the interviewer records the number '3' and the time period 'week'. This would be too complex for respondents on a self-administered questionnaire, and so a list of responses ranging from, say, 'more than twice a day' to 'never or less than once a week' would be needed. Secondly, self-administered question-naires are often used for large studies which use automated data capture systems (e.g. optical scanning), many of which can only read closed-ended responses (e.g. marks in boxes).

The alternative answers offered in a closed-ended question should be simple and brief, and mutually exclusive if only one is to be selected. If more than one response could be selected, it may be best to seek explicit 'yes/no' responses for each of the categories. If the response categories provided are not exhaustive of all possible responses, a final open category (e.g. 'Other. Please give details _____') should be given.

As noted above, respondents are reluctant to place themselves in the extreme category of an undesirable behaviour. When categories are needed, for example for alcohol intake, it may be appropriate to add an extra extreme category (e.g. 6+ a day) to encourage response to the penultimate category.

One decision in selecting responses to closed-ended questions is whether to include 'don't know' as an option. A 'don't know' response should be offered only if the possibility exists that some respondents would truly not know the answer. For example, in asking about family history, a 'don't know' response is needed for those who are adopted and do not know their biological family. However, generally a 'don't know' response category should not be given, because a greater percentage of subjects will answer the question if an explicit 'don't know' is not given. For example, a study by Poe *et al.* (1988) has shown that, in approaching the next of kin of dead subjects for data on demographic variables and aspects of health history and health-related behaviour, exclusion of the 'don't know' option gave an appreciably higher proportion of usable responses for many items without adversely affecting response rate or intramethod reliability.

The response list should be in a logical sequence, because subjects will often stop reading the answers after they find the appropriate one. For the same reason, specific definitions should be given before general ones. For example, for a question on type of spread used at the table, the response 'Low-fat spread or diet margarine' should be before 'Regular margarine'. Then subjects would read the 'low-fat' response before deciding whether the 'regular margarine' response applied to them.

It is also important in closed-ended questions to limit the number of response categories as far as is reasonably possible. A large number of alternative responses increases respondent burden, increases the probability of non-response to the question (Leigh and Martin 1987), and may increase the probability that one of the response options listed first will be selected (Krosnick and Alwin 1987).

Question content

Questions may be about:

- *knowledge* (what people know)
- *attitudes* (what people say they want or think)
- *beliefs* (what people say is true)
- *experiences* (what has happened to people)
- *behaviours* (what people do, have done, or will do)
- *attributes* (what people are).

Generally, only experiences, behaviours, and attributes are relevant to exposure measurement in epidemiology. However, most of the research on question content and questionnaires has related to questions about knowledge, attitudes, and beliefs. This research will be drawn on and, as far as possible, described in terms of its relevance to exposure measurement through questionnaires.

Like the subject matter as a whole, the content of individual questions is largely determined by the objectives of the study. Therefore it is not possible to be prescriptive on this subject, but some general advice can be given.

Before developing questions on a particular topic, the investigator should become thoroughly familiar with it by reading and by discussions with experts. It is advisable to obtain copies of questionnaires that have been used previously by experts to cover the subject matter of interest and to make prudent use of them, within the limits of any copyright restrictions that may apply and provided that due acknowledgement is given.

The use of standard questions has a number of advantages.

- The questions will usually have been used extensively and proved satisfactory in use.
- The questions may have been assessed for reliability and/or validity and, even if they have not, sufficient results may be available from their use to permit validity to be inferred.
- Their use will permit comparison among datasets and possibly the combining of datasets.
- It is an easy way of drawing on the expertise of others, and it can substantially facilitate the task of questionnaire design.

All that said, it is important for the investigator to evaluate questions obtained from other sources in terms of the adequacy of their design, their appropriateness to the objectives of the current study, and their suitability for use in the population on which the study will be conducted. It should also be noted that questions developed for use in a face-to-face interview may require modification in their wording or format if they are to be used in a telephone interview or a mailed self-administered questionnaire.

One source of questionnaires is a website developed by the US National Cancer Institute (http://dceg.cancer.gov/QMOD/qmod_categories.htm). This includes questionnaires for a range of exposures that have been used in studies of cancer.

Question wording

There are two important issues to be considered in question wording.

◆ How does one arrive at a suitable wording in the first place?

◆ Are small changes in wording likely to lead to differences in response?

The latter issue is particularly relevant to comparisons between populations and over time when the same basic data have been sought by slightly different questions.

Table 6.1 gives a list of questions that should be asked about the wording of each question in a questionnaire.

The words

The words used in a questionnaire should be the usual 'working tools' of the respondents. They should be neither too difficult (be suspicious of words

Table 6.1 Questions that should be asked about the wording of each question in a questionnaire[a]

◆ Will the words be uniformly understood by the subject population?

◆ Does the question contain abbreviations, unconventional phrases, or jargon?

◆ Is the question vague?

◆ Is the question too precise?

◆ Is the question biased?

◆ Is the topic sensitive?

◆ Does the question contain a double negative?

◆ Are the answer options mutually exclusive (or if not, is *'Answer all that apply'* stated)?

◆ Are the answer options exhaustive, i.e. is there an appropriate response for all respondents?

◆ Is an unambiguous time reference provided?

◆ Does the question contain more than one concept?

◆ Does the question require a calculation?

◆ Is the concept too complex?

[a] Adapted from Dillman (2000).

more than seven letters in length) nor too simple. Difficult words may not be understood, and simple words (where better but more difficult words could have been used) may appear condescending, may not convey the right meaning, and may needlessly lengthen the questionnaire. Where doubt exists, however, there is a virtue in simplicity. Abbreviations, unconventional phrases, and jargon present the same problems as difficult words; they may not be understood or, perhaps worse, they may be misunderstood.

These general principles may be illustrated by some examples. The question

HAVE YOU EVER HAD AN ECG?

includes an abbreviation that is also technical jargon. In addition, the abbreviation used in some English-speaking countries is EKG, not ECG. Nonetheless, the abbreviation is likely to be familiar to many subjects, and perhaps more familiar than any alternative terms. The solution here is to offer some alternative terms in the question, for example

HAVE YOU EVER HAD AN ECG, THAT IS, A 'HEART TRACING', EKG, OR ELECTROCARDIOGRAPH?

In the particular circumstance of quantifying sensitive behaviour (e.g. sexual activity or the use of alcohol or illicit drugs), asking the respondent to supply words that he/she is accustomed to using to describe the behaviour may increase the accuracy of reporting (Blair *et al.* 1977). Two forms of question were asked about drunkenness:

IN THE PAST YEAR, HOW OFTEN DID YOU BECOME INTOXICATED WHILE DRINKING ANY KIND OF ALCOHOLIC BEVERAGE?

and

SOMETIMES PEOPLE DRINK A LITTLE TOO MUCH BEER, WINE, OR WHISKY SO THAT THEY ACT DIFFERENTLY FROM USUAL. WHAT WORD DO YOU THINK WE SHOULD USE TO DESCRIBE PEOPLE WHEN THEY GET THAT WAY, SO THAT YOU WILL KNOW WHAT WE MEAN AND FEEL COMFORT ABLE TALKING ABOUT IT?
IN THE PAST YEAR, HOW OFTEN DID YOU BECOME (*RESPONDENT'S WORD*) WHILE DRINKING ANY KIND OF ALCOHOLIC BEVERAGE?

The second form of the question consistently increased the reporting of this and other sensitive behaviours. Because socially undesirable behaviours tend to be under-reported, an increase in reporting is assumed to mean reduction in error.

There are no data to suggest that particular terms familiar to the subjects should be used for other than sensitive behaviours and, in general, slang or vulgar terms should not be used in questionnaires. Their use may lead to misunderstanding, the appearance of condescension, and, for some subjects, offence.

Vague questions

Questions may contain vague words—words that vary substantially in their meaning among different people. 'Usually', 'normally', and 'regularly' are three commonly used vague descriptors of frequency. In many circumstances they can be replaced by more precise quantifiers. For example,

HOW OLD WERE YOU WHEN YOU FIRST BEGAN TO SMOKE CIGARETTES REGULARLY?

could be made more precise by asking

HOW OLD WERE YOU WHEN YOU FIRST SMOKED ONE OR MORE CIGARETTES A DAY FOR ONE MONTH OR LONGER?

The latter wording eliminates uncertainty about the meaning of 'regularly'.

Similarly, it would be better to ask subjects about their 'usual' intake of alcoholic beverages over a specific period of time (e.g. the past 12 months) than simply to ask about their 'usual' intake.

Questions that are too precise

While precision is desirable, particularly when estimating amount or duration of exposure, respondent burden may be increased unduly if too much precision is requested. For example, in precisely quantifying dose rate and cumulative exposure to cigarette smoke, it might be tempting to ask smokers to estimate their average daily cigarette consumption for each year of their smoking life. This would be unreasonably burdensome and prone to substantial error in recall. A better approach would be to ask subjects about major changes in daily cigarette intake (e.g. an increase or decrease of 10 or more cigarettes a day), and document the time of each of these changes.

Biased questions

Biased questions are questions that suggest to the respondent that a particular answer is preferred from among all possible answers. 'Leading' questions are well known, and should be easily avoided. 'Loaded' questions are more likely to turn up in questionnaires seeking attitudes or beliefs than more factual data. The question

DO YOU THINK THAT SMOKING SHOULD BE BANNED IN PLANES?

would be more likely to bias responses because of use of the strong negative word 'banned' than would the more neutral, and balanced,

DO YOU THINK THAT SMOKING SHOULD BE PERMITTED OR NOT PERMITTED IN PLANES?

A significant influence of question wording has been shown in surveys of attitudes to public assistance to the poor in the USA (Smith 1987). In six surveys spanning 17 years, the proportion of Americans in favour of more spending on welfare was substantially less when the word 'welfare' was used in the question than when the question referred to 'assistance to the poor'. Smith (1987) concluded that this difference was due to a connotation of 'welfare' with waste and bureaucracy that 'assistance to the poor' did not have, or at least not to the same degree.

Sensitive questions

Sensitive or threatening questions are questions that '. . . ask respondents about behaviours that are illegal, contra-normative [deviant] or generally not discussed in public without tension, or relate to issues of self-preservation' (Blair *et al.* 1977). They fall into two distinct classes: those that ask about behaviours or attributes that are socially desirable, and those that ask about socially undesirable behaviours or attributes. The threat of questions about socially desirable behaviours arises from the possibility that a person does not wish to admit that he/she does not practise the behaviour (e.g. giving to charity or, of more direct relevance to epidemiology, exercising regularly). These behaviours tend to be over-reported. Socially undesirable behaviours or attributes (such as past history of sexually transmitted disease and alcohol drinking) tend to be under-reported. Questions about income, savings, and assets are threatening, although they are not readily categorized as either socially desirable or undesirable. A question can be considered as potentially threatening if subjects can possibly feel that there is a right or wrong answer to it (Sudman and Bradburn 1983).

Eliciting accurate answers to sensitive questions can be enhanced by selection of a more impersonal mode of administration (see Chapter 2), by interviewer training if a personal interview is to be used (see Chapter 7), and by the wording of questions (covered below).

A number of techniques have been used to maximize reporting of socially undesirable behaviours, two of which have already been mentioned: use of words familiar to the respondent, and open-ended questions. Reporting of undesirable behaviours was also increased by use of a long introduction to the question (Blair *et al.* 1977). For example, the following introduction was added to the question on drunkenness:

OCCASIONALLY PEOPLE DRINK ON AN EMPTY STOMACH OR DRINK A LITTLE TOO MUCH AND BECOME (INTOXICATED *OR RESPONDENT'S WORD*). IN THE PAST YEAR, HOW OFTEN . . .

This introduction exemplifies another technique for dealing with question threat—deliberately loading the question. In this case the use of 'occasionally', 'drink on an empty stomach', and 'a little too much' all tend to minimize the significance of the behaviour so that the respondent will be more willing to report it. The threat may also be reduced by *embedding* the sensitive question in a list of questions on related topics, some of which are more threatening and some less so. Questions on past history of sexually transmitted disease, for example, can be asked in a series of questions on past disease history.

Reporting of socially undesirable behaviours increases if explicit assurances of confidentiality are given before the interview or before the sensitive question (Frey 1986; Singer 1985). In an in-person interview, socially undesirable questions can often be phrased in a straightforward way, with reliance on the accepting demeanour of the interviewer to yield accurate answers.

There is a difference between strategies appropriate to reducing over-reporting of socially desirable behaviour and those appropriate to increasing reporting of socially undesirable behaviour. Use of a long introductory statement, for example, is likely to encourage rather than discourage over-reporting of desirable behaviours, unless it loads the question against reporting the behaviour. A question on walking might be asked as follows:

MANY PEOPLE FIND IT DIFFICULT TO FIND TIME TO GET REGULAR EXERCISE, LIKE WALKING. IN THE PAST YEAR DID YOU WALK FOR EXERCISE AT LEAST ONCE A WEEK?

The significance of the behaviour may also be minimized by use of the phrase: 'Did you happen to . . .'

IN THE LAST MONTH, DID YOU EVER HAPPEN TO FORGET TO USE A CONDOM?

This might be best asked after the question 'Do you usually use a condom?' to allow a socially desirable response first, which might help to obtain more accurate answers to the question of actual interest above.

A final approach appropriate for questions about socially desirable behaviours, as with socially undesirable behaviours, is to reduce the threat by embedding them in a sequence of questions about non-threatening behaviours.

For example, intake of fat-free milk could be included in a list of questions on frequency of drinking types of milk.

Double negatives

A double negative can arise whenever a question that is phrased negatively can have a negative answer. Dillman (2000) gave the following example:

SHOULD THE CITY MANAGER NOT BE RESPONSIBLE TO THE MAYOR?

Yes ☐
No ☐

The question was asked because the city council was contemplating a change from the city manager being responsible to the mayor to him/her not being responsible to the mayor. It is unnatural to say 'yes' when the answer really means 'no' (that the city manager should *not* be responsible to the mayor), and so answers to this question would be ambiguous. The solution in this case was to ask to whom the city manager should be responsible—the mayor or the city council. Double negatives are probably more common in questions on attitudes and beliefs than in questions likely to be asked in epidemiological studies.

Mutually exclusive answers

A subject could reasonably select more than one answer to the following question:

WHAT SPREAD DO YOU USE ON BREAD?

BUTTER ☐
LOW-FAT SPREAD
  OR DIET MARGARINE ☐
REGULAR MARGARINE ☐
OTHER SPREAD ☐
  PLEASE GIVE DETAILS

_____

Therefore the subject is uncertain about which alternative to choose, and there is a risk of non-response. The problem could be solved by asking 'What spread do you *usually* eat on bread?', by instructing respondents to '*Mark all that apply*', or, preferably, by asking about the frequency of use of all the spreads individually.

Response for all participants

Response lists should also be exhaustive, i.e. all respondents should be able to find an appropriate response. Response categories are sometimes omitted because the researcher has made an assumption that would not apply to all respondents. For example, the following question assumes that all respondents eats steak:

HOW DO YOU LIKE YOUR STEAK TO BE COOKED?

> **RARE** ☐
> **MEDIUM** ☐
> **WELL DONE** ☐

If this assumption is wrong, at best the respondent will not answer the question (in a self-administered questionnaire), and at worst the respondent may find the assumption about his/her behaviour to be offensive. The solution is to add the response alternative '*I don't eat steak*', or to ascertain first whether or not the respondent eats steak and skip to a succeeding question if he/she does not.

An unambiguous time reference

Any period referred to in a question should be clear and unambiguous. The question described above on walking 'in the past year' might have been asked as follows:

DO YOU WALK FOR EXERCISE AT LEAST ONCE PER WEEK?

This question, while most likely referring to the present, has no clear time reference. Different subjects would be likely to refer to different periods of time in the past in answering it.

In a case–control study, it is usually desirable to specify a time for each case somewhat before onset of disease beyond which the exposure will not be recorded to avoid eliciting behaviour which has been influenced by the onset of disease, and a similar date for controls (see Chapter 1). For example:

IN 2002, DID YOU WALK FOR EXERCISE AT LEAST ONCE PER WEEK?

A specific *reference date*, usually the date of diagnosis of the case (or diagnosis date minus a year or two to account for a time when symptoms may have influenced behaviours), is assigned to each case and his/her matched controls. The use of this reference date is usually explained at the beginning of the interview or questionnaire, and questions relating to it usually begin: 'Before [reference date], did you . . .', etc.

One potential solution to problems of ambiguity in the time reference of a question is for the interviewer to have, or the questionnaire to include, a calendar on which the period referred to in that question, or a number of related questions, is marked (see the section below on aids to recall).

More than one concept

A question that has more than one concept should not be posed. For example:

THINK ABOUT YOUR DIET OVER THE PAST YEAR. HOW OFTEN DID YOU EAT A SERVING OF FRUITS OR VEGETABLES? *DO NOT INCLUDE JUICES, SALADS, POTATOES, OR BEANS.*

While fruit and vegetable intake may form a single exposure in a study, most subjects would consider fruits and vegetables as separate categories. Subjects would typically think through the answer by adding the number of times they eat vegetables to the number of times they eat fruit. This is an example of *decomposition*, which is a method used by subjects in formulating an answer to a question by breaking it down into more manageable parts (Bradburn *et al.* 1987). Thus the above question should be asked as two questions, one on fruits and one on vegetables. One can learn which questions subjects decompose and how they decompose them through 'think aloud' interviews, described below in the section on pre-testing questionnaires. The researcher can use this information to break down a complex question into simpler components.

Questions that require calculations

Certain questions which may appear to be a simple concept may actually require the subject to perform a calculation to derive an answer. For example:

IN THE PAST YEAR, ABOUT HOW MANY HOURS PER WEEK DID YOU WALK FOR EXERCISE?

To answer this question, most subjects would need to break it down into the number of times they walked each week and the minutes they walked per session, and then multiply these together (and then convert to hours!). In this case, it would be better to ask separate questions:

IN THE PAST YEAR, ABOUT HOW MANY TIMES PER WEEK DID YOU WALK FOR EXERCISE?

and

HOW MANY MINUTES DID YOU WALK EACH SESSION?

Complex concepts

Some exposures have complex definitions, which would be burdensome for the subject to comprehend. For example, to be classified as 'exposed' in a study, a subject might need to have both a sufficient dose and duration of exposure. For example, the researcher may want to define walking for exercise as walking at least once a week for at least 20 minutes per session and at least at a moderate pace. Then the question might be phrased as:

OVER THE PAST YEAR, DID YOU WALK FOR EXERCISE AT LEAST ONCE A WEEK FOR 20 MINUTES OR MORE PER SESSION? *DO NOT INCLUDE CASUAL WALKING.*

If the question were phrased this way, it would certainly annoy some respondents with its complexity. Instead, part of the concept in the question can be incorporated into the answers to sub-questions. The above question could be phrased: '*Over the past year, did you walk for exercise at least once a week?*' Then, sub-questions would ask about sessions per week, minutes per session (with the lowest response category 'less than 20 minutes'), and pace (with the lowest category 'casual or strolling'). Then, when the algorithm for energy expenditure from walking is developed, those who walked for less than 20 minutes per session or who walked at a casual pace could be coded as not walking for exercise.

Question order

General principles

Beliefs about the order in which questions should appear in a questionnaire have been summarized by Sudman and Bradburn (1983). Questions about a particular topic should be grouped together, and proceed from the general to the particular within a group. This approach, by focusing first in a general way on a particular behaviour or experience, assists and allows more time for recall of the specific details. It is sometimes suggested that questions using a particular response scale should be grouped together, but this is probably undesirable because it may tend to promote a *response set*—a tendency to give the same response to each question regardless of what the correct response should be.

The order in which questions are asked can influence the responses obtained. The evidence for this statement derives mainly from research into questions on attitudes and beliefs (e.g. Helsing and Comstock 1975; McFarland 1981; Schuman *et al.* 1981), but the possibility exists that similar effects could be observed for some questions relating to experiences, behaviours, or attributes. Thus for comparative studies between populations and over time, the order of the questions in the questionnaire should be kept constant as far as possible. Any new questions that are added should go at the end of the questionnaire. Alternatively, any change in question order might be evaluated by comparison of the old and new questionnaires in a single population.

The first question

It is common practice to place the demographic questions at the beginning, but this is not a good idea. These questions are of comparatively low interest to the respondents, and some of them are threatening (see below). Instead, the questionnaire should begin with a question or questions which relate directly to the topic of the research and will command the subject's interest. For example, in a study of sun exposure in relation to skin cancer, it is appropriate to begin with questions on recreational pursuits involving sun exposure.

Sensitive questions

Sensitive questions should be placed towards the end of the questionnaire, in order of increasing threat. This reduces the likelihood that they will precipitate early termination of the interview, or failure to complete the questionnaire. The degree of threat presented by particular questions can be determined empirically by asking subjects 'how uneasy most people' would feel about particular topics of questioning in a questionnaire. In a questionnaire mainly about leisure and sporting activities, the degree of threat of particular topics, from least to greatest, was (Blair *et al.* 1977):

- general leisure and sporting activity
- alcohol drinking
- gambling with friends
- income
- petting and kissing
- drunkenness
- use of stimulants and depressants
- sexual intercourse
- use of marijuana
- masturbation.

Although sensitive questions should be placed near the end of a questionnaire, they should not appear on the last page of a self-administered questionnaire. Questions on the last page are highly visible if the subject peruses the questionnaire.

Demographic questions (e.g. about race, religion, or income) are sometimes threatening and usually not interesting, and therefore are appropriately asked at the end of the questionnaire. If, for some reason (e.g. to select particular respondents), it is necessary to place them at the beginning, some explanation for their position should be given to the respondent.

Logical sequence

Within any topic, questions should follow a logical sequence—the sequence that the respondents might be expected to follow in thinking about the topic. Thus, for example, in collecting residential or job histories, it is usual to proceed chronologically beginning with the present residence or occupation and proceeding to successively earlier ones. The 'backwards' chronological approach also gives the respondent more time to recall the events of the more distant past (Bradburn *et al.* 1987). Other topics, such as pregnancy outcomes, might be more easily recalled in chronological order.

Questionnaire structure

In addition to the questions, every questionnaire should contain:

- an introduction
- instructions (for self-administered questionnaires), including skip patterns
- linking phrases between topics
- a conclusion.

Introduction and instructions

In an interview, the introduction takes the form of a standard statement read by the interviewer. For a self-administered questionnaire it is usually part of the letter soliciting their cooperation. The introduction serves both to elicit participation and to discharge the investigator's ethical obligations to the subjects. The items to be included in the introduction are discussed in Chapter 11 in the section on response rates and their maximization.

General instructions will usually be only necessary in a self-administered questionnaire. Such instructions should be short and simple; an example is given in Figure 6.1. General instructions for interviewers will form part of interviewer training and an interviewer's manual rather than the questionnaire. Instructions relating to specific questions should appear with those questions in the body of the questionnaire, whether it is for self-administration or interview. Figure 6.1 provides examples of question-specific instructions given in italics after some questions. These include instructions to 'mark all that apply' when more then one response may be appropriate, skip instructions (discussed below), and instructions about the meaning of specific questions.

Linking statements

Linking statements break the subject's concentration on a particular topic, provide a brief pause, and establish his/her concentration on a new topic. They may also be used to break the monotony of a long series of questions on

Figure 6.1 Example of instructions and format of a self-administered questionnaire.

one topic. They should not be unnecessarily long, appear to be demanding, or give unwarranted importance to the succeeding questions. Nor should they contain words or phrases that may bias the succeeding responses. The following are some examples.

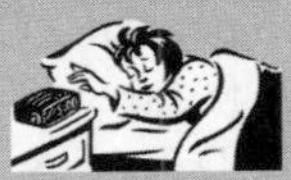

◆ To signify a major change in questioning:

THE FOOD WE EAT IS AN IMPORTANT PART OF OUR EVERYDAY LIVES. I WOULD NOW LIKE TO ASK SOME QUESTIONS ABOUT THE FOODS THAT YOU USUALLY EAT AND THE AMOUNTS OF THEM THAT YOU EAT.

- ◆ To break the monotony of a series of food frequency questions:

  NEXT, I WOULD LIKE TO ASK ABOUT BREAD AND BREAKFAST CEREALS.

- ◆ To introduce the demographic questions at the end of the questionnaire:

  FINALLY, I WOULD LIKE TO ASK A FEW QUESTIONS ABOUT YOU FOR STATISTICAL PURPOSES.

Skips or branches

It is commonly necessary to make 'skips' or branch points in a questionnaire where some succeeding questions are not applicable to all respondents. Computer-assisted interviewing has greatly reduced missing data due to failure to follow the proper skip patterns (Nicholls *et al.*1997). However, paper and pencil questionnaires must still rely on good instructions and navigational aids for the interviewer or subject to follow the skip patterns. This is especially true for self-administered questionnaires, where failure to follow the skip patterns correctly is a major source of missing data (De Leeuw 2001).

Probably the most important requirement of skip instructions is that they are placed immediately after the *answer* that leads to the branch point in the questionnaire. Skip instructions should always be worded positively ('Go to question 4') rather than negatively ('Skip question 3'). Figure 6.1 (question 4) provides an example of skip pattern instructions for a self-administered questionnaire, using arrows and instructions to show the skip pattern and using arrows and boxes to show the sub-questions. It is more important to make the path clear for those who are to complete the sub-questions, as was done in the example, than for those who should skip them. Complex branching designs are usually only possible in interviewer-administered questionnaires.

A device that may be used to avoid skips in a self-administered questionnaire is the inclusion of a specific 'inapplicable' category among the alternative answers, as in the following example:

HOW OFTEN DO YOU CUT THE FAT OFF MEAT BEFORE YOU COOK OR EAT IT?

NEVER	☐
LESS THAN HALF THE TIME	☐
MORE THAN HALF THE TIME	☐
ALWAYS	☐
I NEVER EAT MEAT	☐

Here, use of 'I never eat meat' as a response category provides an alternative answer for everyone and eliminates the need for a skip.

Conclusion

The conclusion of either a self-administered questionnaire or an interview should include an expression of appreciation and should provide an opportunity for the respondent to make comments. A self-administered questionnaire could also include a request for the respondent to check that all questions have been answered (or that all pages have been completed, for a long questionnaire). The conclusion should also contain the address for the return of a mailed questionnaire; while an addressed return envelope will usually be included, it may have become separated from the questionnaire. Interviewer-administered questionnaires should also provide for the entry of the interviewer's comments.

Questionnaire format

Formatting questions

The principles of formatting individual questions are summarized in Table 6.2. Examples of formatting interviewer-administered questions have been given in some of the questions shown in the preceding pages. Figure 6.1 gives examples of formatting self-administered questions.

Table 6.2 Principles of formatting individual questions (for self-administered questionnaires and interviews)

- Identify separate parts of questions with different typefaces

  For interviewer-administered questionnaires:

    CAPITAL LETTERS for the question
    Bold face for the alternative responses that are not to be read to respondent
    BOLD CAPITAL letters for the alternative responses to be read
    Italics for instructions not to be read
    CAPITAL ITALICS for instructions to be read

  For self-administered questionnaires:

    Bold face for questions
    Regular typeface for alternative responses
    Italics for instructions

- Include specific instructions and prompts (for interviewers) with the question as needed

- Record responses to closed-ended questions by check boxes

- Use vertical answer formats (except for scales)

- Provide spaces or boxes for coding open-ended questions

- Consider data capture methods when making design decisions, e.g. if key entry is to be used, precode closed-ended responses

---

The principles require little explanation. The different typefaces for questions, responses, and instructions help to lead the interviewer or respondent to the correct parts of the question. The use of capital letters (of the appropriate typeface) provides a consistent cue to the interviewer of what is to be read aloud. Putting any specific instructions or prompts (for interviewers) next to the question eliminates the need for complex initial instructions and serves as a reminder at the time the instruction is needed. The use of checkboxes for closed-ended questions is easy to understand, and a vertical format for the alternative responses makes it clear which box goes with which response. An exception to this is response scales or ratings (e.g. a scale for an attitude or for degree of pain). These categories may be better visualized on self-administered questionnaires if they are on a horizontal line (e.g. question 3 in Figure 6.1). Coding boxes or spaces are also needed for open-ended questions, including those that will be coded after the interview (e.g. occupational coding).

Finally, the method of data-capture needs to be considered when making formatting decisions. When the responses to a questionnaire are to be key-entered, the response options need to be precoded into numbers that are printed on the form to facilitate key-entry. For example:

Yes $\square_1$
No $\square_2$

It is also helpful to the key entry personnel if the responses to be entered are consistently placed on the right hand margin, rather than throughout each page of the questionnaire. Formats need to be tailored to the specific requirements of other data-capture methods, including computer-assisted interviews, web surveys, and self-administered questionnaires that will be processed by optical mark or character recognition. Dillman (2000) provides a detailed description of additional format considerations when designing web surveys and surveys to be processed by optical recognition.

Formatting self-administered questionnaires

Presentation of the questionnaire is particularly important if it is to be self-administered, both for ease of use and to give an authoritative appearance that will encourage response. Dillman (2002) proposed a Tailored Design Method, based on decades of experience and on numerous studies conducted by him and others. This is outlined in Table 6.3.

The questionnaire should be printed in booklet form so that will open flat on a table. The first page should have the title of the project and instructions for completing the questionnaire. A graphic illustration may make it more attractive to the target population. Use of coloured paper may increase

Table 6.3 Formatting self-administered questionnaires[a]

- ◆ Use a booklet format
- ◆ Put title of project and instructions on first page
- ◆ Include a graphic and/or colour for visual interest
- ◆ Consider coloured background with white response boxes
- ◆ Use a two-column format
- ◆ Consecutively number pages and questions
- ◆ Make skip patterns clear, e.g. through use of arrows after response and instructions

---

[a] Adapted from Dillman (2000).

response rates by a small degree (Edwards *et al.* 2002). Missing data may be reduced if subjects are asked to write their answers, either open-ended or check marks, in white boxes which stand out from a coloured background. A two-column format for the questions is easier to read because participants may skip words when reading longer lines of text. Two columns also allows more questions per page. Use of the vertical answer format will generally increase the amount of space between questions, and it is important that the questionnaire is not too congested. An example of many of these principles is given in Figure 6.1.

It is important for the respondent to be able to see the path of questions easily. Pages and questions should be numbered consecutively, and subsections of questions should be indented and identified with letters rather than numbers. Question numbers should extend to the left of questions to stand out. As far as possible, questions should not extend over more than one page. As discussed above, clear skip patterns are particularly important in self-administered questionnaires.

As noted in Table 6.2, the questions should be in bold typeface, the closed-ended response list should be in regular typeface, and italics are often used for instructions. Certain visual changes, such as underlining words or using capital letters, can be used to emphasize a change in concept, for example when the time frame differs between questions. However, such visual changes should not be over-used.

Matrix formats

The collection of data about a number of exposures of interest to epidemiology is done most efficiently in the form of a matrix. For example, all places of residence, all occupations, or all uses of a particular medication can be recorded on one axis, and a number of specific details regarding each episode or period of exposure can be recorded on the other. The conversion of such matrices to a vertical single-column format increases the length of question-naires substantially and is tedious to the interviewer or respondent. Therefore it is desirable to retain the matrix form in the questionnaire if possible. However, a matrix adds complexity to a self-administered questionnaire, and this may increase respondent burden and lead to missing data.

Figure 6.2 shows a matrix that was used to collect occupational information in a self-administered questionnaire. The data sought were limited in scope,

12. Have you ever worked in the timber or woodworking industries?

☐ No → *Go to question 13, next page*
☐ Yes
↓

If yes, describe your work with wood or timber in the spaces below.
Here is an example:

Jobs in timber or woodworking	Type of industry	Your job	Year job began	Year job ended
Last job	*furniture making*	*french polisher*	*1996*	*2006*

Now describe your work here:

Jobs in timber or woodworking	Type of industry	Your job	Year job began	Year job ended
Last job				
Job before that				
Job before that				
Job before that				
Job before that				
Job before that				

If there is not enough space, please detail the additional jobs on a separate sheet of paper and attach it to questionnaire.

Figure 6.2 An open-ended question with matrix response intended for use in a self-administered questionnaire.

and the matrix was kept small enough to fit on one page. The example included in the question was intended to show the respondent the form and detail of response that was desired, in the hope that instructions for the question could be kept to a minimum.

Asking about behaviours that vary over time

Epidemiologists are often interested in exposures occurring over many years or decades. A behaviour which varies appreciably over the time period of interest often presents difficulty in the design of questionnaires. It will rarely be sufficient to summarize it by way of a simple question on its 'usual' frequency, both because this summary is likely to introduce error and because the pattern of variation of the behaviour with time may be important (see Chapter 1). It may be unreasonably burdensome on the respondent to attempt to elicit a usual pattern for the behaviour (e.g. smoking) for each year of what is considered to be the aetiologically relevant time period. One solution is division of that period into larger but arbitrarily determined intervals of time (e.g. 0–4 years before diagnosis, 5–9 years before diagnosis, etc., or decades of age).

Another approach to measuring time-variable behaviour is to focus on obtaining details of the behaviour in periods of life in which it has been reasonably stable. Because this approach is complex, it would only be suitable for interviewer-administered questionnaires. Essentially, data are collected in a matrix format, except that reported changes in the subject's pattern of exposure over time determine when a new row is to be completed. This approach has been used in the Lifetime Drinking History described by Skinner and Sheu (1982), in which subjects are first asked about their alcohol consumption in the first year that they drank on a regular basis. Major changes in their drinking patterns are then identified chronologically. For each pattern, questions are asked about the frequency of drinking, typical and maximum quantity consumed per occasion, types of beverage, and when this pattern of drinking changed.

This approach has also been used to document exposure to the sun in a case–control study of skin cancer conducted following a survey of the prevalence of skin cancer in the town of Geraldton, Western Australia (Kricker *et al.* 1991). Subjects first completed, on their own, a life calendar covering each change of residence, school, occupation, and the number of days they worked each week. At interview, they were asked to identify, on the calendar, years in which major changes in their outdoor activity took place. They were prompted with the suggestion that these changes '. . . could've been due to things like changes in where you lived, changes in the sport you played, changes of school, different jobs, changes in the number of days you worked, and by marriage'. Having identified these years of change and, by inference, periods of comparatively stable outdoor activity, subjects were asked detailed questions about outdoor activity in each period. These questions included the typical numbers of hours outdoors between 9 a.m. and 5 p.m. and 10 a.m. and 2 p.m., on working and non-working days, in both cooler and warmer months of the year, and during summer holidays, frequency of sunbathing, extent of suntan, frequency and severity of sunburn, use of sunscreen preparations, and wearing a hat.

Aids to recall

Disease may be influenced by exposures which occurred many years or decades before diagnosis. Therefore epidemiologists have long used a variety of approaches to improve recall of past exposures by subjects. These include use of lists of alternative answers, use of a life events calendar, and lead-in questions to help the participant recall a specific time period or event. These approaches are now supported by an increasingly strong body of research on memory (Bradburn *et al.* 1987; Jobe and Mingay 1989; Schwarz and Sudman 1996; Tourangeau *et al.* 2000).

The most commonly used aid to recall is the list of alternative answers supplied as part of a self-administered questionnaire. In an interview, this list may be provided in the form of a card given to the respondent. A list of possible answers may also be given for open-ended questions (e.g. a list of recreational physical activities), but it is essential that it be as comprehensive as possible or it may bias response. Where the list of possible answers to an open-ended question is very long, a list of headings under which all responses might fall can be used instead to stimulate recall.

In questions about use of the oral contraceptive pill, it is common to show the respondent photographs of all present and past formulations to assist her in eliciting the brand actually used. The photographs include the pill itself, the packaging, and the name. Similarly, Beresford and Coker (1989) found that six out of 14 women who had used post-menopausal hormone replacement therapy for 6 months or more were assisted in their recall of the name and dose by reference to photographs of preparations which had been in use over the preceding 15 years.

Another effective aid to recall is the *life events calendar*, on which subjects are asked to place personal landmarks (e.g. marriage, birth of children) and/or job and residential histories. As a means of improving recall of use of birth control methods, Daling and colleagues (Holt *et al.* 1989; J. Daling, personal communication) have used a simple month-by-year matrix calendar on which marriages and periods of 'living as married' were first recorded by use of a black marker pen, pregnancies were recorded by use of a blue marker, and periods of birth control use were recorded, with reference to the other details on the calendar, by use of a red marker. Details for each of the periods of birth control use were then sought and recorded on the main data form. Engel *et al.* (2001) were able to elicit more jobs from study participants, particularly jobs from the distant past, by use of a life events calendar than from questions on recall of job history alone. Use of a calendar of residences, schools, and jobs to assist in recall of outdoor activities has been described earlier in this chapter.

Use of a life events calendar also improves the accuracy of recall of the *dates* of events, as well as recall of the events (Means and Loftus 1991). Research on memory has shown that most events are not stored with dates. Instead, people attach dates to events by relating them to datable events (e.g. marriage) and time periods (college, jobs, places of residence).

The use of a life events calendar is one example of the use of autobiographical sequences to aid recall (Bradburn *et al.* 1987). *Autobiographical sequences are groups of events clustered in time*, and often organized within some wider framework (e.g. a job or an illness), within which memory appears to be organized. Thus any means of entry into an autobiographical sequence, whether by way of calendar time, place lived, or through some highly salient event, such as childbirth or an illness, may assist in recall of events or behaviours of low salience. Thus, for example, asking first about illnesses which may have been indications for the use of particular medications may assist in recall of those medications. In two studies it was found that open-ended questions about prescription drug use during pregnancy without aids to recall only yielded 40–65 per cent of drugs eventually recalled. Additionally, drugs were recalled when questions were then cited on use of drugs for specific indications, and another 15–40 per cent of drugs were recalled only when the specific drug was named (Mitchell *et al.* 1986; de Jong-van den Berg *et al.* 1993).

A simple aid to recall is simply allowing the subject some time to think about the question. Thus longer introductions or redundant wording would allow a few more seconds for retrieval of information. Telephone interviews are at a disadvantage with regard to recall because silent pauses are more awkward on the telephone, and subjects might respond too quickly to retrieve the memory fully.

Recall may also be aided by asking the subject to refer to his/her personal records where they may be relevant. This is more easily done in a mailed questionnaire, where the respondent can refer to the records at leisure, than it is in a personal interview. However, these records may be made available in an interview by notifying the subjects in advance of the proposed lines of questioning and asking that they collect together whatever records they may have.

Pre-testing questionnaires

Overview

Pre-testing is an essential part of the development of all questionnaires, regardless of whether or not they have been substantially based on previous questionnaires. The objectives of pre-testing are to identify questions that are poorly understood, are ambiguous, or evoke hostile or other undesirable responses. Some of the questions that a pre-test should answer are (Dillman 2000) as follows.

* Are all the words understood?
* Are the questions interpreted similarly by all respondents?
* Does each closed-ended question have an answer that applies to each respondent?
* Are some questions not answered?
* Do some questions elicit uninterpretable answers?

Table 6.4 lists techniques of pre-testing questionnaires These include traditional methods such as expert reviews, debriefing meetings with interviewers after they have conducted a number of interviews, and analysis of the distribution of item responses, including percentage non-response. Also listed in the table are newer cognitive and behavioural approaches to questionnaire design and pre-testing that have been developed in the field of survey research (Schwarz and Sudman 1996; Esposito and Rothgeb 1997; Jobe 2003). These include cognitive or intensive interviews with respondents, interactive coding of interviewer and respondent behaviours during the interview, and testing different questionnaire versions in small experiments. Each of these methods is described in more detail below.

Pre-testing typically involves several of these methods applied to different versions of the questionnaire as it is revised and gets closer to its final form. Some of the techniques, such as expert reviews, cognitive interviews, and experiments, are more appropriate for earlier stages of pre-testing, while others, such as item response distribution analysis and validity studies, would be done on questionnaires which are closer to finalization. (Some authors use the word *pre-test* for the early testing of the questionnaire and the phrase *pilot test* for later testing of the study field methods, including selecting subjects, recruitment, and data collection). Some of the methods, such as intensive interviews and interactive coding, might be too costly in terms of time and money for most epidemiological studies. However, even when time and budget are restricted, one should at a minimum seek expert review of the questionnaire (e.g. from colleagues), conduct a pre-test on at least 20 test subjects followed by debriefings (of respondents for self-administered

Table 6.4 Methods of pre-testing questionnaires (for self-administered questionnaires and interviews)

EXPERT/PEER REVIEW for content, wording, and format

COGNITIVE/INTENSIVE INTERVIEWS WITH RESPONDENTS to see how items were understood and answered

    Think-aloud techniques

    Paraphrasing the question by respondent

    Specific probes about how question was answered

INTERVIEWER DEBRIEFINGS to identify items with problems

    Debriefing questionnaires

    Group sessions

RESPONDENT DEBRIEFINGS to identify items with problems

    Debriefing questionnaires or interviews

    Focus groups

OBSERVATION OF INTERVIEWS and POSSIBLE INTERACTION CODING to identify interviewer and respondent behaviours for each question, such as rewording of question by interviewer or uncertainty about the answer expressed by respondent

ITEM RESPONSE DISTRIBUTION ANALYSIS

    Distribution of valid responses

    Percentage 'don't know"

    Percentage missing

EXPERIMENTS, e.g. comparison of two versions of question wording

RELIABILITY AND VALIDITY STUDIES to quantify repeatability and accuracy

questionnaires or of interviewers for interviewer-administered questionnaires), and perform an item distribution analysis. Interviewer debriefing sessions and monitoring of the distribution of item responses should also be done at the beginning of actual data collection and, if necessary, further changes made to the questionnaire or protocol to resolve problems.

Ideally, the subjects in questionnaire pre-tests should be similar to the target population of the parent epidemiological study in terms of age, education, and study eligibility criteria. However, for a first pre-test, one could use a small sample of convenience such as co-workers, friends, or relatives of the interviewers. The mode of administration (self-administration, telephone, or in-person interview) should be the same as it will be in the parent epidemiological study.

Expert reviews

A good first step in pre-testing is to ask experts in the content areas or in questionnaire development to review the questionnaire and make comments.

Often one's professional colleagues can fill this role. They can help determine whether all necessary items have been included to meet the aims of the study, as well as providing advice on wording, format, etc. The study statistician and data processing supervisor also need to review the content and format of questionnaire to identify problems, before data collection begins, which might otherwise arise at the data processing and analysis phase.

Cognitive/intensive interviews

Cognitive interviews are a useful tool in refining questions on new or complex exposure areas. Cognitive or intensive interviews with participants gather detailed information about how the respondents formulate their answers to key questions (Belson 1981; Willis *et al.* 1991; Schwarz and Sudman 1996; Willis *et al.* 1999). Responding to a question involves several cognitive steps: understanding the question, retrieving the information from memory, judgement (such as estimation when an exact number cannot be recalled), censoring the response (typically to be more socially desirable), and providing an answer in the response format requested (Tourangeau *et al.* 2000). In *cognitive interviews*, the interviewer asks respondents to 'think out loud' while they are coming up with their response, or to explain how they came to their response after the answer has been given. This can aid the researcher in understanding whether a question is misunderstood by some subjects or whether it is complex and needs to be decomposed into simpler questions. Respondents can also be instructed to state when any question is difficult, annoying, or embarrassing to answer. *Intensive interviews* have the same elements as cognitive interviews, but also ask the subject to paraphrase the question after it is asked and give a confidence rating of the accuracy of their answer.

Cognitive interviews can also use item-specific probes to understand how specific concepts are understood. For example, for the question, 'How many people are there in your household?', the following questions (among others) would be appropriate.

+ Did the respondent include him/herself in the count?
+ To what period did the respondent think the question related, i.e. if a household member had been temporarily away, would he/she have been included?
+ How did the respondent interpret the term household?

This is a demanding form of pre-test; Belson (1981) suggested that each respondent should be asked in detail about only three or four questions. However, this method has the potential to uncover problems in questions that might otherwise be missed.

Interviewer and respondent debriefings

Debriefings can be interviews, questionnaires, or group meetings conducted immediately or soon after the questionnaire is completed. Debriefings can be with the interviewer or respondent.

Interviewers should always be debriefed after they have pre-tested the questionnaire on a number of participants. They can be asked which items caused the most problems in terms of obtaining adequate answers from participants, and for those items, about what percentage of the time there was a problem. Experienced interviewers are very knowledgeable about which questions are misunderstood by respondents or are too taxing for the respondent to answer. Interviewer debriefing can take the form of a debriefing questionnaire or a group session with several interviewers where problem questions and possible modifications are elicited.

Respondent debriefings can be interviews, questionnaires, or focus groups. Respondents should be told that they are pilot participants before they complete the questionnaire or interview, and that their help is needed to identify any problems with the questionnaire. In the debriefing, they should be asked about which questions were confusing or hardest to answer and why, for which questions the answer they wanted to give was not an alternate response, whether any questions were offensive to them, and whether they found it easy to follow the skip patterns. Questions should also be asked about specific items about which the researcher has concerns; for example, did the participant notice that the time reference changed for a particular question? If the debriefing is an interview, the respondent should be asked why he/she skipped any questions that the interviewer notes should have been answered. Finally, respondents should be asked for any additional comments and suggestions.

Interaction or behaviour coding

In *interaction or behaviour coding*, a monitor listens to the interview (usually a tape recording) and codes specific behaviours of the interviewer and the respondent for each question (Schwarz and Sudman 1996; Dykema *et al.* 1997). An example of a behaviour coding scheme is given in Table 6.5. Length of pause between the end of the question and the answer (reaction time or response latency) is sometimes coded as an indicator of difficulty in answering the question. By analysing the frequencies of behaviours for each question, one can determine problem questions, for example which questions interviewers do not read as worded (often to attempt to improve the meaning of the question). Questions with a moderate proportion (e.g. 10 per cent or more) of respondent codes for uncertainty, uncodeable answers,

Table 6.5 Interviewer–respondent interaction coding scheme[a]

INTERVIEWER BEHAVIOURS in question-asking (assign one code only)	
Substantive change	Makes a substantive change in reading question as written
Incorrect prompt	Repeats question not as written or suggests an answer
Skips question	Skips applicable questions
Reads wrong question	Reads question that was not supposed to be read
RESPONDENT BEHAVIOURS (code all that apply)	
Interrupt	Interrupts question with an answer
Uncertain	Expresses uncertainty about question, requests clarification
Qualified	Qualifies answer
Uncodeable	Response does not meet question objectives, uncodeable
Don't know	Offers a 'don't know' response
Refusal	Refuses to answer

[a] Adapted from Dykema *et al.* (1997).

or interruptions can also be used to identify problematic questions which could be phrased better.

Dykema *et al.* (1997) tested the usefulness of behaviour coding in predicting questions with large measurement error. They recorded interviewer–respondent interaction codes (as shown in Table 6.5) for each question in a health-related questionnaire. They then evaluated the accuracy of the subjects' answers by comparing the responses in the health interview with medical records to establish whether the behaviour codes indicated inaccuracies. The interviewer behaviours were not associated with inaccuracy (see Chapter 7). However, if any of the respondent behaviours occurred for a question, that question was more likely to be inaccurately answered by that respondent. In particular, initial 'don't know' and qualified answers were associated with inaccuracy. Thus if these codes occur frequently for a question, it may be an indication that the question as phrased is difficult to answer accurately.

Item non-response and response distributions

After a reasonable number of representative pilot participants have completed the pre-test questionnaire/interview, the distribution of responses to each question should be reviewed. The percentage of non-response for each question is a particular concern. There are two types of non-response: missing/refusal and explicit 'don't know'. A major source of missing data in self-administered questionnaires is subjects not following the skip patterns. Improving the format of the questionnaire to make the skip pattern clearer could reduce the amount of missing data. Another reason for missing/refusal is the sensitivity of the question. The techniques presented earlier in this chapter for asking sensitive questions might reduce the amount of non-response.

The second purpose of reviewing item response distributions is to review the frequency of each response category when questions are closed-ended. Response categories should be changed if some responses were selected by a very low or high percentage of respondents. An exception to this is when certain extreme response categories are given to encourage reporting of socially undesirable behaviours.

Experiments

As part of pre-testing, two (or more) versions of each question can be tested, usually with each questionnaire version given to a different group of subjects. The versions of each question can be different phrasing of the question or different categories for the answers for closed-ended questions. The two versions can be compared based on interviewer debriefings, respondent debriefings, item analysis, behaviour coding, or comparison with more accurate measures of the exposure (e.g. records or diaries). Interviewer debriefing questions could include: Which form of the questionnaire was easier to administer? Why was this form easier and the other more difficult? From this information, the researcher can select the best alternative of each question for the final questionnaire.

Reliability and validity studies

Conducting a validity or reliability study to evaluate the accuracy of an exposure measurement can be an important part of pre-testing. If one determines before an epidemiological study begins that the exposure is not measured with reasonable accuracy, then the researcher can continue to search for or develop a more accurate method. Chapter 4 covers the design, analysis, and interpretation of validity and reliability studies.

Revising the questionnaire

Typically a questionnaire is tested and revised several times before being used in the field. Once problems are identified during a pre-test, they can be resolved through changes in questionnaire wording, questionnaire format, or interviewer training. However, often a revised question which solves problems identified by some respondents will lead to problems for other respondents. For many questions, there will be at least a small percentage of respondents who have trouble understanding the question, or who have personal circumstances which make the question difficult for them to answer. Often adding explanations to make the question clearer to some respondents will make the question longer, more burdensome, or even confusing to others. Thus it seems reasonable to modify only questions that are problematic for a moderate proportion of subjects (e.g. 10 per cent or more) and/or have a simple solution. For example, in pre-testing the self-administered question 'How many flights of stairs do you climb each day at home, work, or elsewhere?', some respondents questioned whether to count going up and down a flight of stairs as one or two flights. Others asked questions such as whether climbing up two floors three times a day counts as two, three or six flights per day, although most seemed to understand that the answer in this case should be six. Rather than adding lengthy explanations to solve these problems for a small percentage of subjects, this question was simply changed to 'How many flights of stairs do you climb *up* each day?'

Translating questionnaires

The conduct of international multicentre epidemiological studies often necessitates the translation of a questionnaire into a language other than that in which it was first developed. Translation may also be required when a population contains ethnic minority groups. There is evidence that the intramethod reliability of some questions in a questionnaire is greater when they are administered in the respondent's mother tongue, even when the respondent is multilingual (Becklake *et al.* 1987).

There are four phases in translation of a questionnaire (Del Greco *et al.* 1987):

* preliminary translation
* evaluation of the preliminary translation
* ascertainment of cross-language equivalence
* assessment of validity and reliability.

The preliminary translation aims at producing a translated questionnaire which is as near as possible in meaning to the original. It is best done by someone who understands both the overall objective of the questionnaire and the intent of each question, as well as being expert in both the original language and the language into which the translation is being made. The usual method of evaluating the preliminary translation is to have it translated back into the first language by someone who has not seen the original version. The back-translated version is then compared with the original version, and further work done on questions that have changed their meaning. Some questions may go through the process of re-translation and back-translation several times before they are considered to have been translated correctly. A complementary approach to back-translation in evaluating the preliminary translation is to have bilingual experts evaluate the translation of each question in terms of its content, meaning, clarity of expression, and comparability to the original question.

Cross-language equivalence is determined by administering both the original and the translated versions of the questionnaire to bilingual subjects, and comparing their responses to each. It is usual to give half the subjects the original questionnaire first and half the translated questionnaire first to minimize order effects. A high correlation between the responses is taken to indicate cross-language equivalence.

Del Greco *et al.* (1987) noted that the reliability and validity of the questionnaire may not be maintained after translation, and it should be re-evaluated in the translated form. However, any change in validity and reliability could be due as much to cultural differences between the two populations as to any problems with the translation.

Where only a few interviews need to be conducted in a foreign language, it may be convenient to use a bilingual interviewer who translates from the original questionnaire as he/she interviews. Alternatively, an interpreter may be used. In either of these approaches, it is much more likely than with a carefully translated questionnaire that the questions will not be translated correctly and erroneous responses will be obtained.

Summary

The objectives of questionnaire design are to obtain, with minimum error, measurements of exposure variables essential to the objectives of the study and to create an instrument that is easy for both the interviewer and subject to use, and is easy to process and analyse.

Open-ended questions should be used as far as possible to seek the simple factual information that is most commonly needed in epidemiological studies. If closed-ended questions are used, the alternative answers offered should be simple, brief, mutually exclusive, and exhaustive.

The words used in questions should be the usual working tools of the respondents; jargon and complex, vague, and loaded words should be avoided. Questions should:

- contain only one concept
- not require any calculations
- have an unambiguous time reference.

Questions that ask about behaviour or attributes which are socially desirable or undesirable present a particular threat to subjects and require special care in wording.

The way in which questions are formatted, the order in which they are presented, the structure of the questionnaire as a whole, and the way it is printed are all important in facilitating its use by interviewers and respondents, in ensuring ease and accuracy of processing data from the questionnaire, and in minimizing error.

Aids may be used to assist subjects in recalling information. They include:

- lists of alternative answers
- photographs of specific agents to which the subject may have been exposed
- a calendar on which key dates are marked
- reference to personal records.

All questionnaires should be pre-tested before their use in the research study begins. The particular objectives of pre-testing are to see whether the questions are understood and elicit appropriate responses and to ensure that, where alternative answers have been provided, they cover the full range of relevant answers. Pre-testing should include, at least, initial evaluation by peers and testing on a sample of subjects from the population to be studied.

References

Aday, L.A. (1996). *Designing and Conducting Health Surveys: A Comprehensive Guide* (2nd edn). Jossey-Bass, San Francisco, CA.

Becklake, M.R., Freeman, S., Goldsmith, C., *et al.* (1987). Respiratory questionnaires in occupational studies: their use in multilingual work forces on the Witwatersrand. *International Journal of Epidemiology*, **16**, 606–11.

Belson, W.A. (1981). *The Design and Understanding of Survey Questions*. Gower, Aldershot, Hampshire.

Bennett, A.E. and Ritchie, K. (1975). *Questionnaires in Medicine*. Oxford University Press, London.

Beresford, S.A.A. and Coker, A.L. (1989). Pictorially assisted recall of past hormone use in case–control studies. *American Journal of Epidemiology*, **130**, 202–5.

Blair, E., Sudman, S., Bradburn, N.M., and Stocking, C. (1977). How to ask questions about drinking and sex: response effects in measuring consumer behavior. *Journal of Marketing Research*, **14**, 316–21.

Bradburn, N.M., Rips, L.J., and Shevell, S. K. (1987). Answering autobiographical questions: the impact of memory and inference on surveys. *Science*, **236**, 157–61.

de Jong-van den Berg, L.T.W., Waardenburg, C.M., Haaijer-Ruskamp, F.M., Dukes, M.N.G., and Wesseling, H. (1993). Drug use in pregnancy: a comparative appraisal of data collecting methods. *European Journal of Clinical Pharmacology*, **45**, 9–14.

De Leeuw, E.D. (2001). Reducing missing data in surveys: an overview of methods. *Quality & Quantity*, **35**, 147–60.

Del Greco, L., Walop, W., and Eastridge, L. (1987). Questionnaire development. III: Translation. *Canadian Medical Association Journal*, **136**, 817–18.

Dillman, D.A. (2000). *Mail and Internet Surveys: The Tailored Design Method* (2nd edn). Wiley, New York.

Dykema, J., Lepkowski, J.M., and Blixt, S. (1997). The effect of interviewer and respondent behavior on data quality: analysis of interaction coding in a validation study. In *Survey Measurement and Process Quality* (ed. L. Lyberg, P. Biemer, M. Collins, *et al.*), pp. 287–310. Wiley, New York.

Edwards, P., Roberts, I., Clarke, M., *et al.* (2002). Increasing response rates to postal questionnaires: systematic review. *British Medical Journal*, **324**, 1183–91.

Engel, L.S., Keifer, M.C., and Zahm, S.H. (2001). Comparison of a traditional questionnaire with an icon/calendar-based questionnaire to assess occupational history. *American Journal of Industrial Medicine*, **40**, 502–11.

Esposito, J.L. and Rothgeb, J.M. (1997). Evaluating survey data: making the transition from pretesting to quality assessment. In *Survey Measurement and Process Quality* (ed. L. Lyberg, P. Biemer, M. Collins, *et al.*), pp. 541–573. Wiley, New York.

Frey, J.H. (1986). An experiment with a confidentiality reminder in a telephone survey. *Public Opinion Quarterly*, **50**, 267–9.

Helsing, K.J. and Comstock, G.W. (1975). Response variation and location of questions within a questionnaire. *International Journal of Epidemiology*, **5**, 125–30.

Holt, V.L., Daling, J.R., Voigt, L.F., *et al.* (1989). Induced abortion and the risk of subsequent ectopic pregnancy. *American Journal of Public Health*, **79**, 1234–8.

Jobe, J.B. (2003). Cognitive psychology and self-reports: models and methods. *Quality of Life Research*, **12**, 219–27.

Jobe, J.B. and Mingay, D.J. (1989). Cognitive research improves questionnaires. *American Journal of Public Health*, **79**, 1053–5.

Kricker, A., Armstrong, B.K., Epglish, D.R., and Heenan, P.J. (1991). Pigmentary and cutaneous risk factors for non-melanocytic skin cancer: a case–control study. *International Journal of Cancer*, **48**, 650–662.

Krosnick, J.A. and Alwin, D.F. (1987). An evaluation of a cognitive theory of response-order effects in survey measurement. *Public Opinion Quarterly*, **51**, 201–19.

Leigh, J.H. and Martin, C.R. (1987). 'Don't know' item nonresponse in a telephone survey: effects of question form and respondent characteristics. *Journal of Marketing Research*, **24**, 418–24.

McFarland, S.G. (1981). Effects of question order on survey responses. *Public Opinion Quarterly*, **45**, 208–15.

Means, B. and Loftus, E. (1991). When personal history repeats itself: decomposing memories for recurring events. *Applied Cognitive Psychology*, **5**, 297–318.

Mitchell, A.A., Cottier, L.B., and Shapiro, S. (1986). Effect of questionnaire design on recall of drug exposure in pregnancy. *American Journal of Epidemiology*, **123**, 670–6.

Nicholls, W.L. II, Baker, R.P., and Martin, J. (1997). The effect of new data collection technologies on survey data quality. In *Survey Measurement and Process Quality* (ed. L. Lyberg, P. Biemer, M. Collins, *et al.*), pp. 221–48. Wiley, New York.

Poe, G.S., Seeman, I., McLaughlin, J., Mehl, E., and Dietz, M. (1988). 'Don't know' boxes in factual questions in a mail questionnaire. Effects on level and quality of response. *Public Opinion Quarterly*, **52**, 212–22.

Schuman, H., Presser, S., and Ludwig, J. (1981). Content effects on survey questions about abortion. *Public Opinion Quarterly*, **45**, 216–23.

Schwarz, N. and Sudman, S. (ed.) (1996). *Answering Questions: Methodology for Determining Cognitive and Communicative Processes in Survey Research*. Jossey-Bass, San Francisco, CA.

Schwarz, N., Hippler, H.J., Deutsch, B., and Strack, F. (1985). Response scales: effects of category range on reported behaviour and comparative judgements. *Public Opinion Quarterly*, **49**, 388–95.

Singer, M. (1985). Mental processes of question answering. In *The Psychology of Questions* (ed. A.C. Graesser and J.B. Black), pp. 121–56. Erlbaum, Hillsdale, NJ.

Skinner, H.A. and Sheu, W.J. (1982). Reliability of alcohol use indices. The lifetime drinking history and the MAST. *Journal of Studies on Alcohol*, **43**, 1157–70.

Smith, T.W. (1987). That which we call welfare by any other name would smell sweeter. An analysis of the impact of question wording on response patterns. *Public Opinion Quarterly*, **51**, 75–83.

Sudman, S. and Andersen, R. M. (1977). Health survey research instruments. In *Advances in Health Survey Research Methods: Proceedings of a National Invitational Conference* (ed. L.G. Reeder), DHEW Publication No. (HRA) 77–3154, pp. 7–12. US Department of Health, Education and Welfare, Washington, DC.

Sudman, S. and Bradburn, N.M. (1983). *Asking Questions: A Practical Guide to Questionnaire Design*. Jossey-Bass, San Francisco, CA.

Tourangeau, R., Rips, L.J., and Rasinski, K. (2000). *The Psychology of Survey Response*. Cambridge University Press.

Willis, G.B., Royston, P., and Bercini, D. (1991). The use of verbal report methods in the development and testing of survey questionnaires. *Applied Cognitive Psychology*, **5**, 175–92.

Willis, G., DeMaio, T., and Harris-Kojetin, B. (1999). Is the bandwagon headed to the methodological promised land? Evaluating the validity of cognitive interviewing techniques. In *Cognition and Survey Research* (ed. M. Sirken, D.J. Herrmann, S. Schechter, N. Schwarz, J. Tanur, and R. Tourangeau), pp. 133–54. Wiley, New York.

7

The personal interview

A series of studies in the early decades of survey research raised the issue of interviewer effects on responses. A classic demonstration was Rice's 1929 study of the causes of destitution. Comparing the results obtained from poverty-stricken respondents by two different interviewers, he discovered that the data collected by one interviewer showed overindulgence in alcohol as the most common cause of destitution while the other interviewer found social and economic conditions the most frequent causes. The case for interviewer bias appeared to be established when it was learned that the first interviewer was a prohibitionist and the second was a socialist ...
(Cannell et al. 1981)

Introduction

The personal interview, whether face-to-face or by telephone, is the most common method of collecting data on exposure in epidemiological studies. The objectives of a research interview are the same as those of a research questionnaire: to obtain measurements of exposure variables essential to the objectives of the study and to minimize error in these measurements.

While it is possible to use essentially identical questionnaires to collect data from study subjects by way of either interview or self-administration, the personal interview differs from the self-administered questionnaire in one very important respect: the presence of the interviewer. On the one hand, the interviewer may reduce error by increasing the response rate, motivating the subject to respond well, and probing to obtain complete data when the responses volunteered fall short of what is desired. On the other hand, the interviewer may increase error if, by his/her appearance, manner, method of administration of the questionnaire, or method of recording of the responses, he/she exerts a qualitative influence on the subject's responses.

This chapter, then, will deal principally with the role of the interviewer in the research interview and the ways in which the benefits of having an interviewer can be maximized and the potential disadvantages minimized. Other subjects covered include types and styles of interviews, the optimal circumstances for an interview, and aspects of telephone interviewing which differ from face-to-face interviewing.

Interviewer error

Types of interviewer error

Interviewer error can take several forms (Hyman *et al.* 1954; Groves 1989; Fowler 2002).

- *Asking errors:* omitting questions or changing the wording of questions.
- *Probing errors:* failing to probe when necessary, biased probing, irrelevant probing, inadequate probing, or preventing the respondent from saying all that he/she wishes to say.
- *Recording errors:* recording something not said, not recording something said, or incorrectly recording what was said.
- *Flagrant cheating:* recording a response when a question is not asked or answered.
- *Interviewer interaction with respondent:* the interviewer's age, sex, race, attitudes, or manner influence the accuracy of the responses given by the subject.

Examples of interviewer error

That these errors do occur has been amply demonstrated in many studies, from which the following examples are drawn.

In a classical study, the American Jewish Committee in association with the National Opinion Research Center studied 15 comparatively inexperienced interviewers. Each interviewer administered a 50-question questionnaire to 12 subjects, four of whom were 'planted respondents'. One of the planted respondents played the role of a 'punctilious liberal', a person incapable of giving an unqualified categorical response to any question, although friendly to the interviewer, and another played a 'hostile bigot' who required considerable persuasion to answer many of the questions and was 'quite vicious' with the interviewer. On average, each interviewer committed 13 asking errors, 13 probing errors, eight recording errors, and four cheating errors in each interview. All except the cheating errors were highly pervasive, being committed to a similar degree by all interviewers. All interviewers cheated at least once when interviewing the 'hostile bigot'. However, four cheated only in a very minor way while another four clearly fabricated large parts of the interview. The interviewers who cheated extensively with the 'hostile bigot' also cheated more than the others when interviewing the 'punctilious liberal', although the overall prevalence of cheating with this respondent was very much less. While the presence of the planted respondents makes these results non-generalizable to the usual interview situation, they do illustrate the extent to which error may arise, especially when the respondent is difficult (Hyman *et al.* 1954).

Another illustration of interviewer error is given by Cannell *et al.* (1977). In the course of studies of the validity of data collected by in-person interview on health service use, they observed that the reporting of contacts with health services fell with increasing experience of the survey by the interviewers. Thus, for example, over five weeks of surveying in the Health Interview Survey (HIS), the proportion of hospitalizations which went unreported rose from 12.4 per cent in the first two weeks to 22.9 per cent in the last two weeks. These and other data were taken to indicate that the interviewers lost interest and enthusiasm for the task over time, and in consequence performed it less well.

Additional relevant data were obtained in the same study in which the regular HIS was compared with the same interview with additional probe questions and a special introductory statement (Cannell *et al.* 1977). The proportions of hospitalizations not reported over 5 weeks of surveys averaged 17.5 per cent for the regular HIS versus 9.0 per cent for the HIS with additional probes. Moreover, the expected increase in under-reporting with increasing duration of the survey because of interviewer fatigue was absent when the interview included additional probes and introductory material. Therefore it appears that these additions may have overcome the effects of the interviewers' loss of enthusiasm for the task, as well as improving overall reporting.

There is evidence that interviewer error may vary with particular personal characteristics of the interviewer. Some more obvious external attributes of interviewers, such as race, sex, age, and social status, are discussed below under 'selection of interviewers'. Other relevant attributes are less obvious, but may underlie subtle effects of the interviewer on the data obtained. For example, in the study described by Blair *et al.* (1977), interviewers who expected the interview to be difficult obtained 4–12 per cent lower reporting of sensitive behaviours than interviewers who did not. Elsewhere, those who expected the behaviours to be under-reported obtained fewer reports of them than those who did not (Bradburn and Sudman 1979). These observations have implications for both the selection and training of interviewers.

It is the opinion of at least some experts that modern methods of survey interviewing (e.g. the stressing of interviewer neutrality in training, the standardization of questionnaire wording and administration, and the development of non-directive probing techniques) have substantially reduced the likelihood that the interviewers' personal attitudes and beliefs affect the responses obtained (Cannell *et al.* 1981; Groves 1989; Fowler and Mangione 1990; Anderson and Olsen 2002).

Measurement of interviewer error

Only a few studies have attempted a statistical quantification of the amount of interviewer error. The two components of interviewer error are *interviewer bias*, i.e. the tendency of some interviewers to systematically promote over- or under-reporting of particular exposures by the survey subjects, and random error by the interviewers. Unfortunately, the random component or the total contribution of systematic and random interviewer error are difficult to measure. Specifically, in a reliability study comparing the same interviewer re-interviewing the same set of subjects or two interviewers on the same set of subjects, much of the disagreement between the two interviews could be due to respondent error rather then interviewer error. These types of studies cannot separate the relative contribution of the interviewer versus the respondent to lack of reliability.

Interviewer bias is more easily assessed than the total interviewer error, particularly in studies in which interviewers are randomly (or at least not systematically) assigned to subjects. As noted in Chapter 5, the researcher should compare the distribution of responses to questions among interviewers during the course of data collection. This could identify systematic differences which may indicate differences between interviewers in implementing certain questions. Another way of quantifying the degree of interviewer bias across interviewers (i.e. the systematic differences between interviewers but not the random component of interviewer error) is by the *interviewer intraclass correlation* ρ_{int}, which is the ratio of the variance between interviewers to the total variance of a measure (Groves 1989) (ρ_{int} can be computed as the intraclass correlation R_3, as described in Chapter 4, except that the repeated measures are repeated subjects for each interviewer, rather than repeated interviews for each subject). A low ρ_{int} indicates low interviewer systematic error.

Groves (1989) summarized seven studies of interviewer bias across hundreds of variables. He reported that, on average, $\rho_{int} = .03$, i.e. 3 per cent of the total variance of the variables of interest was due to interviewer systematic bias. However,several studies have reported interviewer effects as high as 20 per cent for some variables. One study used characteristics of the survey question to predict the magnitude of the interviewer variability. The difficulty of the question (cognitive burden) was the main question characteristic which increased variability between interviewers. Difficult opinion questions led to more interviewer variability than factual questions.

Types and styles of interview

Interviews may be structured or unstructured. A *structured interview* is one in which all the interviewer's tasks and the exact wording of questions are delineated. Structuring may extend not only to the questions to be asked but also to the introductory statement, the prompts to be used in particular circumstances, and even the 'feedback' to be given (if any) in response to answers of particular types.

While there is some disagreement about the advantages of the structured interview (Groves and Magilavy 1986; Fowler and Mangione 1990; Beatty 1995; Dykema *et al.* 1997; Fowler 2002), much of the available empirical evidence suggests that highly structured interviews are associated with the lowest rates of error. Such interviews require a highly professional and business-like approach by the interviewer. The emphasis conveyed by the interviewer to the subject is on the task to be done and the need to obtain complete and accurate data.

Some of the objections to structured interviewing could be lessened by improvements to the interview itself (Beatty 1995) rather than by adopting a more informal style. The objection raised most commonly in regard to highly structured business-like interviews is that they inhibit the interviewer's development of rapport with the subject. Rapport is presumed to be important to the subject's continuing cooperation and to his/her provision of accurate data. In one study, interviewers trained in a personalized interactive style of interviewing elicited more information in response to several open-ended questions on health status than interviewers using a business-like manner (Henson et al. 1976). However, this study did not allow feedback to the respondent in the business-like interviews, and prompts and feedback *should* be used in structured interviews to improve complete reporting. In contrast, in a study of telephone interviews, Rogers (1976) reported that, for interviewers who were perceived as 'warm', respondents were less consistent in reporting education, less willing to report family income, and more likely to give socially desirable and 'don't know' responses.

One aspect of the structured interview, the exact reading of questions as worded, has not been shown to increase accuracy (Groves and Magilavy 1986; Dykema *et al.* 1997). In fact, in one study rewording of certain questions by interviewers increased accuracy (Dykema *et al.* 1997), perhaps because the interviewer's changes made the question's objective clearer to the respondent.

However, rather than allow interviews to reword questions to make them clearer, the questions should be fully pre-tested. Then the revision of questions which interviewers feel are problematic during pre-testing should reduce their tendency to rephrase questions during the conduct of the study.

The optimal circumstances for an interview

The optimal circumstances for an interview are determined by time and place.

Time

Two considerations are relevant (Gorden 1975): the time of the interview in relation to the respondent's usual responsibilities, and the time of the interview with reference to the time when the exposures of interest occurred. In the first case, the time should be chosen to minimize, as far as possible, competing demands on the respondent and to find the respondent in the optimal place for the interview (see below). Appointments are usually made for in-person interviews. However, to increase response rates for telephone interviews, a request for immediate interview should be made on the first contact telephone call (Harlow and Hartge 1983), and an interview appointment is arranged only if that is not possible.

Day of the week is important in determining whether or not a respondent will be contacted and an interview obtained. In a telephone survey of US Veterans conducted in 1985 and 1986, Weeks *et al.* (1987) found that weekday evenings, Saturdays any time, and Sunday afternoons and evenings were the best times to obtain both an answer to the call and an interview. The evenings gave the highest answer and interview rates. These results applied for both first calls and repeat calls.

To maximize the accuracy of recall, the interview should take place as near as possible in time to the occurrence of the exposures of interest. The sensitivity of recall to delay is illustrated by studies of under-reporting of visits to doctors and periods of hospitalization by the time since they occurred (Cannell 1985). Within 10 weeks of discharge, only 3 per cent of hospital admissions went unreported, but this proportion increased to 42 per cent at 51–53 weeks. Similarly, after a delay of 1 week, 15 per cent of physician visits were not reported, while after 2 weeks 30 per cent were missed. This suggests an effect of salience on the persistence of recall, a suggestion that was confirmed by the finding that long periods of hospitalization were recalled better, at all time intervals, than short periods. In practice, in chronic disease epidemiology, and especially in case–control studies, moderate delay in interviewing will add little to the time since the period of aetiologically relevant exposure.

Therefore, for ethical reasons and to minimize the effects of illness on responses, it is usual to delay the interview until after the subject has recovered from the diagnosis and initial treatment of his/her disease.

Place

The place of interview should be chosen for its convenience to the subject and, as far as possible, to minimize inhibitors of communication (Gorden 1975). In practice, the vast majority of face-to-face interviews are carried out in the subject's home. Within the home, the location for the interview should be chosen so that it is away from distractions which remind subjects of their other obligations in life. This objective may be achieved through time (e.g. when children are at school or after they have gone to bed) as well as through location. The place of interview should be quiet and comfortable. The interviewer should be able to sit facing the respondent (so that the respondent cannot read the questionnaire), ideally at a table for the interviewer's portable computer and/or papers. Privacy is also important although, like the other ideals, it is not always attainable. If the respondent may be asked to refer to records during the interview, it will be necessary to interview in the place where the records are kept, or to make arrangements for them to be brought to the interview.

There are some empirical data on the effect of the presence of 'third parties' on responses at interview. It was noted that a third party was present in a quarter of interviews despite instructions to interviewers to the contrary (Bradburn and Sudman 1979). Thus, where there is a major concern about the privacy of the interview, special efforts may have to be made to obtain a private location, or telephone interviewing may be the preferred mode. The presence of another person has been observed to modify respondent's answers to questions about sensitive behaviours. In one study, refusal to answer questions on frequency of petting or kissing, sexual intercourse, and masturbation in the past month increased some threefold, from 3–6 per cent to 6–18 per cent, in the presence of a spouse (Bradburn and Sudman 1979). In another study, men reported lower alcohol consumption when a third party was present (Edwards and Slattery 1998).

The interviewer's task

Depending on the nature of the investigation, the interviewer's task may include all or most of the sample selection, initial contact with the respondent, elicitation of cooperation, asking questions and obtaining answers, recording answers, and editing and coding the completed questionnaires.

Sample selection

The interviewer may be required to select subjects for the study if they are identified by random household survey or random digit dialling. Alternatively, if these are the sampling methods (as for selection of controls in a population-based case–control study), a two-step procedure may be adopted in which identification and selection of respondents is done by one field worker and the interviews by another. The choice between these alternatives will be determined by economic and logistic as well as scientific considerations. If interviewers select subjects for the samples, they cannot be blind to their disease status (as is desirable, for example, in a case–control study).

If sample selection is a component of the interviewer's task, details of the sampling scheme and its operation will form part of interviewer training.

Securing the interview

Whether or not the subject has already been contacted by a member of the survey team and an appointment made for the interview, the interviewer must take care to ensure the subject's cooperation. The interviewer should establish his/her identity by showing an official ID card from the institution conducting the research and make the introductory statement that has been prepared by the investigators (see Chapter 11). It is important that this statement, and any subsequent information that the interviewer gives, should not be too specific regarding the purposes of the study so as not to bias the respondent or increase the salience of the study to a particular class of respondents (e.g. cases in a case–control study or subjects exposed to a particular agent). The interviewer should adopt a positive manner, assuming that the interview will not be refused.

The interviewer should be prepared to answer specific questions put by the respondent. Some that commonly arise, and for which prepared answers should be given to the interviewer, are listed in Table 7.1. It is important that the answers given are honest and that they will not bias the interview. It is quite acceptable to give incomplete answers for explicit scientific reasons. For example, in response to 'Who gave you my name?,' it would be reasonable to answer: 'The names of some people in the study were given to us by their doctors because they have recently been ill and the doctors want to help find out the causes of disease. The names of others have been selected at random from [sampling frame]. I don't know which of these groups you belong to. It is important that I don't know because knowing which group you belong to may affect the way I ask you the questions.' This statement both answers the question and impresses on the respondent the care with which the research is being conducted.

Table 7.1 Questions commonly asked by respondents for which answers should be prepared and given to the interviewer[a]

- I've never heard of your organization—where did you say you were from?
- How did you get my name/address/phone number?
- I don't know anything about the subject.
- Why don't you talk to my spouse? He/she knows more about this than I do.
- What's the purpose of this interview?
- Who is sponsoring this?
- I'm not interested. I'm too busy.
- What good will this do?
- What else am I going to have to do?
- Why do you need my name?
- Who will see this information? What happens to all my personal answers?
- Why do you want to know that?
- What are you going to do with these answers anyway?

---

[a] Adapted from SRC (2002).

It has also been found to be helpful for the interviewer to have available material that establishes the reputation of the research team (e.g. press clippings that refer to its work, copies of reports of previous work, and other material that demonstrates the value of the work to the community) to assist in establishing his/her bona fides, should that be necessary.

If it appears that the respondent is going to refuse to be interviewed, the positive reasons for participation should be restated (the significance to the community of the research and the reasons why *each* respondent is important) and any implied questions behind the refusal should be answered. As far as possible, a refusal should not be accepted until it is explicit. On occasions, it may be better for the interviewer to withdraw before the refusal has been made explicitly ('I see that I've caught you at a bad time. . .') and while it may still be possible for a more experienced interviewer to return and obtain the respondent's cooperation.

Training and motivating respondents

Another important interviewer task is training and motivating the respondent immediately before the interview begins. Fowler (2002) suggests that a standardized instructional and motivating script be read. This includes a description of the types of questions to be asked and the types of answers sought. It also includes encouragement to respondents to answer the questions as accurately as possible, to take their time, and to ask the interviewer to clarify anything that they do not understand.

Asking questions and obtaining answers

Asking questions

Rules for asking questions in a structured interview are listed in Table 7.2. These rules are largely self-explanatory; their objective is to ensure that a uniform stimulus to response is received by all respondents. The ideal reading speed is about two words per second, rather slower than we would naturally read. Reading the questions slowly not only allows the respondents more time to think about the answers, but has been shown to encourage them to spend more time over the answers and therefore to answer more fully.

Questions should be read with correct intonation and emphasis. While 'correct intonation and emphasis' is rather difficult to define in the general case, it will be achieved by an interviewer if he/she fully understands the intended meaning of the question. This understanding will come as a consequence of careful training. Cannell (1985) observed, after listening to many recordings of interviews, that interviewers were placing the emphasis on different parts of questions and thus giving them different meanings. He found that underlining words that were to be emphasized increased the degree of standardization of question asking.

Table 7.2 Rules for asking questions in structured interviews[a]

◆ Ask the questions exactly as they are worded in the questionnaire.

◆ Read each question slowly, about two words per second.

◆ Use correct intonation and emphasis.

◆ Ask the questions in the order in which they are presented in the questionnaire.

◆ Ask every question that applies to the respondent (all inapplicable questions will be identified as such by skip instructions in the questionnaire).

◆ Use response cards when provided.

◆ Repeat questions in full that are misheard or misunderstood.

◆ Only use allowable probes.

◆ Read all linking or transitional statements exactly as they are written.

◆ Do not add apologies or explanations for questions unless they are printed in the questionnaire.

◆ Provide positive feedback for acceptable respondent performance.

[a] Adapted from Brenner (1985) and SRC (2002).

As noted in Table 7.2, when a respondent mis-hears or misunderstands a question it should be repeated in full. When the respondent is still unsure of the meaning of a question after repetition, the interviewer should not attempt to explain it but say something neutral like 'Whatever it means to you' (see other permissible probes below). If that does not solve the problem, the question should remain unanswered and the reason for the difficulty noted on the questionnaire.

Probing

Probes are additional questions asked or statements made by the interviewer when the answer given by a respondent is incomplete or irrelevant. Probing has two major functions: to motivate the respondent to reply more fully and to help the respondent focus on the specific content of the question. It must fulfill these functions without biasing the respondent's answers.

The ability to probe an unsatisfactory answer is one of the most important advantages of the personal interview, but it is also a method whereby bias can easily be introduced (e.g. by the interviewer summarizing his/her understanding of the response to the subject when an unclear response has been given, or offering some alternative interpretations of the response from which the respondent can choose). In a highly structured questionnaire, permissible probes for each question and the circumstances under which they can be used may be printed in the questionnaire. Alternatively, a list of acceptable non-directive probes may be given to the interviewers, and their use explained, during the course of training. In either case, it is important to stress the significance of neutral inflection to avoid influencing the respondent, particularly for attitudinal questions.

Table 7.3 provides a list of acceptable probes that the interviewer can use when the respondent gives a vague or incomplete answer (SRC 2002). These include the following.

- *Repeat the question*. Vague answers may be a consequence of misunderstanding or mis-hearing the question, or may arise because the respondent has not had long enough to think about the answer. All that may be required to obtain clarification is to repeat the question after an appropriate introduction like: 'I am not sure that I understand you. Let me just ask the question again so that I can be sure to get your answer right. . . .?'

- *The expectant pause*. Waiting expectantly tells the respondent that the interviewer is looking for more information than has been given already.

- *Repeat the reply*. Repeating the reply aloud while recording it may stimulate the respondent to provide more details.

Table 7.3 also lists neutral questions or comments which can be used as probes for particular purposes, such as clarification, specificity, or completeness.

Table 7.3 Acceptable probes by interviewers when respondent gives a vague or incomplete answer[a]

NON-DIRECTIVE PROBES

- *Repeat the question*
- *Use an expectant pause*
- *Repeat the reply*

....

NEUTRAL QUESTIONS OR COMMENTS WHICH MAY BE USED AS PROBES FOR PARTICULAR PURPOSES

For clarification

- 'What do you mean exactly?'
- 'What do you mean by. . . .?'
- 'I don't think that I quite understand. Could you explain that a little?'
- 'In what way?'

....

For specificity

- 'Would you tell me what you have in mind?'
- 'Could you be more specific about that?'
- 'Can you be any closer about the [date]?'
- 'Can you be more exact?'
- 'Which would be closer?' (when the respondent has proposed two options)

....

For completeness

- 'Anything else?'
- 'What else can you think of?'
- 'Can you tell me more about it?'
- 'Are there any other reasons why you feel that way?'

---

[a] Adapted from SRC (2002).

It is usual to probe 'don't know' responses. Often they are given because the respondent did not understand the question, or because he/she needs more time to think about the answer. Thus, repetition of the question or an expectant pause may be particularly useful techniques to try. Sometimes some assurance may be necessary like: 'There are no right or wrong answers to these questions, just give whatever answer you think is the right one for you (or the closest one).'

Providing feedback

The provision of feedback by the interviewer to the respondent about his/her performance of the response task has been the subject of some research. It was observed that, after asking questions, provision of unprogrammed feedback to respondents formed the highest proportion of interviewer behaviour (Cannell *et al.* 1981). The feedback phrases were almost invariably positive or encouraging to the respondent; they included phrases such as 'uh huh, I see', 'okay', 'that's good', 'all right', 'that's interesting', etc. Moreover, the probability of feedback was greatest in response to poor respondent behaviour; for example, when the respondent said 'I don't know'.

As a consequence of these observations, Cannell and his colleagues hypothesized that accuracy and completeness of response could be increased by providing feedback that was contingent on the nature of the subject's responses. Thus, precise and apparently complete responses would be rewarded by feedback like 'Uh huh, I see, this is the kind of information we want', 'Thanks, you've mentioned four things', 'Thanks, we appreciate your frankness', or 'Uh huh, we're interested in details like these', while vague or incomplete responses would be discouraged by phrases like 'You answered that quickly', 'Sometimes its easy to forget. . .Could you think about it again?' or 'That's only two things'. Subsequent studies showed that the use of contingent feedback in health-related surveys increased the amount of reporting of most events (e.g. number of doctor visits) and the precision in reporting of some (e.g. dates of medical events). The feedback phrases and the contingencies under which they were to be used were printed in the questionnaire.

Recording responses

The task of recording responses is generally simplified by highly structured interview questionnaires in which the only open questions are those which seek simple factual information. Table 7.4 gives rules for the recording of responses.

Table 7.4 Rules for recording responses in interviews[a]

- Make sure that you understand each response.
- Make sure that each response is adequate.
- Do not answer for the respondent (i.e. do not infer a response from an incomplete or inadequate reply).
- Record all responses during the interview.
- Begin recording the response as soon as the respondent begins talking (the respondent's interest may be held by repeating the response aloud as you are writing).
- Use the respondent's own words and record the answers verbatim.
- Include everything that pertains to the question's objectives.
- Note the nature and place of important probes used.
- If a response is wrong, strike it out and enter the correct response and note the source of the error (RE, respondent error; ME, my (interviewer) error).
- Record 'refused' beside any question that the respondent refused to answer.
- Ensure that the respondent's comments and your own can be distinguished visually by using parentheses or other demarcation.

[a] Adapted from Brenner (1985) and SRC (2002).

Their application is generally to the recording of answers to open-ended questions rather than to closed-ended questions, which present few problems.

The emphasis of these instructions for recording responses is on accuracy and completeness. Accuracy means recording exactly what it was that the respondent said. Completeness includes providing all relevant information, including additional things that the respondent may have said which pertain to the objectives of the question, who made the error if an error was made, and whether missing information was a consequence of refusal to answer the question, lack of respondent knowledge of the answer, or some other reason.

Editing and coding

The questionnaire should be edited as soon as possible after the interviewer (or respondent) leaves the place of interview and, preferably, before another interview is undertaken. The objectives of editing are to ensure that all entries are legible, any abbreviations used are explained, interviewer comments are in parentheses (to distinguish them from the respondent's replies), all unclear responses are clarified by parenthetical notes, and reasons are given (again parenthetically) for all missed responses. If editing uncovers missed questions or a missed section of the questionnaire, the interviewer should return to the respondent, with appropriate apologies, and complete them. The cover sheet should be edited to ensure that all identifying data are correctly entered and all other sections (interview start and finish times, call record, etc.) are correctly completed.

Coding of open-ended questions (e.g. classifying occupations or reasons for taking a specific drug) might also be the task of the interviewer. However, often the study editor or supervisor codes all interviews. The interviewer should not be required to code responses to open-ended questions during an interview, except when the number of possible responses is very small. More details about coding systems are given in Chapter 5.

Advantages of computer-assisted interviewing

Computer-assisted interviewing (CAI) is now common, including computer-assisted personal interviewing (CAPI) using a portable computer in the respondent's home and computer-assisted telephone interviewing (CATI). CAI can aid the interviewer in several of his/her tasks, including the following (de Leeuw and Nicholls 1996; Nicholls *et al.* 1997).

- The question-specific or general instructions can be invoked on screen by the interviewer.
- CAI can be programmed to ensure that the proper skip pattern is followed and that no applicable questions are missed.

- CAI is superior to traditional interviews for items that require the interviewer to tailor the wording of questions based on prior responses by the subject. For example, the subject could be given a list of recreational activities and asked which ones he/she participated in at least 12 times over the last year. Once the activities selected by the respondent are entered into the computer, appropriate detailed questions on the frequency and duration of each activity can appear on the screen.

- Simple coding can occur during the interview via look-up tables.

- Range and logic checks can occur concomitantly with the interview. This can lead to immediate queries to the interviewer to clarify with the respondent an out-of-range response or a response that was inconsistent with prior responses. These computerized edits can eliminate the need for an editor to review each interview.

- CAI can automate certain record keeping, such as length of interview and response rates.

- CAI eliminates the need for key entry of data and therefore yields data immediately ready for the next stage of processing.

Studies of data quality suggest that CAI information may be slightly more reliable than 'paper and pencil' interview data (Nicholls *et al.* 1997). When accurately programmed, CAI can virtually eliminate missing data due to interviewer errors in skipping items that are applicable to the subject (but not due to refusals or 'don't know' responses) (Nicholls *et al.* 1997).

Some computer-assisted 'interviewing' techniques do not include an interviewer! Specifically, audio and video computer-assisted self-interviewing (ACASI and VCASI) methods have been developed. One advantage of these techniques is that they may lead to less social desirability bias in answering sensitive questions (Kissinger *et al.* 1999; Metzger *et al.* 2000). While these methods have several of the advantages listed above, they have more in common with self-administered questionnaires than with the interviewer techniques discussed in this chapter.

Selection, training, and supervision of interviewers

Selection

Interviewers need good reading and speaking skills and some computer skills, and the flexibility to work at weekends and in the evening. There is empirical evidence that interview tasks are performed better by women than by men, by college graduates than by those with less education, and by persons under 40 years of age (USBC 1972). However, other studies suggest that older interviewers have higher response rates and less item non-response

(Fowler and Mangione 1990). College students have the reputation of being poor interviewers, although this may be due to lack of training and experience rather than their young age (Cannell and Fowler 1977). Interviewer productivity increases and technical error rates decrease with increasing experience, reaching a plateau after about 2 years. As noted above, however, experience in a particular interview task may be associated with a fall in the quality of data obtained from respondents (Cannell *et al.* 1977). This observation is an argument for a continuing programme of on-the-job motivation and training, rather than firing experienced interviewers and hiring inexperienced ones.

Much consideration has been given to matching the interviewer to the respondent on characteristics such as sex, age, race, and socio-economic status. This is probably a more important issue in research into opinions and attitudes than it is for most epidemiological research. Even for opinions and attitudes, matching appears to be important only if the topic of the study is highly related to interviewer or respondent characteristics and the respondent has not arrived at a firm position on it. For example, white respondents are more likely to express pro-black attitudes if interviewed by a black interviewer than if interviewed by a white interviewer (Groves 1989). An interviewer's apparent social class was shown to influence reporting of social and political opinions by working-class respondents (Cannell *et al.* 1981). The sex of the interviewer appears to have little effect on attitudes, but is commonly matched in interviews seeking a detailed sexual history. Matching of race may be beneficial in securing the interview (Moorman *et al.* 1999). It is clearly important to employ interviewers who are fluent in the language usually used by the respondents.

It has been common in epidemiological studies to employ nurses or other health professionals to act as interviewers, because of their probable familiarity with the subject matter of the research. They may also be necessary if blood or other biological specimens are to be collected. However, the employment of health professionals for the US Health Interview Survey is discouraged because they 'may tend to diagnose or interpret rather then merely record' (Koons 1973). No empirical data were offered to support this position.

Certain personality traits may enhance interviewer performance. Hox *et al.* (1991) reviewed the empirical evidence and concluded that interviewers who obtain the most valid responses are self-confident, have more social skills, and are less socially dependent. The latter two traits imply that the interviewer has good interpersonal skills, but not a social disposition (e.g. a tendency to help the respondent answer), which leads to more interviewer variance.

Certain personality traits may also be helpful for obtaining high participation rates, one of the most challenging and important tasks of the interviewer (see Chapter 11). For this task, interviewers need a positive, confident, and assertive manner, to convey that there is no doubt that the participant will cooperate with the study (Fowler 2002). Enlisting cooperation cannot be performed by simply reading a predefined script. Instead, interviewers need to engage each potential participant personally and be responsive to their concerns. It is difficult to train interviewers in these skills, and often difficult to identify these traits in the hiring process. Unfortunately, this means that to ensure that the interviewer staff have the requisite skills, new interviewers should be hired on a provisional basis (e.g. for 3 months) so that those who achieve poor response rates can be terminated.

The interviewers' manual

Each study requiring the collection of data by personal interview should have an interviewers' manual. An interviewers' manual is a specific form of the

Table 7.5 Contents of a typical interviewers' manual[a]

The sample survey
When is a survey conducted?
What kinds of questions are asked?
How is survey information used?
Types of surveys
Conducting a survey
Overview of the role of the interviewer
Using the questionnaire
Introduction to the format of questionnaires
Asking the questions
Skip patterns
Complex questions
Probing and other interviewing techniques
Probing
The use of feedback
Recording answers
Editing the questionnaire
Telephone interviewing

Table 7.5 (continued) Contents of a typical interviewers' manual[a]

Computer-assisted interviewing—using the software

Sampling principles and procedures

　Sampling methods

　Selecting the respondent's household

　Selecting the respondent

Tracking hard to find participants

Call and call-back strategy

　Making contact

　Making an interview appointment

　Dealing with reluctant respondents ('refusal aversions')

Administrative procedures, forms, and records

Ethical principles for interviewers and the maintenance of confidentiality

Interviewer safety

[a] Adapted from SRC (2002).

general procedures manual outlined in Chapter 5. It contains material general to all interviews and also material specific to the particular study for which it has been prepared. Table 7.5 outlines the topics applicable to interviewing in epidemiological research which are covered in a general manual prepared by the Survey Research Center of the University of Michigan (SRC 2002).

The interviewers' manual should also include a copy of the questionnaire, and often includes a question-by-question (Q-by-Q) explanation and instructions for the interviewer. An example of a page from a Q-by-Q section of an interviewers' manual is shown in Figure 7.1.

Training

Training of interviewers has been shown empirically to improve their performance, particularly in reducing under-reporting of information and item non-response (Billiet and Loosveldt 1988). Fowler and Mangione (1990) found that interviewers with two or more days of training, as compared with those with only half a day, performed much better in reading questions as worded, recording answers to open-ended questions, and being non-biased in their approach. Over 80 per cent of interviewers were rated as excellent or satisfactory on these tasks after two days of training. For probing open-ended questions, which was the most difficult task for interviewers, only 44 per cent of trainees reached an excellent or satisfactory rating with two days of training, and only

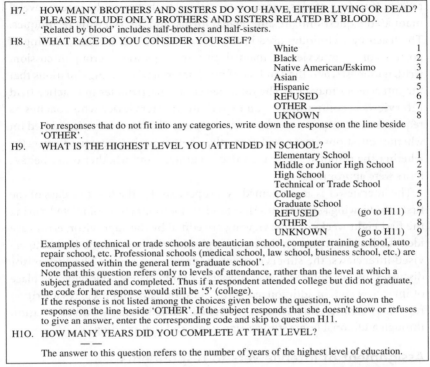

H7. HOW MANY BROTHERS AND SISTERS DO YOU HAVE, EITHER LIVING OR DEAD? PLEASE INCLUDE ONLY BROTHERS AND SISTERS RELATED BY BLOOD. 'Related by blood' includes half-brothers and half-sisters.

H8. WHAT RACE DO YOU CONSIDER YOURSELF?

White	1
Black	2
Native American/Eskimo	3
Asian	4
Hispanic	5
REFUSED	6
OTHER _____	7
UKNOWN	8

For responses that do not fit into any categories, write down the response on the line beside 'OTHER'.

H9. WHAT IS THE HIGHEST LEVEL YOU ATTENDED IN SCHOOL?

Elementary School		1
Middle or Junior High School		2
High School		3
Technical or Trade School		4
College		5
Graduate School		6
REFUSED	(go to H11)	7
OTHER _____		8
UNKNOWN	(go to H11)	9

Examples of technical or trade schools are beautician school, computer training school, auto repair school, etc. Professional schools (medical school, law school, business school, etc.) are encompassed within the general term 'graduate school'.
Note that this question refers only to levels of attendance, rather than the level at which a subject graduated and completed. Thus if a respondent attended college but did not graduate, the code for her response would still be '5' (college).
If the response is not listed among the choices given below the question, write down the response on the line beside 'OTHER'. If the subject responds that she doesn't know or refuses to give an answer, enter the corresponding code and skip to question H11.

H10. HOW MANY YEARS DID YOU COMPLETE AT THAT LEVEL?
__ __

The answer to this question refers to the number of years of the highest level of education.

Figure 7.1 Example of question-by-question instructions to interviewers adapted from an interviewers' manual used in a multicentre collaborative case–control study of uterine sarcoma and cervical adenocarcinoma. (Fred Hutchinson Cancer Research Center, Stephen Schwartz PhD, with permission.)

69 per cent with 10 days of training (much longer than a typical training program).

A carefully planned and structured programme of training of interviewers is essential to the success of epidemiological studies. A general approach to the training of field workers has been outlined in Chapter 5. The contents of the interviewers' manual (e.g. Table 7.5) would serve as the outline for the didactic part of the training sessions. The training should also include demonstrations and practice in eliciting agreement from respondents to be interviewed and in administering the questionnaire. An excellent example of interviewer training (for US Health Interview Survey interviewers), has been outlined by Koons (1973). Briefly, new interviewers are first given a package of self-study materials which includes administrative materials, a copy of the questionnaire, an interviewers' manual, and copies of letters sent to respondents. Interviewers then receive five days of classroom instruction which covers the interviewers' manual, the questionnaire and related forms, and interviewing techniques. The teaching techniques used in the classroom include lectures, reading of portions of the interviewers' manual, answering questions, group discussion, written exercises, and the conduct of mock interviews covering situations that the interviewer may face. The interviewer also participates in practice field interviews accompanied by an experienced interviewer who coaches as required and completes an observation report. The interviewer is assessed on whether questions were asked correctly, whether probes were used correctly, whether the responses were recorded accurately, and whether other behaviours were appropriate.

The interviewer is accompanied by a supervisor for the first two days of the first interviewing assignment. All interview questionnaires completed during the first eight weeks of interviewing are edited by the supervisor, errors are identified, and a report on the errors is given to the interviewer. In the supervised interviews, the supervisor acts as an observer only. The supervisor discusses his/her notes with the interviewer immediately on leaving the place of interview and, in addition, edits the questionnaire and prepares a written report. Thereafter, interviewers receive continued training and motivation through additional home study assignments and staff meetings.

Assignment of interviewers to respondents

As noted earlier in this chapter, different interviewers may elicit a different distribution of responses from respondents (interviewer bias). Therefore it is important in case–control studies to assign each interviewer the same proportion of cases and controls in order to avoid inducing differential measurement error. To do this, one needs to interview cases and controls contemporaneously; otherwise, if the research begins with case interviews only, there is a risk that some interviewers may leave the study before they have conducted their share of control interviews. Another way to avoid introducing differential interviewer measurement error is to blind the interviewers to the case–control status of the subjects when feasible.

Supervision

The general principles of quality control during the course of collection of epidemiological data in the field have been outlined in Chapter 5. With respect to interviewing, they include the following.

♦ prompt editing by a supervisor or editor of the work completed by each interviewer, or computerized editing concomitant with interviewing using CAI

♦ concomitant or timely performance of range and logic checks by computer

- periodic observation of the work of each interviewer
- re-interview of a proportion of subjects by a supervisor or other experienced interviewer
- comparison of the distribution of variables among interviewers
- analysis of trends in the variables over time.

The importance of observation or re-interview is emphasized by the fact that only 12 per cent of interviewer errors could be identified by a careful examination of the completed questionnaires (Cannell et al. 1975). Tape recording of interviews is an acceptable alternative to supervisor observation of interviewers (Cannell et al. 1975). A simple request to the respondent, 'The University has asked me to tape this interview for quality assurance, if that's agreeable to you', is usually sufficient to obtain his/her consent to the recording. The recorder should be placed on the table between the interviewer and the respondent, and thereafter forgotten as far as possible.

Random call-backs to respondents are important to reduce the risk of the most egregious type of error—the fabrication of entire interviews by interviewers. Knowing that this monitoring is taking place should reduce the likelihood that interviewers will falsify interviews. The call-back can be a short telephone call with questions such as 'Was the interviewer polite at all times?' and with repeated questions from the interview for a few key items.

It is important that these quality control procedures are carried out in a timely fashion and that there is prompt feedback to interviewers, either by way of direct supervisory communication or through staff meetings. Where problems have been identified and corrected, continuing surveillance should be maintained to ensure that the correction has been successful. It may be necessary to terminate the services of an interviewer who persistently presents work which fails the quality control checks.

Special aspects of telephone interviewing

Differences between telephone and face-to-face interviewing

The differences between telephone and face-to-face interviews are covered in Chapter 2. Some of the disadvantages of telephone interviewing are that the questions must be less complex and the use of visual aids, such as 'show cards', is impossible on the telephone and must be compensated for in questionnaire design. Telephone interviews also need to be designed to be shorter, because an interviewer cannot build rapport and maintain motivation as well by telephone as in person. It is also more difficult for the interviewer to establish the legitimacy of the interview on the telephone.

Another difference which affects several aspects of telephone interviewing is that non-verbal communication, both from interviewer to respondent and from respondent to interviewer, is absent. The telephone interviewer may not be able to probe as effectively because he/she cannot see visual cues from the respondent. The 'expectant pause' cannot be used as effectively as a probe for additional information on the telephone. The pace of the interview may be faster (because of the need to keep talking), leading to hurried and, perhaps, less thoughtful responses. There is evidence that these differences lead to response differences. In comparing identical questionnaires administered by telephone and in person, telephone interviews tended to be shorter, respondents gave less information in response to open-ended questions, and subjects responded to fewer items on a list (de Leeuw and van der Zouwen 1988; de Leeuw 1992). In addition, when a list of responses is read by telephone, respondents are more likely to choose the first or last response than when they can see the list (Sudman *et al.* 1996). However, there is no clear evidence that the accuracy of answers elicited in telephone interviews is worse or better than by face-to-face interview, including no clear difference for sensitive questions (de Leeuw 1992). On the positive side, the telephone interview should eliminate most biasing by others present in the home (because others in the home can only hear the response not the question), are lower cost, and have other practical advantages (see Chapter 2).

Supervision of telephone interviews

Telephone interviewing offers considerable advantages in its ease of supervision. The interviewers may all be working together in the same building as the supervisor, and it is a comparatively simple matter for the supervisor to listen to and code interviewer behaviour in selected interviews without influencing either interviewer or respondent behaviour (subject, of course, to any legal or ethical constraints on such procedures).

Computer-assisted telephone interviewing

Computer-assisted telephone interviewing (CATI) has the same advantages as computer-assisted interviewing listed above. In addition, CATI has the following capabilities (Nicholls 1988):

- administrative management of the sample
- on-line call scheduling and selection of subjects to be called as each interviewer becomes free
- on-line monitoring of interviews by a supervisor who can see the computer screen currently visible to the interviewer as well as hear the interview

◆ automatic record keeping with respect to calls, response rates, interviewer productivity, etc.

Evidence of the advantages of CATI is somewhat mixed. Harlow *et al.* (1985) conducted a study of data obtained by telephone from proxy respondents for cases and controls in a case–control study of colorectal cancer based on death certificates. They found no differences in the proportions of unresolved 'don't knows' and the quality of the interview, as assessed by the interviewer, between CATI and 'hard-copy' telephone interviews. The CATI interviews took longer and were associated with less recording of comments and use of probes by the interviewers. However, the mean differences between CATI and hard-copy interviews on these variables were much less than the differences between means for individual interviewers. The finding that CATI interviews are, on average, longer appears to be consistent (Groves and Mathiowetz 1984; Catlin and Ingram 1988). Groves and Mathiowetz (1984) found only small differences in response rates, reactions of interviewers and respondents, and the values of the health statistics sought between CATI and hard-copy interviewing. Interviewer variability was less with CATI, and there were fewer skip errors.

Summary

The personal interview is the most common method of collecting data on exposure in epidemiological studies. It differs principally from other methods by the presence of the interviewer—a presence which can have many positive and a few negative effects on the quality of the data obtained.

The interviewer's tasks may include sample selection and establishment of initial contact with the subject, as well as asking questions and obtaining answers, recording responses, and initial editing and coding of the question-naire. Whatever the initial approach to subjects, the interviewer must be skilled in obtaining the cooperation of the subjects. Interviewers should be provided with an appropriate introductory statement and model answers to questions that subjects are likely to ask.

Interviews may be structured or unstructured. Available evidence suggests that the former, in which the interviewer's tasks and words are set out in detail on the questionnaire, are associated with the least error.

When asking questions, interviewers should read them slowly, with correct intonation and emphasis and exactly as they are worded in the questionnaire. Questions should be asked in the order that they are presented in the questionnaire; all questions relevant to each subject should be asked; and all linking and transitional statements should be read exactly as written. Probing should be non-directive and aimed at obtaining more complete and more relevant responses. Provision of feedback to respondents which is contingent on the quality of the response can be used to improve the quality of responses.

The emphasis in recording responses should be on accuracy in recording exactly what the respondent said and completeness in providing all relevant information. The questionnaire should be edited as soon as possible after the interview or concomitantly with the interview using computer-assisted interviewing.

The best interviewers are generally female college graduates. Interviewer productivity increases and technical error rates decrease with increasing experience of the interviewer. Training improves the performance of interviewers and should be carried out in accordance with a carefully planned programme of instruction which includes practice in the field. As part of their training and for ongoing maintenance of standards, interviewers should be provided with a specific study manual. A programme of continuing training, motivation, and supervision is advisable.

The principles that apply to face-to-face interviewing generally also apply to interviewing by telephone. Telephone interviewing offers considerable advantages in ease of supervision.

References

Anderson, A.-M.N. and Olsen J. (2002). Do interviewers' health beliefs and habits modify responses to sensitive questions? *American Journal of Epidemiology*, **155**, 95–100.

Beatty, P. (1995). Understanding the standardized/non-standardized interviewing controversy. *Journal of Official Statistics*, **11**, 147–60.

Billiet, J. and Loosveldt, G. (1988). Improvements of the quality of responses to factual survey questions by interviewer training. *Public Opinion Quarterly*, **52**, 190–211.

Blair, E., Sudman, S., Bradburn, N. M., and Stocking, C. (1977). How to ask questions about drinking and sex: response effects in measuring consumer behavior. *Journal of Marketing Research*, **14**, 316–21.

Bradburn, N.M. and Sudman, S. (1979). *Improving Interview Method and Questionnaire Design*. Jossey-Bass, San Francisco, CA.

Brenner, M. (1985). Survey interviewing. In *The Research Interview: Uses AND Approaches* (ed. M. Brenner, J. Brown, and D. Canter), pp.9–36. Academic Press, London.

Cannell, C. F. (1985). Overview: response bias and interviewer variability in surveys. In *Survey Interviewing, Theory and Techniques* (ed. T.W. Beed and R.J. Stimson), pp. 1–23. George Allen and Unwin, Sydney.

Cannell, C.F. and Fowler, F.J. (1977). Interviewers and interviewing techniques. In *Advances in Health Survey Research Methods: Proceedings of a National Invitational Conference* (ed. L.G. Reeder), DHEW Publication No. (HRA) 77–3154, pp. 13–23. US Department of Health Education and Welfare, Washington, DC.

Cannell, C.F., Lawson, S.A., and Hausser, D.L. (1975). *A Technique for Evaluating Interviewer Performance*. Institute of Social Research, University of Michigan, Ann Arbor, MI.

Cannell, C.F., Marquis, K.H., and Laurent, A. (1977). A summary of studies of interviewing methodology. *Vital and Health Statistics*, Series 2, No. 69, DHEW Publication No. (HRA) 77–1343. US Department of Health Education and Welfare, Washington, DC.

Cannell, C.F., Miller, P.V., and Oksenberg, L. (1981). Research on interviewing techniques. In *Sociological Methodology 1981* (ed. S. Leinhardt), pp. 389–437. Jossey-Bass, San Francisco, CA.

Catlin, G. and Ingram, S. (1988). The effects of CATI on costs and data quality: a comparison of CATI and paper methods in centralized interviewing. In *Telephone Survey Methodology* (ed. R.M. Groves, P.P. Biemer, L.E. Lyberg, J.T. Massey, W.L. Nicholls, and J. Waksberg), pp. 437–50. Wiley, New York.

de Leeuw, E.D. (1992). *Data Quality in Mail, Telephone, and Face to Face Surveys.* Amsterdam, TT-Publikaties.

de Leeuw, E. and Nicholls, W. (1996). Technological innovations in data collection: acceptance, data quality and costs. *Sociological Research Online*, **1**. Available online at: www.socresonline.org.uk/socresonline/1/4/leeuw.html.

de Leeuw, E.D. and van der Zouwen, J. (1988). Data quality in telephone and face-to-face surveys: a comparative meta-analysis. In *Telephone Survey Methodology* (ed. R.M. Groves, P.P. Biemer, L.E. Lyberg, J.T. Massey, W.L. Nicholls, and J. Waksberg), pp. 283–99. Wiley, New York.

Dykema, J., Lepkowski, J.M., and Blixt, S. (1997). The effect of interviewer and respondent behavior on data quality: analysis of interaction coding in a validation study. In *Survey Measurement and Process Quality* (ed. L. Lyberg, P. Beimer, M. Collins, *et al.*), pp. 287–310. Wiley, New York.

Edwards, S.L. and Slattery, M.L. (1998). Measurement errors stemming from nonrespondents present at in-person interviews. *American Journal of Epidemiology*, **8**, 272–7.

Fowler, F.J. (2002). *Survey Research Methods* (3rd edn). Sage, Thousand Oaks, CA.

Fowler, F.J. and Mangione, T.W. (1990). *Standardized Survey Interviewing*. Sage, Newbury Park, CA.

Gorden, R.L. (1975). *Interviewing: Strategy, Techniques and Tactics*. Dorsey, Homewood, IL.

Groves, R.M. (1989). *Survey Errors and Survey Costs*, pp. 357–406, Wiley, New York.

Groves, R.M., and Magilavy, L. J. (1986). Measuring and explaining interviewer effects. *Public Opinion Quarterly*, **50**, 251–6.

Groves, R.M. and Mathiowetz, N.A. (1984). Computer assisted telephone interviewing: effects on interviewers and respondents. *Public Opinion Quarterly*, **48**, 356–69.

Harlow, B.L. and Hartge, P. (1983). Telephone household screening and interviewing. *American Journal of Epidemiology*, **117**, 632–3.

Harlow, B.L., Rosenthal, J.F., and Ziegler, R.G. (1985). A comparison of computer-assisted and hard copy telephone interviewing. *American Journal of Epidemiology*, **122**, 335–40.

Henson, R., Cannell, C.F., and Lawson, S. (1976). Effects of interviewer style on quality of reporting in a survey interview. *Journal of Psychology*, **93**, 221–7.

Hox, J.J., de Leeuw, E.D., and Kreft, I.G.G. (1991). The effect of interviewer and respondent characteristics on the quality of survey data: multilevel model. In *Measurement Errors In Survey* (ed. P.P. Biemer, R.M. Groves, L.E. Lyberg, N.A. Mathiowetz, and S. Sudman), pp 439–61. Wiley, New York.

Hyman, H., Cobb, W.J., Feldman, J.J., Hart, C.W., and Stember, C.H. (1954). *Interviewing in Social Research*. University of Chicago Press, Chicago, IL

Kissinger, P., Rice, J., Farley, T., *et al.* (1999). Application of computer-assisted interviews to sexual behavior research. *American Journal of Epidemiology*, **149**, 950–4.

Koons, D.A. (1973). Quality control and measurement of nonsampling error in the Health Interview Survey. *Vital and Health Statistics*, Series 2, No. 54, DHEW Publication No. (HSM) 73–1328. US Department of Health Education and Welfare, Washington, DC.

Metzger, D.S., Koblin, B., Turner, C., *et al.* (2000). Randomized controlled trial of audio computer-assisted self-interviewing: utility and acceptability in longitudinal studies. *American Journal of Epidemiology*, **152**, 99–106.

Moorman, P.G., Newman, B., Millikan, R.C., Tse, C.K., and Sandler, D.P. (1999). Participation rates in a case–control study: the impact of age, race, and race of interviewer. *Annals of Epidemiology*, **9**, 188–95.

Nicholls, W.L. (1988). Computer-assisted telephone interviewing: a general introduction. In *Telephone survey methodology*, (ed. R.M. Groves, P.P. Biemer, L.E. Lyberg, J.T. Massey, W.L. Nicholls, and J. Waksberg), pp. 377–85. Wiley, New York.

Nicholls, W.L., Baker, R.P., and Martin, J. (1997) The effect of new data collection technologies on survey data quality. In *Survey Measurement and Process Quality* (ed. L. Lyberg, P. Beimer, M. Collins, *et al.*), pp. 221–48. Wiley, New York.

Rogers, T.F. (1976). Interviews by telephone and in person: quality of responses and field performance. *Public Opinion Quarterly*, **40**, 51–65.

SRC (Survey Research Center) (2002). *Interviewers' Manual* (revised edn). Institute of Social Research, University of Michigan, Ann Arbor, MI.

Sudman, S., Bradburn, N.M., and Schwarz, N. (1996). *Thinking About Answers: The Application of Cognitive Processes to Survey Methodology*. Jossey-Bass, San Francisco, CA.

USBC (US Bureau of the Census) (1972). Investigation of census bureau interviewer characteristics, performance and attitudes: a summary. Working Paper No. 34. US Government Printing Office, Washington, DC.

Weeks, M.F., Kulka, R.A., and Pierson, S.A. (1987). Optimal call scheduling for a telephone survey. *Public Opinion Quarterly*, **51**, 540–9.

8

Use of records, diaries, and proxy respondents

> Anyone who has ever worked with medical records knows that they are an imperfect source of scientific data. The records contain all the idiosyncrasies and errors that can occur in the communication of human observations ... The recorded data often consist of anecdotal generalities rather than precise specifications; the statements often represent opinions or interpretations rather than descriptions of observed evidence; important information may sometimes be absent or unobtainable; and the remarks made by one doctor may sometimes contradict those made by another.
>
> *(Feinstein et al. 1969a)*

Introduction

In this chapter we consider the use of records, diaries, and proxy respondents, all of which are important methods of exposure measurement in epidemiology.

Use of records

Scope of records

The term *record* will be used here to describe data recorded for a purpose other than the epidemiological study of interest. Records useful for epidemiological research include medical (inpatient and outpatient), pharmacy, disease registry, birth certificate, death certificate, and environmental records. From the standpoint of exposure measurement, records come in one of two formats. The first comprise paper records or electronic records composed primarily of text, such as medical records. These types of record need *record abstraction* to yield coded data that can be analysed. The second comprise records that are already in an electronic format as coded variables, such as death records and disease registries.

A common element in the use of records is that part or all of the data collection has already been carried out. To gain insight into the accuracy of the information, the researcher should become familiar with the process of data recording that has already occurred.

For example, in the USA, the information on birth certificates is recorded at each hospital, usually by the medical records staff or the obstetric nursing staff. The National Center for Health Statistics has published a procedure manual (NCHS 2002a), but generally there is no uniform training of recorders. The personal information (mother's age, education) is recorded on the birth certificate from a questionnaire developed by each hospital, which is administered during the mother's hospital stay and placed in the mother's hospital chart. The medical information (method of delivery, months of prenatal care, complications) is abstracted from the mother's and infant's inpatient records and the prenatal records if they are available. The attending physician verifies the accuracy of the medical information and signs the form, and the state or local vital registration office checks for completeness and queries incomplete or inconsistent certificates.

In most countries the medical information on death certificates is recorded by a physician or coroner. However, the doctor signing the form may not be the decedent's primary physician, and may be unfamiliar with the decedent's past medical history or the circumstances surrounding the death. In many countries, the funeral director is responsible for recording personal items concerning the decedent (age, marital status, usual occupation, type of business or industry) through an informant. The informant, usually a relative, is named on the certificate. In the USA, the National Center for Health Statistics provides procedure manuals (NCHS 2002b) for physicians and funeral directors, which may be modified by individual states to meet their needs. Formal training in completion of death certificates is provided by some medical schools and by some state or local vital record offices. State or local record departments review the records, and provide informal training to physicians and funeral directors during call-backs to clarify information.

The information in hospital records may include an admission form completed by a clerk, handwritten or electronic notes by physicians, nurses, and other health workers, results of diagnostic tests (X-rays, laboratory tests); reports from consultations with sub-specialists, operation reports or reports of other therapeutic procedures, and a discharge summary. The notes by the healthcare providers include information volunteered by or solicited from the patient, information from the physical examination of the patient, medical diagnoses, and prescribed medicines or other therapeutic procedures.

These examples highlight some of the limitations of the use of records compared with data collection by structured interview. When a structured interview is used, the researcher attempts to collect the same information in the same manner for all subjects. In contrast, when records are used, the researcher has little control over how questions are phrased, the definition of terms, what items are recorded, and the order in which they are recorded. Moreover, records are often produced by a large number of recorders with little uniform training. Records are also subject to many of the same sources of error as interviews, including erroneous reports by the subject (e.g. self-report of alcohol use) or errors in the entry of information into the record. Further, treatment information in outpatient records may indicate only the intended treatment; for example, a record of a drug prescription does not necessarily mean that the prescription was filled or was taken (Christensen *et al.* 1994).

Advantages of the use of records

The use of records has several advantages over other methods of data collection. The study costs are usually low, and the study time is reduced because some or all of the data collection has been carried out by others.

More importantly, despite the limitations of records, the accuracy of selected data items can be better than that obtained by personal interview. One of the primary advantages of records is that they can provide prospectively recorded information collected on exposures in the past. The prospective nature of records minimizes errors due to poor recall of the exposure or to lack of knowledge of the exposure by the subject. For example, use of pharmacy records in a case–control study of prescription drug use could overcome lack of recall or knowledge by subjects of the names and doses of drugs taken. Moreover, differential exposure measurement error between those with and without disease is unlikely to affect prospectively recorded records, provided that the exposure information used from the records is limited to that recorded before the onset of disease (or other outcome) or symptoms of the disease. Thus case–control studies which use records to assess exposure are much less likely to have bias due to differential error than case–control studies which rely on retrospective interviews.

Medical records are generally assumed to be more accurate than subject interview for medical conditions, diagnostic procedures, and prescription drug use. Indirect support for the superiority of records comes from the poor to moderate agreement between questionnaire data and medical records.

The concordance between medical diagnoses in records and reports by subjects varies widely across conditions and between studies. In a study of older men and women, the sensitivity of self-report compared with medical record ranged from 0.18 for congestive heart failure to 0.81 for diabetes (Fowles *et al.* 1998). Subject reports of X-ray procedures appear to be poor. Tilley *et al.* (1985) found $\kappa = 0.37$ for agreement between physician records and mothers' recall, after more than 10 years, of trunk X-ray during pregnancy. Studies of drug use have focused on oral contraceptive use and post-menopausal oestrogen use and suggest moderate agreement. For agreement between personal interview and physician records of use of exogenous oestrogen (ever versus never), κ ranged from 0.51 to 0.74 across three studies (Horwitz *et al.* 1980; Paganini-Hill and Ross 1982; Goodman *et al.* 1990) with a reported correlation of 0.54–0.63 for total duration of use (Paganini-Hill and Ross 1982; Goodman *et al.* 1990).

Records may be less vulnerable than retrospective interviews to certain sources of error. Telescoping of exposures from the past into a more recent time period may affect records less than interviews. Walter *et al.* (1988) found that women report more Pap smears over the previous five years than their medical records suggest, and report their last one as more recent than indicated in their outpatient records. Records may also be less influenced by social desirability bias; in one study, psychiatric diagnoses were reported twice as often in medical records as in interviews (NCHS 1973). A final advantage of the use of records is the potential for a high response rate. The use of birth records affords a complete sample of births within an entire state. Computerized pharmacy records of a health maintenance organization (Stergachis 1989) may offer near-complete data on a well-defined population. Response rates can be particularly high if subject contact is not required to permit use of the record. In such studies, information can be obtained even when the subject is dead or his/her current address unknown. Approval from human subject review committees for such studies can often be obtained if confidentiality can be assured; for instance, if personal identifying information such as name and address are not abstracted from the records and abstractors sign a commitment to confidentiality.

Unfortunately, not all studies which make use of medical records achieve a high response. In some studies, subjects or next of kin must recall the names of healthcare providers before medical records can be obtained. Permission or a written response from the provider or hospital is often required. Response rates from physicians can be low (Stolley *et al.* 1978; Tilley *et al.* 1985); in one study, 31 per cent of hospitals refused access to their records (Savitz and Grace 1985).

Finally, records can be lost or no longer available, for example when the physician has died.

Reliability and validity of record information

Studies of the agreement between medical records and questionnaire data, such as those cited above, provide only indirect information on the validity of records because they were interpreted under the assumption that discrepancies between the two methods were due to errors in the interview data. Of course medical record data are also subject to error, but direct studies of the reliability and validity of record information are difficult to conduct.

A few studies of the accuracy of the types of measurements that are documented in medical records have been reported. A comprehensive study of the reliability of physical examination information was conducted among Vietnam veterans (CDC 1989). Subjects had a second examination by a different physician on the same day as their first examination. The inter-physician κ for agreement on common conditions (conditions affecting at least 5 per cent of subjects) ranged from a high of 0.47 for ear canal abnormalities and 0.45 for abnormal heart sounds (murmurs, systolic clicks, or gallop sounds) to a low of −0.05 for prostate abnormalities (enlargement or tenderness). The correlation between blood pressure readings was 0.54–0.73 for systolic and 0.45–0.73 for diastolic blood pressure. Biochemical analyses of blood from repeated blood samples (analysed in the same batch) were highly reproducible; correlations ranged from 0.87 for albumin to 0.99 for cholesterol.

Further information on the validity of medical records comes from studies in which records were compared with a more accurate source of data, such as direct observation or video recording of the patient–physician visit. Based on such studies, it appears that for most medical tests and medication prescriptions, the information in the medical record has only moderate sensitivity. Compared with direct observation, medical records only included notations for 49 per cent of hormone replacement prescriptions, 86 per cent of clinical breast examinations, 78 per cent of PSA (prostate-specific antigen) tests ordered, and 64 per cent of cholesterol tests ordered (Stange *et al.* 1998). Overall, the range of sensitivity for laboratory tests and screening services was 62 per cent (for mammography) to 92 per cent (for ECG). Specificity was high, with a range of 94–100 per cent. In a similar study among patients with chronic obstructive pulmonary disease the proportion of drugs prescribed that were noted in the medical record (sensitivity) ranged from 0.60 to 0.82 (Gerbert *et al.* 1988). In a study which compared medical records of antihypertensive medications with a computerized pharmacy database in a health maintenance organization, the sensitivity was high (92–95 per cent), but 30 per cent did not agree on dosage (Christensen *et al.* 1994).

Certain exposures in records, such as alcohol use, smoking, and occupation, originate from self-report by the subject. For these exposures, comparison of records with interviews provides some information about the validity of the records because the interview may be the more accurate source. Brownson *et al.* (1989) compared information in hospital medical records (abstracted for a cancer registry) with that obtained by a telephone interview with the subject. In comparison with the interview, hospital medical records could be used to classify 57 per cent of alcohol drinkers correctly (sensitivity) and 96 per cent of the non-drinkers correctly (specificity). A similar comparison for smoking led to a sensitivity of 0.80, a specificity of 0.91, and a Spearman rank correlation coefficient of 0.93 across four levels of packs smoked per day. Exact agreement of US Census three-digit occupational codes was achieved for 70 per cent of occupations and 72 per cent of industries. However, these statistics may be somewhat misleading as they were based only on records with information that could be coded. They do not reflect the problem of missing data, which is discussed below.

Certain information reported on death certificates has a further source of error: the information is provided by a proxy respondent. The accuracy of this variable is discussed in the section on proxy respondents below.

Sources of error and quality control procedures for record abstraction

Records should be selected as the method of exposure measurement only after consideration has been given to the quality of the data collection process that has already been carried out. Then, quality control procedures should be applied to the remaining steps of data collection. If one is using electronic records that are already in coded variable format, range and logical checks on the data items should be performed as a minimum requirement. For uncoded records (paper or electronic text), the challenge is to reduce an unstructured text into a well-defined set of coded variables. Explicit criteria are needed to minimize the need for judgement and interpretation by the abstractor.

When data are to be abstracted from records, most of the general quality control procedures outlined in Table 5.3 can be applied to the abstraction process. These include the design of a clear abstraction form which is easy to use, development of a detailed protocol for abstraction of the information, thorough training of abstractors, and pre-testing of the protocol. Figure 8.1 gives an example of a data abstraction form and Figure 8.2 shows an example of the protocol for coding some data items from an abstractors' manual. Quality control during

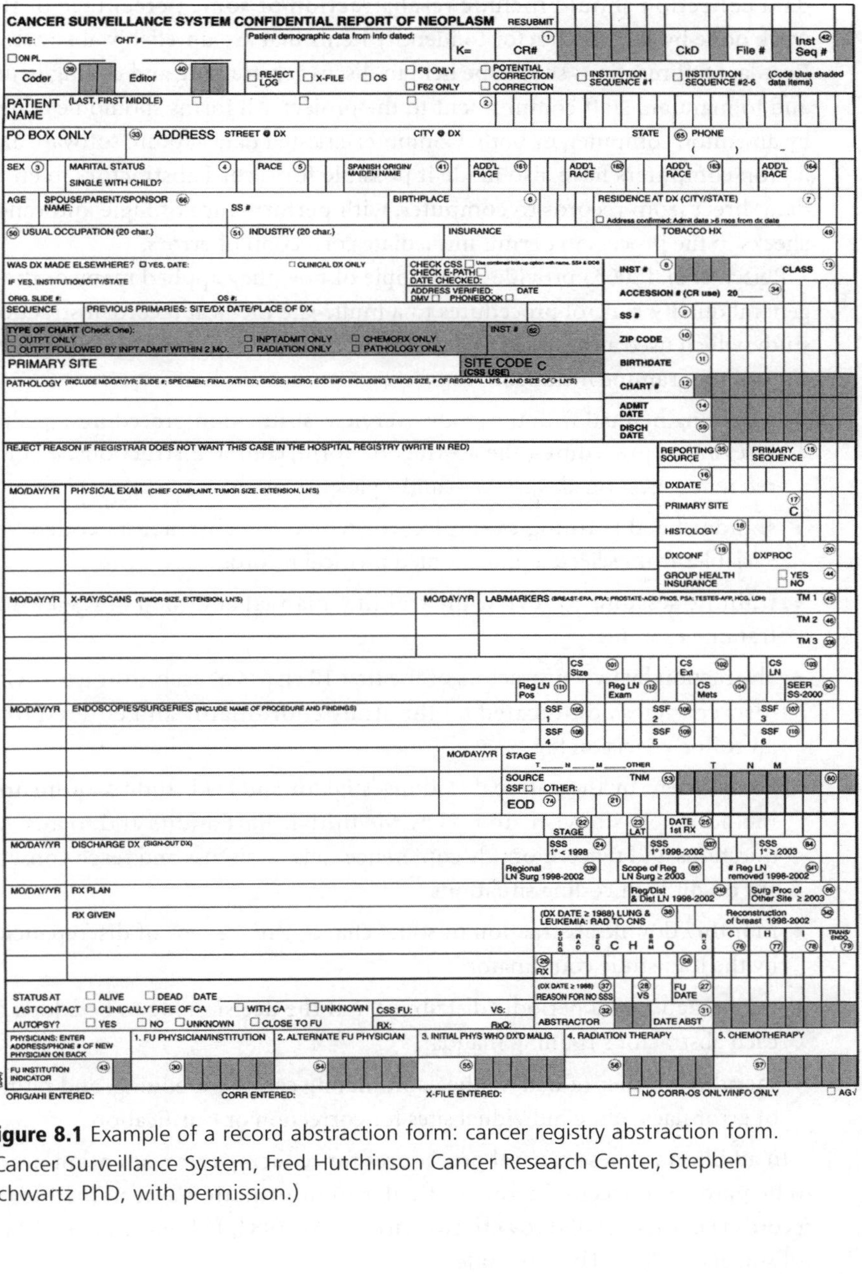
CANCER SURVEILLANCE SYSTEM CONFIDENTIAL REPORT OF NEOPLASM RESUBMIT

NOTE: CHT #: Patient demographic data from info dated: K= CR# CkD File # Inst Seq #

ON PL

Coder Editor REJECT LOG X-FILE OS F8 ONLY F62 ONLY POTENTIAL CORRECTION CORRECTION INSTITUTION SEQUENCE #1 INSTITUTION SEQUENCE #2-6 (Code blue shaded data items)

PATIENT NAME (LAST, FIRST MIDDLE)

PO BOX ONLY ADDRESS STREET @ DX CITY @ DX STATE PHONE ( ) -

SEX MARITAL STATUS SINGLE WITH CHILD? RACE SPANISH ORIGIN/ MAIDEN NAME ADD'L RACE ADD'L RACE ADD'L RACE ADD'L RACE

AGE SPOUSE/PARENT/SPONSOR NAME: SS # BIRTHPLACE RESIDENCE AT DX (CITY/STATE) Address confirmed: Admit date >6 mos from dx date

USUAL OCCUPATION (20 char.) INDUSTRY (20 char.) INSURANCE TOBACCO HX

WAS DX MADE ELSEWHERE? YES, DATE: CLINICAL DX ONLY CHECK CSS CHECK E-PATH DATE CHECKED: INST # CLASS

IF YES, INSTITUTION/CITY/STATE

ORIG. SLIDE #: OS #: ADDRESS VERIFIED: DATE DMV PHONEBOOK ACCESSION # (CR use) 20

SEQUENCE PREVIOUS PRIMARIES: SITE/DX DATE/PLACE OF DX SS #

TYPE OF CHART (Check One): OUTPT ONLY OUTPT FOLLOWED BY INPT ADMIT WITHIN 2 MO. INPT ADMIT ONLY RADIATION ONLY CHEMORX ONLY PATHOLOGY ONLY INST # ZIP CODE

PRIMARY SITE SITE CODE (CSS USE) C BIRTHDATE

PATHOLOGY (INCLUDE MO/DAY/YR; SLIDE #; SPECIMEN; FINAL PATH DX; GROSS; MICRO; EOD INFO INCLUDING TUMOR SIZE, # OF REGIONAL LN'S, # AND SIZE OF LN'S) CHART # ADMIT DATE DISCH DATE

REJECT REASON IF REGISTRAR DOES NOT WANT THIS CASE IN THE HOSPITAL REGISTRY (WRITE IN RED) REPORTING SOURCE PRIMARY SEQUENCE

MO/DAY/YR PHYSICAL EXAM (CHIEF COMPLAINT, TUMOR SIZE, EXTENSION, LN'S) DXDATE PRIMARY SITE C HISTOLOGY DXCONF DXPROC GROUP HEALTH INSURANCE YES NO

MO/DAY/YR X-RAY/SCANS (TUMOR SIZE, EXTENSION, LN'S) MO/DAY/YR LAB/MARKERS (BREAST-ERA, PRA; PROSTATE-ACID PHOS, PSA; TESTES-AFP, HCG, LDH) TM 1 TM 2 TM 3

CS Size CS Ext CS LN Reg LN Pos Reg LN Exam CS Mets SEER SS-2000

MO/DAY/YR ENDOSCOPIES/SURGERIES (INCLUDE NAME OF PROCEDURE AND FINDINGS) SSF 1 SSF 2 SSF 3 SSF 4 SSF 5 SSF 6

MO/DAY/YR STAGE T N M OTHER T N M

SOURCE TNM SSF OTHER:

EOD

STAGE LAT DATE 1st RX

MO/DAY/YR DISCHARGE DX (SIGN-OUT DX) SSS 1° < 1998 SSS 1° 1998-2002 SSS 1° ≥ 2003

Regional LN Surg 1998-2002 Scope of Reg LN Surg ≥ 2003 # Reg LN removed 1998-2002

MO/DAY/YR RX PLAN Reg/Dist & Dist LN 1998-2002 Surg Proc of Other Site ≥ 2003

RX GIVEN (DX DATE ≥ 1988) LUNG & LEUKEMIA: RAD TO CNS Reconstruction of breast 1998-2002

SURG RAD SEQ C H BRM O RXO C H I TRANS/ENDO

RX

STATUS AT LAST CONTACT ALIVE DEAD DATE CLINICALLY FREE OF CA WITH CA UNKNOWN (DX DATE ≥ 1988) REASON FOR NO SSS VS FU DATE

AUTOPSY? YES NO UNKNOWN CLOSE TO FU CSS FU: VS: RX: RxQ: ABSTRACTOR DATE ABST

PHYSICIANS: ENTER ADDRESS/PHONE # OF NEW PHYSICIAN ON BACK 1. FU PHYSICIAN/INSTITUTION 2. ALTERNATE FU PHYSICIAN 3. INITIAL PHYS WHO DX'D MALIG. 4. RADIATION THERAPY 5. CHEMOTHERAPY

FU INSTITUTION INDICATOR

ORIG/AHI ENTERED: CORR ENTERED: X-FILE ENTERED: NO CORR-OS ONLY/INFO ONLY AG√

Figure 8.1 Example of a record abstraction form: cancer registry abstraction form. (Cancer Surveillance System, Fred Hutchinson Cancer Research Center, Stephen Schwartz PhD, with permission.)

data collection should include re-abstraction of some percentage of the work done by each abstractor to identify items that are unreliably abstracted. Regular staff meetings should be held to discuss abstracting and coding issues and to maintain staff commitment to the project. All forms should be edited by an editor, computer, or both. Computer-assisted data capture software and laptop computers have also made it possible for record abstractors to enter data direct from records to computer, with performance of logic and range checks in the process to permit immediate correction of errors.

Reisch *et al.* (2003) provide an example of how they applied many of these general quality control procedures to a multi-site medical record abstraction study, which used a computerized abstraction form. Their training and quality control programme included:

- a training manual with the study overview, abstraction procedures, quality assessment procedures, the abstraction form, coding instructions, a quick reference sheet on all variables, and a glossary of terms
- standardized training examples, for which the abstractors coded key variables from selected photocopied medical records
- training sessions to review the training manual and then to review the training examples
- abstraction by two abstractors of the first 10 charts of each abstractor, with discrepancies adjudicated by the study coordinator and entered into an editor's decision log
- involvement by the national lead investigator and lead study coordinator, including on-site visits to review the initial chart audits and to answer questions and twice-monthly conference calls to discuss and reach consensus on difficult coding situations
- monthly double abstraction of some charts, with review of discrepancies by the lead study coordinator
- maintenance and periodic distribution of the decision log to be added to each abstractor's training manual
- monthly transfer of data to the coordinating centre for editing, and return of error flags to the individual sites for correction or clarification.

In addition to these general procedures for reducing error, attention needs to be paid to sources of error particular to information ascertained from records (Feinstein *et al.* 1969a,b; Horwitz and Yu 1984; Hilsenbeck *et al.* 1985; Allison *et al.* 2000). These include:

- difficulty in blinding abstractors to the disease status of subjects
- lack of complete coverage by records of the time period of interest

FOR BREAST CASES (site C50.0-C50.6, C50.8-C50.9)
FIELDS 45/46 ERA/PRA

Beginning with January 1, 1990 breast cancer diagnoses, SEER collects Estrogen
Receptor status (ERA) as Field 45 and Progesterone Receptor status (PRA) as Field 46.

Field 45/46 Codes for ERA/PRA

    0 Not done
    1 Positive/elevated
    2 Negative/normal; within normal limits
    3 Borderline; undetermined whether positive or negative
    8 Ordered, but results not in chart
    9 Unknown; no information

NOTES

1. Code ERA/PRA status as done only if done on the primary tumor; if done on other than the primary tumor, code status to 0.
2. If abstract clearly indicates per clinician/pathologist "No ERA PRA" or "ERA PRA not done" code to 0. If there is no indication this is a physician's statement, code to 9.
3. Code '0' for all "Autopsy Only" cases;
   Code '9' for all "Death Certificate Only" cases.
4. Assign codes 1, 2 and 3 on the basis of lab-specific determinations of normal range as noted in the laboratory report.
5. Tumors too small to evaluate by the conventional estrogen/progesterone receptor assays may be measured by immunostaining. The procedure is based on an antigen-antibody reaction. Include these results when conventional procedures are absent.
6. If a value from an ERA/PRA done using only immunocytochemical (ICC) or immunohistochemical (IHC) technique is converted to ERA/PRA status (e.g. UW lab: >30% = positive), it is codeable in fields 45-46. ICC and IHC use the same method which is based on monoclonal antibody techniques. They provide semi-quantitative results that will be expressed either as a % of cells that stain (e.g. >30%) or the intensity of the staining (e.g. 2+). Both can be done on either fresh or fixed tissue. They are usually performed on tissue but can be done on cells.
7. A statement of "immunoreactive" is equal to positive.
8. If more than one ERA/PRA is done using the same technique and the results differ, code positive over negative.
9. If an ERA/PRA is done on both femtomoles/mg and ICC/IHC technique, code the femtomoles/mg over the ICC/IHC.
10. If a status is given as positive or negative along with a statement that a false positive or negative cannot be ruled out, code the status given (e.g. ERA/PRA status: neg; cannot R/O false neg. Code to negative).
11. If an ERA/PRA result is stated as "<u>negative</u> with positive internal control", this should be coded as negative (a positive internal control is used to check on whether it might be a false negative).
12. If the ERA/PRA results differ on the in situ and infiltrating components for the same primary, code to the infiltrating tumor results (e.g. PRA – positive for the intraductal ca; PRA – negative for the infiltrating ca. Code to negative).
13. If there is a ductal/lobular primary and the ERA/PRA status of the ductal tumor differs from that of the lobular tumor, bring the case to the Coding Supervisor.

Figure 8.2 Example from a record abstraction protocol: coding of oestrogen receptor assay. (Cancer Surveillance System, Fred Hutchinson Cancer Research Center, Stephen Schwartz PhD, with permission.)

- missing information on the exposure or covariates of interest
- lack of uniform order of information in the record
- ambiguous or inconsistent information within and between records.

These sources of error are described in more detail below, together with quality control procedures which may reduce them.

The emphasis of the following sections is on abstracting data from written medical records. However, many of the sources of error and quality control procedures described apply to other types of records as well, and some also apply to electronic records.

Blinding abstractors to disease status of subjects

In most epidemiological studies which use medical records, the records of the cases will have information on their diagnosis of the disease. Thus special efforts need to be taken to blind the abstractor to case–control status. Typically, a reference date (date of diagnosis or some earlier time point for cases and a comparable date for controls) is established, and the abstractor is instructed not to go beyond that date. Masking of the diagnosis can be achieved by having the data collection supervisor mark the reference date with a clip and by covering summary pages which indicate diagnoses or vital status. Alternatively, only the relevant pages can be photocopied for the abstractor to work from.

Incomplete coverage of the time period of interest

Records should only be selected as the method of exposure measurement if the data required are expected to be available for a large proportion of subjects; additionally, the completeness of coverage within the records themselves should also be considered.

The time period covered by the record may not be the complete time period of interest. Outpatient medical records cover only the time period that a subject has been with the provider or clinic. Medical conditions or personal information, such as occupation, relevant to earlier time periods may be only variably recorded. A related problem is the use of multiple providers during a given time period. For example, a subject may have seen several physicians or used multiple pharmacies, and the researcher may not have access to all providers. In one study, the agreement on use of oral oestrogens was substantially higher for interview compared with medical records than interview compared with pharmacy records ($\kappa = 0.51$ and $\kappa = 0.21$, respectively) (Paganini-Hill and Ross 1982). The authors attribute this to subjects' use of pharmacies other than the community medical centre pharmacy that was surveyed.

One concern with incomplete coverage is that differential misclassification can be introduced if the time periods of coverage are systematically different between cases and controls. Suppose that a case–control study were to be conducted of myocardial infarction in relation to certain medications within a health maintenance organization. If cases had been enrolled for an average of 10 years and randomly selected controls had been enrolled for an average of 5 years, this selection of controls would almost certainly have led to differential measurement error in medication history. To minimize this bias, cases and controls should be matched or stratified on the date of commencement of their records and on length of time with the provider.

Finally, records or certain volumes of records may be missed, lost, or otherwise unavailable (Horwitz and Yu 1984). A system of recording volume numbers should be used to ensure that all volumes of a subject's medical record are obtained.

Missing information in records

Information of interest to the researcher is often missing in records. As noted earlier, even patient care information such as drug prescriptions is sometimes not recorded in medical records (Gerbert *et al.* 1988; Stange *et al.* 1998). Symptoms, health behaviours, family history, and physician counselling about diet, exercise, and smoking may be even less consistently noted in medical records (Gilliland *et al.* 1997; Stange *et al.* 1998). Moreover, there is a greater tendency to omit negative findings than to omit positive ones. For example, no information in a record on smoking could mean either that the question was not asked, or that it was asked and a negative answer was obtained but not recorded.

A particular problem with the use of records is that they may have been selected for the availability of information on the primary exposure, but information on potential confounders may not be recorded for many subjects, or may be recorded in insufficient detail. For example, Brownson *et al.* (1989) found that among records of cancer patients, 15 per cent had missing information on smoking, 25 per cent on alcohol consumption, and 36 per cent on occupation. These deficiencies would lead to an inability to control fully for the effects of confounding variables.

An additional problem is that missing information may be related to the disease or exposure under study. For example, the physician may be more likely to ask a question on family history of breast cancer among women with benign breast disease, which would lead to more reports of a positive history even in the absence of any true association. The selection of an appropriate reference date may lessen the problem of differential recording of exposures between those with and without the disease. A reference date for each case before the onset of symptoms of the disease could be selected, and a similar date assigned to each control. Information recorded after that date would not be abstracted. As noted above, this procedure also helps to blind data abstractors to the disease status of subjects.

Supplemental data collection is one solution to missing data. Certain exposures may be measured by record review and others by interviews conducted with the subject, the physician, or the next of kin. For example, if the primary exposure in a study were use of a particular class of drugs, pharmacy records might be used, but information on smoking, occupation, etc., would be ascertained by personal interview. Alternatively, interviews could be conducted only for those subjects with missing items in the record. However, this approach should be used cautiously; any difference in the proportion of missing data between cases and controls would lead to a difference in exposure measurement methods between groups, which could produce differential measurement error.

The coding of missing information in records can present problems. For each item of data, the researcher must decide whether no mention of the item in the record implies that the exposure is absent or that it should be treated as missing data. Sometimes when a data item is missing in a medical record, it can be assumed with reasonable confidence that the condition is absent. For example, if a woman's obstetric and delivery record has no mention of placenta praevia, it is unlikely to have occurred. Items such as this could be coded on the abstraction form simply as 'yes' or 'no', with no mention of the condition in the record coded as 'no'. On the other hand, if there is any doubt about the meaning of missing information, such as missing information on smoking, it should be coded as 'missing' so that its further treatment can be considered at the time of analysis. Additional detail about missing information might be useful; for example, a 'missing' laboratory test result might be coded as 'not done', 'ordered but results not in chart', or 'no information'. The protocol in Figure 8.2 gives an example of the detailed coding of missing information for oestrogen receptor status.

Unfortunately, differentiating 'missing information' from 'condition absent' may be difficult for abstractors. In two studies of coding errors made by well-trained data abstractors, miscoding of 'missing' as 'no' was a common mistake (Herrmann et al. 1980; Horwitz and Yu 1984)

Lack of uniform order of information in records

Another common source of error in record abstraction stems from the lack of uniform order of information in the medical record. Information on certain items may appear in different places in records of different subjects, and may be missed by the abstractor. The usual approach is for the abstractor to review the entire medical record or to read major sources of information such as the hospital admission form, the history and physical examination, the discharge summary, and laboratory reports (in some specified order), and to record the information on the data collection form as it is found. This contrasts with a personal interview, where the interviewer can collect information in the order that the items appear on the questionnaire.

This variation in where the requisite information appears in the record leads to the information sometimes being missed by abstractors (Horwitz and Yu 1984). In a study of medical intervention surrounding delivery (Caesarean section delivery, electronic fetal monitoring, amniotomy, etc.), abstractors coded as absent 10 per cent of the events that were recorded in the chart (Hewson and Bennett 1987). Errors in the opposite direction were rare; almost no absent events were coded as present. Similarly, birth records, which are abstracted from medical records, have incomplete ascertainment of complications of pregnancy (Kristensen et al. 1996; Dobie et al. 1998).

This unique aspect of medical record abstracting needs to be taken into consideration in the design of the data collection form and the training of abstractors (Hilsenbeck et al. 1985; Horwitz and Yu 1984). If possible, the data collection form should be on a single page, so that abstractors do not need to flip pages forward and back to record information as it is found. Use of two columns of items on the page and use of abbreviations for item descriptions can help to limit the form to a single page. Instructions and lists of responses usually found on an interview form can be omitted from the abstraction form and included in the abstractors' manual instead. Figure 8.1 gives an example of a one-page abstraction form.

The data abstraction form should be structured in a way that is logically related to the structure of the record. Items that are likely to be grouped together in the record should be in the same section of the form. For example, the subject's age and sex would first appear on the hospital admissions form, and these items might form the first section of the abstraction form. Abstractors should be familiar with the organization of medical records, and have the ability to scan large amounts of information. In addition, the training of abstractors and the data collection manual should specify in which parts of the record each item is likely to be found.

Use of check lists for items of interest leads to fewer missed items than if open-ended questions are used. In the state of Washington, when birth certificates were formatted with an open-ended question on birth complications, only 33 per cent of Caesarean section deliveries and 52 per cent of breech presentations were recorded in comparison with hospital reports of these conditions (Frost et al. 1984). When a format was introduced that listed each complication of interest, over 90 per cent of Caesarean sections and breech presentations were recorded.

After abstraction is complete but before returning the record, abstractors should completely review the data form to search for data items that were missed. Use of a coloured pen on a black-and-white form helps in detecting missed items. Computer-assisted abstraction should be programmed to query the abstractor about missing items before the subject's record can be closed.

Uncertainties and inconsistencies in records

A final problem in record abstraction is the handling of uncertainties and inconsistencies in the records. Records often include information recorded with an indication of uncertainty. For example, 'possible asthma' may be recorded in a chart based on the patient's report of history of attacks in the absence of signs at the time of the visit, with no subsequent follow-up information. How should qualifiers such as 'possible', 'probable', or 'consistent with' affect the coding of the condition? Or, how should a test value of '<20' be recorded? Decisions such as these should be made by the researcher and specified in the abstractors' manual rather than left to the abstractor's judgement. The existence of such difficulties, if not anticipated, should be uncovered during pre-testing of the abstraction form.

Inconsistencies occur when conflicting information is recorded within a subject's record, or when technical terms are used differently between records. One source of inconsistencies within and between records is the large number of data recorders. Information in hospital records, in particular, is likely to be recorded by multiple providers—the primary physician, residents, specialists, and nurses—and this can lead to conflicting information on the same item (Herrmann et al. 1980; Horwitz and Yu 1984). Even standardized tests such as the Apgar score of infant condition at birth can be applied differently by different healthcare providers. In a study of uncomplicated births at five hospitals, the proportion of infants who scored a perfect 10 on the five-minute Apgar test ranged from 58 per cent at one hospital to none at another (Hewson and Bennett 1987).

Medical terms are interpreted differently not only between providers, but also between abstractors. Herrmann et al. (1980) found that inter-abstractor agreement was poorest for items which required judgement on the part of the abstractors. In particular, among six pre-existing conditions abstracted from hospital records of trauma patients, the inter-rater agreement was lowest for obesity ($\kappa = 0.41$).

To minimize inconsistencies, the aim of the abstractors' manual and the emphasis of the training of abstractors should be on the standardized extraction of information from records. Abstractors should be familiar with medical terminology and, more importantly, well trained in the definition of terms used in the study. The coding procedures shown in Figure 8.2 give examples of ways to provide the abstractors with guidance to terminology and the handling of inconsistencies in the medical record. Boyd *et al.* (1979) found that when physician-abstractors were provided with explicit definitions of terms, the inter-rater κ values for measures of several symptoms of Hodgkin's disease were higher (0.75–0.93) than when physicians worked without the use of explicit criteria (0.29–0.59). When feasible, abstractors should code the quantitative measures that lead to the diagnoses of interest, in addition to the diagnoses. For example, pre-diagnostic fasting blood glucose levels could be recorded for diabetes, and height and weight could be recorded for obesity.

Feinstein *et al.* (1969a) suggest separating abstracting from coding to promote the uniform application of coding rules. First, abstractors record all items requiring coding as words and abbreviations, and then coders code the items numerically. This allows one or more staff members to specialize as coders, and enables coding to be checked without re-accessing the records. On the other hand, this two-step process could increase study costs, has not been demonstrated to reduce error, and could conceivably introduce error through misunderstanding of the abstract by the coder. Therefore it may only be appropriate for variables with complex coding rules. The form in Figure 8.1 was designed for this two-step procedure.

Feinstein *et al.* (1969a) also suggest ranking the sources of information in priority order to resolve conflicts within records. For example, data from the primary source (e.g. the laboratory) should be abstracted in preference to secondary sources (e.g. laboratory values in the medical notes). Conflicting information in a record can also reflect true change over time in a patient (even over a very short time, such as in a trauma patient). The record abstraction instructions should make clear the preferred time to which the observation should relate, relative to the start of the record, the disease diagnosis, or the reference date.

A final source of inconsistency within or between records is that laboratory tests often differ between hospitals or over time in analytical method, units of measurement, and upper and lower limits of detection or reporting. Consideration needs to be given to handling differing units of measure (e.g. birth weight may be recorded in pounds in some records, grams in others) and various laboratory analytical techniques. Abstractors should not perform conversions. Instead, for example, an abstraction form might include two items for birth weight—one if it is recorded in pounds, and another if it is recorded in grams.

Summary

The prospective nature of records makes them an attractive source of information which may be less subject to the biases of retrospective interview. However, their use in exposure measurement has limitations. In particular, the researcher has little control over the availability of records for each subject for the time period of interest, the items recorded, the definition of terms used, and the order of information in the records. Careful design of the record abstraction form, precise definition of terms, and abstractor training can reduce some of these sources of error. Additional quality control procedures include matching cases and controls with respect to length of time with the healthcare provider, use of a reference date, making preferential selections when conflicting information appears in a record, and using codes to distinguish 'missing information' from 'condition absent' when appropriate.

Use of diaries

Scope of diaries

Diaries refer here to detailed prospective records of exposure kept by the subject. This method has been used to measure physical activity (La Porte *et al.* 1979), sexual activity (Kunin and Ames 1981; Hornsby and Wilcox 1989), alcohol consumption (Hilton 1989), and other frequent exposures. Diaries are also used to measure dietary intake; these are usually termed *food records* (Freudenheim *et al.* 1986; Witschi 1990; Dolecek *et al.* 1997; Buzzard 1998). *Health diaries* are used to measure symptoms, minor illnesses, medication use, and medical care (Verbrugge 1980, 1984).

Diaries are generally open-ended and take the form of a booklet in which the subject records each occurrence of a particular behaviour at the level of detail requested by the researcher. Open-ended diaries usually take the form of a journal with one entry per line, with columns indicating the details needed. Figure 8.3 gives an example of a diet diary; this form is designed for a new page to be started each day and one food or ingredient to be recorded per line, with columns for recording the meal, the place of food preparation, the food description, and the amount. The diary booklet should also incorporate detailed instructions for recording the required information. An example of general instructions for keeping a food record and specific instructions for recording foods is given in Figure 8.4. For a food record, instructions for measuring the amount of food would also be given (not shown), and a sample completed page (Figure 8.3) is helpful for most types of diaries. Diaries also need to have spaces for coding, for example where a coder converts each recorded recreational activity into a numeric code. (The diary form in Figure 8.3 does not include a column for coding of foods, because the coded information is directly entered electronically into a nutrient analysis program.)

Diaries can also take other forms. They can be closed-ended or partly closed-ended. For example, types of physical activities may be printed on the form, with columns for the subject to prospectively record his/her daily frequencies of the listed activities. Open-ended diaries allow more accurate specification of the type of exposure, but closed-ended diaries reduce the amount of coding required. Diaries in which few or no entries are expected for most days, such as a diary of doctor's visits, can take the form of a monthly calendar. When disparate behaviours are being recorded (e.g. both symptoms and doctor's visits), diaries can have a ledger format with separate sections for the different types of entries (Verbrugge 1980).

A method related to diaries is *short-term recall of exposure*, i.e. telephone or face-to-face interviews covering the behaviour in question over short periods of time (hours or days). For example, subjects may be telephoned, once or several times, and asked to report all foods eaten in the last 24 hours (Buzzard 1998). This method is a hybrid between the personal interview and the self-completed diary, and shares some of the advantages and limitations of each method.

Technology has greatly expanded data collection techniques which could also be considered to be forms of diaries. *Electronic diaries* can be used instead of paper-and-pencil diaries in many situations. Daily data collection can be accomplished via touch-tone telephones or hand-held electronic devices ('palm' computers) (Searles *et al.* 1995; Mundt 1997; Carney *et al.* 1998; Shiffman and Stone 1998; Raymond and Ross 2000). These can be used for frequent simple behaviours, such as drinking or use of medication, or for subjective measures such as symptoms. Some devices can be programmed to 'beep' to remind subjects to record information in their diary (Kubey *et al.* 1996). These are particularly useful for diaries of pain or symptoms that are to be recorded at specified or random times during the day, rather than diaries that are to be recorded after specific behaviours such as drinking. Some electronic or mechanical devices can automate data capture with little subject involvement, such as pill containers that monitor medication compliance or motion sensors that record physical activity (Berg *et al.* 1998; Bassett *et al.* 2000). These could be considered a hybrid of diaries and objective measures.

Place Prepared H= Home R= Restaurant O= Other			Day: Saturday		Date: 08/ 04 / 06	
Meal B= B'fast L= Lunch D= Dinner S= Snack	↓		*The following sample pages show you how to record a day's food intake. To begin to record your own food intake, turn to page 12.*			
	↓	↓	**Foods And Beverages**			**Amount**
1	B	R	Pancakes, buttermilk 6" d			2
2			Butter, whipped			2 TB
3			Pancake syrup			1/4 cup
4			Breakfast sausage, pork, 3" links			2
5			Coffee, with caffeine, brewed			2 cups
6			Cream, unknown type			2 TB
7						
8	L	H	Ham Sandwich:			
9			Rye bread (standard slice)			2 sl
10			Ham, boiled, deli (1 slice=4"L x 4"W x 1/4"TK)			1 sl
11			Cheese, American, Kraft Deluxe Slices			1 sl
12			Best Foods Mayonnaise, low fat			2 tsp

Figure 8.3 Example of an exposure diary: food records sample page. (Nutritional Assessment Shared Resource, Fred Hutchinson Cancer Research Center, Alan Kristal DrPH, with permission.)

General Instructions For Keeping a Food Record	Instructions For Recording of Foods

• Remember do **not** change your eating habits!
 	
• Please use ink and write clearly.
 	
• Record **everything** you eat and drink (except water), preferably **right after** it is eaten. This includes any and **all snacks**.
 	
• Fill in the **Meal** and **Place Prepared** columns for each meal or snack.
 	
• Write each food or ingredient on a **separate line**.
 	
• **Skip** a line after each meal or snack.
 	
• Start each **new day** on a **new page**.
 	
• If more space is needed for the same day, use the next page.
 	
Use the **recipe pages** starting on page 39 to describe homemade recipes. List all ingredients and their amounts. Under "Prep" **briefly** tell us how the recipe was prepared. You may attach copies of your recipes, noting any variations.
	Please keep the following things in mind when you write down the foods you eat.
	
	• **Fully describe** foods and beverages.
	  <u>Examples</u>: chicken thigh, skin eaten
	       French dressing, low fat
	
	• Record **brand names**.
	
	• Include the food label (nutrition information and/or list of ingredients) if possible.
	
	• Explain how foods are **prepared**.
	  <u>Example</u>: Is meat fried, broiled, baked, breaded, etc?
	
	• For foods **prepared with fat**, write down the type (butter, margarine, oil, etc.) and the amount used.
	  <u>Example</u>: fried in margarine (brand name), 2 TB
	
	• Include items you add at the table. List them on **separate lines**.
	  <u>Example</u>: baked potato 1 med
	           with butter 1 TB
	
	• For sandwiches, salads and mixed dishes: List **each ingredient and amount**. Use pages 39-43 to record recipes.
	
	• Record **exact** amounts. **Measure** all foods in cups, teaspoons, tablespoons, or size in inches. The following pages explain how to measure, weigh, and estimate portion sizes.

Figure 8.4 Example of diary recording instructions for subjects: food records. (Nutritional Assessment Shared Resource, Fred Hutchinson Cancer Research Center, Alan Kristal DrPH, with permission.)

Advantages and limitations of diaries

Diaries are assumed to be highly accurate in measuring current behaviour because they do not rely on memory. In particular, the use of prospective recording eliminates telescoping and facilitates the collection of information on events of low salience that are quickly forgotten, such as foods eaten. Diaries also allow the collection of greater detail about the exposure than is possible by questionnaire. For example, foods can be weighed or measured by the subject before consumption, or recreational physical activities can be timed.

A further advantage is that diaries do not require the subject to summarize his pattern of behaviour, while questionnaires often ask about 'usual' behaviour. For example, the pattern of alcohol drinking can vary greatly from day to day or from week to week (Alanko 1984). A diary kept for a sufficient time period can capture this kind of variation. Another example comes from a comparison between a diary estimate of frequency of sexual intercourse and a question on usual frequency (Hornsby and Wilcox 1989). The reported usual frequency was overestimated by almost 50 per cent compared with the diary. The authors attributed this to a tendency to consider 'usual' frequency as being that in the absence of menses, travel, illness, or other transient factors.

The primary limitation of the use of diaries is that only current exposure can be measured. Diaries are a measure of past exposure only if current and past behaviour are highly correlated. Furthermore, diaries are accurate measures of average current behaviour only if a sufficient number of days or weeks are captured (discussed below).

In addition, diaries generally demand more time and skills from subjects than do other methods. Subjects need basic measurement and recording capabilities. The training of subjects in the skills needed to keep an accurate diary can be time consuming for both subjects and study staff. Moreover, subjects need the motivation to maintain the diary over the required time period.

These limitations may make it difficult to recruit a representative sample of the population of interest and to obtain a high response rate. A review of response rates across studies of health diaries found a range of 50–96 per cent (Verbrugge 1980). Participation rates and rates of full completion of diaries among participants have been found to be lower for those with less than a high-school education, those of lower social class, those who are over age 65, and those who have experienced recent stressful life events (Marr 1971; Gersovitz et al. 1978; Verbrugge 1984).

Another disadvantage of diaries is the complexity of processing the information. For diet diaries, for example, each food item recorded must be numerically coded, food portions must be standardized, and a computer program and associated database are needed to convert the wide range of foods to nutrients. Some systems have as many as 15 000 food codes (Willett 1998, p. 30).

The training and monitoring of subjects and the lengthy coding procedures tend to make the use of diaries expensive. Roghmann and Haggerty (1972) estimated that seven hours of interviewers' and coders' time were spent per family for an initial interview plus a 28-day health diary, including an average of 2.6 personal visits and 2.5 telephone calls.

These disadvantages have led to limited use of diaries in epidemiology. They have been used primarily as a comparison method for validation studies of questionnaires or other methods. However, diaries could be an appropriate method for exposure measurement in prospective cohort or cross-sectional studies. The advantage of increased accuracy needs to be weighed against the disadvantages of subject burden and the large costs of participant training and staff monitoring, review and coding. However, one study has tested streamlining some of these procedures to reduce costs, and reported only a small decrease in accuracy (Kolar *et al.* 2005). This suggests that diaries might be able to be used in large-scale studies.

Reliability and validity of measures from diaries

Diaries are generally more accurate than questionnaires if they are collected over a sufficient time period. Verbrugge (1980) reports that health diaries are clearly superior to interview, with some studies showing twice as many minor illnesses reported in the diary as by interview. Willett *et al.* (1985) reported that the validity of nutrients computed from a one-week diet diary is somewhat greater than that of a retrospective food frequency questionnaire, using as the standard three other one-week diaries completed over a one-year period. The correlation of calorie-adjusted fat intake from the one-week diary with the standard was 0.64, while the correlation of fat intake from the questionnaire with the standard was 0.52. McKeown *et al.* (2001) found that a seven-day diet diary was much more accurate than a food frequency questionnaire when each was validated against urinary nitrogen and potassium ($r = 0.55$–0.67 for the diary versus $r = 0.29$–0.32 for the questionnaire). However, Hilton (1989) has argued that a retrospective interview on alcohol use is nearly as accurate as a diary and is easier to administer. Among a sample of moderate to heavy drinkers he found a correlation of 0.89 between the two methods, with minimal under-reporting in the interview (59 drinks/month on average in the interview compared with 61 in the diary).

Automated diary methods are generally thought to be more accurate than paper diaries. Electronic diaries are more accurate for pain or symptoms because they allow the time of data entry to be captured, whereas paper diaries can be filled in retrospectively hours (or days) after the instructed times of diary entries (Shiffman and Stone 1998). Completeness of record keeping (e.g. as measured by number of completed diary days) has also been found to be higher with electronic diaries (Jamison *et al.* 2001). In a comparison of medication adherence by self-completed diaries versus an electronic monitoring device, compliance was less (and presumably more accurate) using electronic monitoring (Berg *et al.* 1998). However, objective 'diary' measures via devices are not always more accurate than self-reported diaries. For example, in studies of measuring physical activity in children, there have been conflicting results as to whether activity monitors (accelerometers) are more accurate than diaries or recalls when each was compared with heart rate monitors (Allor and Pivarnik 2001; Coleman *et al.* 1997).

Sources of error and quality control procedures for diaries

Although diaries are generally more accurate than questionnaires, they are still subject to a range of errors. Most of the quality control procedures outlined in Table 5.3 can be applied to diary studies to improve the validity of the exposure measurement. The development of a detailed study procedure manual, pre-testing of the procedures, and monitoring of data collection are important in any data collection effort. In addition, several sources of error specific to diaries need to be considered (Marr 1971; Roghmann and Haggerty 1972; Gersovitz *et al.* 1978; Verbrugge 1980; Sempos *et al.* 1985; Gibson 1987; Dolecek *et al.* 1997; Buzzard 1998). These include the following.

- The time period covered by the diary may not be sufficient to reflect the subject's 'true exposure'.
- The act of keeping the diary may affect the behaviours being recorded.
- Errors may be introduced because the subjects serve as the primary data collectors.
- The coding of diaries may be more complex than for other methods.

These issues and suggested quality control procedures are discussed below.

Selection of diary recording period

Although diaries can only directly measure a few days or weeks of exposure, they are usually intended to reflect the subject's exposure over some longer period of time. Thus, while a one-day diary might be perfectly accurate as a measure of exposure during that day, the validity of that measure depends on how well it captures the true variable of interest, for example exposure over the preceding year. The diary should include a sufficient number of days and a sufficient spread of days over time to account for day-to-day, weekday-to-weekend, month-to-month, or season-to-season variation in exposure. For example, nutrient intake has been shown to differ on weekends compared with weekdays and to vary by season (Marr 1971).

The formulae in Chapter 5 offer guidance as to the number of randomly selected days that each subject should keep a diary. Formulae are given for determining the number of parallel measures needed per subject to achieve a specified validity (Equation 5.6) or to minimize study costs (Equation 5.7). Related formulae are given by Liu *et al.* (1978), Beaton *et al.* (1979), and Sempos *et al.* (1985).

For example, suppose that calcium intake is to be studied prospectively in relationship to bone loss. Calcium intake will be measured by a diet diary, and the number of diary days needs to be determined. Assume that a pilot study demonstrated that for calcium intake measured on two random diary days $(X_1$ and $X_2)$, the reliability coefficient $\rho_{X_1 X_2}$ was 0.41. Then under the assumption that X_1 and X_2 are parallel measures, the validity coefficient ρ_{TX_1} for a one-day diary would be estimated as $\sqrt{0.41} = 0.64$ (from Equation 4.4). Equation 5.6 could then be used to determine the number of days (k) needed to achieve a validity coefficient ρ_{TA} of, say, 0.8 for the diary measure A (calcium intake averaged over k days):

$$k = \frac{0.8^2(1 - 0.41)}{0.41(1 - 0.8^2)} = 2.6.$$

This result indicates that three random days of diary per subject would be needed. Similar computations show that two days would be needed to achieve a validity coefficient of 0.7, and seven days would be needed for a validity of 0.9. These results are similar to those of an empirical study which assessed validity against a standard of 64 days of food records per subject on average (Freudenheim *et al.* 1987).

Selecting the time period for a diary involves practical as well as statistical considerations. Randomly selecting days over the entire time period of interest is statistically the most efficient approach to capturing variation in exposure over time. However, for convenience, diary days are usually consecutive for some time period (2 days to 1 month) and then repeated once or more if necessary to capture month-to-month variation. For example, two or more one-week diaries spread over a year may be needed to measure recreational physical activity. Distribution over a whole year is important for measurement of behaviours that vary seasonally.

The assumption of equal and uncorrelated errors in the equations that yield number of diary days (see Chapter 5) is unlikely to hold when X_1 and X_2 represent measured exposure on two consecutive days. In this situation, the errors may be correlated either positively or negatively. For example, if there were seasonal variation in dietary intake, the errors in X_1 and X_2 might be positively correlated since both reflect the same season. Conversely, higher than average recreational physical activity one day may tend to be followed by no activity on the next day, i.e. the errors may be negatively correlated.

One approach to selecting the number of consecutive days of recording is similar to the approach for selecting the number of random day diaries. The equations in Chapter 5 can be used, but with X_1 and X_2 representing two multiple-day diaries. A reliability study could be conducted in which subjects complete, for example, two seven-day diaries, with the two seven-day periods randomly selected throughout a year. Then variables X_1 and X_2 can be created so that they represent two one-day diaries from random times in the year, or two two-day diaries, etc. The researcher can then estimate how many one-day, two-day, three-day, ... records spread over a year would be needed to achieve a certain level of validity. For example, this might indicate that three one-day records or two two-day records were equally accurate, and the two two-day diaries might be selected by the researcher as more convenient to administer.

Reactivity

Diaries are intended to measure the subject's usual behaviour over some time period. One concern with diaries is that the act of keeping a diary may lead to a change in behaviour (Verbrugge 1980; Sempos *et al.* 1985). This is an example of *reactivity*, i.e. that 'the process of measuring may change that which is being measured' (Campbell and Stanley 1963). Record keeping may sensitize subjects to their actions or feelings, or may lead them to change towards more socially desirable or health-conscious behaviours. For example, recording recreational exercise might lead to an increase in physical activity during the diary period, or recording symptoms may sensitize a subject to recognize minor symptoms which might otherwise go unnoticed. Reactivity may be a particular problem in randomized trials, because participants may be particularly compliant with the intervention on diary days. Forster *et al.* (1990) reported that, during a sodium reduction trial, sodium intake as reported on a one-day diet record declined to a greater degree than urinary sodium excretion.

Subjects may also change behaviours in order to reduce record keeping. In studies in which subjects were questioned about completing food records, 30–50 per cent reported that they had changed their eating habits while keeping the records, in part to lessen the burden of recording the information (Forster *et al.* 1990; MacDiarmid and Blundell 1997). There is also empirical evidence that the number of items recorded in diaries drops over time, although this may be due to under-reporting of behaviours due to fatigue with the study rather than subjects actually modifying their behaviour. Rebro *et al.* (1998) found that middle-age women recorded significantly fewer foods on day 4 of a four-day food diary compared with day 1, and Gillmore *et al.* (2001) reported that college-age subjects reported less drinking and smoking over the course of an eight-week diary. Verbrugge (1980) noted that reported health events such as illnesses and physician visits tended to drop over time independently of any seasonal effects.

Discussion of the problem of reactivity during training of subjects might reduce this source of error. Subjects could be told that for scientific reasons it is important to assess their usual behaviour. For example, part of the written instructions for a diet diary could include the following.

- Don't change what you usually eat.
- Eat as you normally do.
- Give a complete, true record.
- No one is judging what you eat.

Inaccuracies due to study subjects as data collectors

When diaries are used to measure exposure, the study subjects themselves are the primary data collectors. Subjects may record information inaccurately because of deception (e.g. under-reporting socially undesirable behaviours), lack of understanding of the recording techniques, or lack of motivation. For example, studies which used an objective measure of energy intake, doubly labelled water, found that food records underestimate actual caloric intake by about 20 per cent (Black *et al.* 1991; Martin *et al.*1996).

Many of the quality control procedures previously outlined to minimize errors by data collectors can and should be adapted to the situation where the subjects are the data collectors. In particular, study subjects should be trained, preferably in person, in the diary recording techniques. An overview of the diary recording methods is presented, followed by detailed specific examples. Examples of topics that would be covered in a training session on keeping a diet diary are given in Table 8.1. The trainers and those who develop the written instructions must be familiar with the coding scheme, so that the level of detail needed for accurate coding of items is recorded by the subjects. For example, if the database for coding food records has different codes for fresh, canned, and frozen vegetables, then subjects must record this information. Subjects should also be taught how to handle any unusual situations, such as illness, or food eaten outside the home which cannot be weighed. The training session would also include review of examples of completed forms, and practice in completing the diary. To reduce the staff time needed to train each subject, part of the instruction could be presented on video.

Detailed written instructions should also be given to each subject (see Figure 8.4). In addition to the material covered in the training session, the instructions should include the date to start the diary, the date to end the diary, and the name and telephone number of the person to call with any questions.

Subjects should also be instructed in how frequently to record information. Frequent recording reduces errors due to poor memory (Kunin and Ames 1981), but increases the subject burden. Diaries requiring periodic entries during the day should take the form of a small booklet or device that can be carried in a handbag or pocket.

Beyond understanding the data recording procedures, subjects need to be motivated to spend the time and effort to record information accurately. Enthusiastic trainers who can explain the importance of each subject's involvement can help to motivate subjects.

After initial training, the data collection needs to be monitored. The quality control principles of continued training and motivation of the data collectors also apply to diaries. Phone calls often need to be made to remind subjects of the day to begin, and then again to ask about any problems within the first few days of keeping the diary. Subjects should be asked to review their records for accuracy and completeness each day. After the diaries are returned, they should be reviewed immediately by a study editor for unclear entries or missing data. Long diaries should be reviewed periodically. The editor should review any specific problems with the subject, and should also discuss any general recording problems the subject appears to be having if future diaries are to be collected.

Table 8.1 Example of topics covered in training subjects to complete a diary: food records

---

Importance of accurate records (to motivate subjects not to change behaviour)

Scope of records
  General instructions to record the type of food, brand name, method of storage (fresh, frozen, canned), method of preparation, and amount eaten
  How and when to record (e.g. record immediately after eating or drinking, list only one food per line)

Recording foods
  Examples of recording milk products, meats, desserts, packaged foods, supplements
  How to weigh or measure foods
  Recording recipes
  Recording in unusual situations: illness, travel, restaurant foods which cannot be weighed or measured

Reviewing records for accuracy and completeness

Importance of subject to study (to motivate subjects to keep accurate diary)

Logistics
  When to start and stop recording
  Whom to call with problems

Review of sample completed diary form

Practice in completing form

As noted in the section above, it is well documented that the number of items recorded in diaries decreases over time. Several well-spaced shorter time periods rather than long recording periods might minimize subject fatigue as well as capture month-to-month variation.

Errors in coding

As noted above, open-ended diaries can yield a large amount of information which requires detailed coding. For example open-ended food diaries require code numbers for thousands of types of foods which relate to a database of nutrients in foods. Because coding of diaries can be a complex task, quality control procedures specific to this step need to be developed (Dennis *et al.* 1980; Dolecek *et al.* 1997). Coders should be selected who are familiar with the exposure (e.g. nutritionists for food diaries) and are meticulous in dealing with details. As in any type of study, there is a need for training of coders and practice sessions, and for monitoring of coders' work by periodic re-coding by another coder. In large-scale studies, coders may be given an examination to become 'certified' in the coding procedures; this improves accuracy and standardization across coders. Coders should refer uncertain situations to the lead coder or editor for resolution, and staff meetings should include exercises and discussion of items that have led to coding problems. The codebook containing the codes and detailed coding procedures should be updated by the lead coder whenever changes are made.

An alternative to manual numeric coding of all diary entries is direct key entry of the text (or appropriate key words). Sophisticated computer programs can then automate the coding and analysis. Willett (1998, p. 30) lists resources for both manual and automated coding of diet diaries.

Reliability studies of coding have identified several sources of error (Youland and Engle 1976; Henry *et al.* 1987):

- incomplete description of items which require coder judgement
- hand conversions by coders (e.g. cups to weight)
- transposed numbers.

Incomplete description of items can be avoided by appropriate training of subjects and by call-backs to subjects. To avoid errors in hand calculation, all calculations should be performed by computer. For example, a program to convert a diet diary to nutrients should have the capability to convert cups to weight or food dimensions to weight when necessary. A check digit can be included in each code, so that transposition errors can be identified by the data entry program (Gibson 1987). Computer range and logic checks on the raw data (e.g. quantity of each food) and the computed variables (e.g. kilocalories per day intake) can also identify some coding errors. In one study of coding four-day diet diaries, continued improvement of documentation, automated conversions, computerized edit checks, and increased experience of coders resulted in an improvement of inter-coder reliability of dietary fat intake from 0.92 to 0.98 (Henry *et al.* 1987).

Summary

The use of diaries may be a highly accurate method of measuring present common behaviours. The limitations of diaries, compared with interview methods, are the greater burden on subjects, which may lead to a poorer response rate, and the greater cost for subject training and for coding of the data. The accuracy of diary information can be enhanced by using multiple diary days spread over a sufficient time period, and by careful training of subjects and coders.

Use of proxy respondents

Advantages and limitations of use of proxy respondents

Proxy or surrogate respondents are people who provide information on exposure in place of the subjects themselves (index subjects). They are used in epidemiology when, for some reason (e.g. death, dementia, youth, lack of knowledge of their exposure), the subjects of study are unable to provide the data required. Their use may allow an increase in the number of subjects available and provide a more representative group for study, rather than, for example, limiting a case–control study to only live cases (Nelson et al.1990). Thus use of proxies might lead to more accurate estimates of exposure–disease associations because of less selection bias. A possible example comes from a case–control study of oral cancer by Greenberg et al. (1986). They found that exclusion from the analysis of those cases for which proxy respondents were interviewed because the case had died or was too ill to be interviewed led to a weakening of the associations between oral cancer and alcohol and tobacco. If this were due to actual greater consumption of cigarettes and liquor among cases diagnosed at an advanced stage (not greater reporting of these exposures by proxies), then use of proxies reduced selection bias and led to a more accurate odds ratio.

However, use of proxies could also lead to less accurate exposure–disease associations because of increases in non-differential or differential measurement error. In most situations, it is likely that proxy respondents are less accurate reporters of exposures than the index subjects would have been. Moreover, proxy reports may be biased (i.e. may systematically over- or under-estimate the true exposure) relative to self-report by the index subjects. This may

lead to differential measurement error (differential bias) if, for example, proxies are used for some or all cases but not for controls, or if proxy responses are
differentially biased (i.e. a different direction or magnitude of the proxy-index
bias between proxies for cases and controls). Several epidemiological
studies have collected the same information from both proxy respondents
and the index cases, and have shown different results when some or all proxies
were used in the analysis. In a case–control study of leukemia and
non-Hodgkin's lymphoma, Johnson *et al.* (1993) reported that occupational
exposures to pesticides were more commonly reported by the proxies
than by the index subjects among the controls, but were more commonly
reported by the index subjects than by the proxies among the cases. Semchuk
and Love (1995) found the same pattern in a case–control study of Parkinson's
disease and herbicide exposure, tobacco use, and history of head trauma. Thus
there was differential measurement error when proxies were used, and in these
two examples the error generally led to weaker odds ratios when the
proxies were used rather than self-reported data from the index subjects
(although, in general, differential measurement error can have any effect on
the odds ratio).

In this section we review evidence on the quality of information provided
by proxy respondents and offer some practical guidance to their use in
epidemiological studies.

Reliability of data provided by proxy respondents

Reliability of data provided by proxies for living subjects

The reliability of data provided by spouses or other relatives as proxies
for living subjects has been documented in a number of studies (Table 8.2).
While the data from these studies are of variable quality, some conclusions
can be drawn. The extent of agreement between subjects and proxies
was highly variable from one exposure variable to another. There was good
agreement on height and weight, and moderate agreement on smoking
history and medical history. Agreement on consumption of specific foods
and on nutrient intake assessed from frequency of consumption of a list of
foods was generally poor.

There was evidence, for some variables, of bias in the responses given
by proxies relative to responses given by index subjects. In three (Herrmann
1985a; Nelson *et al.* 1994; Reed and Price 1998) of four (Poulter *et al.* 1996)
studies that examined the issue, proxies underestimated the weight of the
index subject. Proxies reported fewer jobs on average than did the index
subjects in several studies (Blot *et al.* 1978; Rocca *et al.* 1986; Colt *et al.* 2001).
This tendency to under-report occupations may extend to the reporting of

specific occupational exposures, as Blot and McLaughlin (1985) noted that proxy respondents in a case–control study of lung cancer were less likely to report occupational exposure to asbestos than subjects who responded for themselves. Several studies suggest that proxies report lower consumption of cigarettes and alcohol than the index respondent (Nelson *et al.*1994; Weiss *et al.*1996; Passaro *et al.* 1997), although two studies found that proxies reported higher cigarette consumption (Kolonel *et al.* 1977; Barnett *et al.* 1997).

The question arises as to whether the extent of disagreement between proxy respondents and index subjects is greater than would be expected in a comparison of the responses of single subjects at two different points in time. In this regard, in a study of recall of medical history and diet, Herrmann (1985a,b) found little evidence to suggest that the agreement of subjects with themselves over an interval of 3 months or more, but with reference to the same time period, was any better than the agreement of subjects with proxies. However, Fryzek *et al.* (2000), in a study of occupational variables, found that after a five-year interval the agreement of subjects with themselves was better than with proxies for most items.

Reliability of exposure data provided by proxies for dead subjects

Several studies have addressed the quality of data provided by proxy respondents after the subject of the study has died, using for comparison information collected, often years earlier, from the index subject before his/her death (Table 8.3). Moderate levels of agreement were observed with respect to estimated height and weight, and the last or usual job. Agreement was poor on number of cigarettes smoked per day, age at starting smoking, frequency of intake of several foods, and exposure to specific occupational hazards. These levels of agreement appeared not to be as good as those observed between proxies and index subjects who were living at the time the proxy was interviewed (Table 8.2); this difference may be explicable, in part at least, by the usually longer recall period when the subject is dead.

With respect to relative bias, there was a tendency for proxies to overestimate height and underestimate weight (Rogot and Reid 1975), and to underestimate the number of jobs that index subjects had had (Lerchen and Samet 1986; see also Pickle *et al.* 1983). Only one (Rogot and Reid 1975) of three studies reported overestimation of cigarette consumption by proxies, and one reported overestimation of age at commencement of smoking only among men (McLaughlin *et al.* 1987).

Table 8.2 Summary of results of studies[a] in which data obtained by personal interview from living subjects were compared with data collected independently from proxy respondents for these subjects

Measurement	Relative bias[b,c]	κ or r[c,d]
Height	Yes/No (4)	0.83–0.94 (4)
Weight	Yes/No (4)	0.93–0.95 (4)
Education	Yes (1)	0.30–0.96 (3)
Number of jobs	Yes (3)	0.49 (1)
Last or present job	NR[e]	0.65–0.86 (1)
Diabetes	NR	0.85–0.89 (5)
Heart disease or heart attack	NR	0.50–1.00 (6)
Hypertension	Yes (1)	0.50–0.74 (7)
Family history of specific medical condition	NR	0.17–0.51 (2)
Oral contraceptive use	No (1)	0.54–0.82 (3)
Hormone replacement therapy use	Yes (1)	0.69 (1)
Smoking	NR	0.33–0.91 (6)
Cigarettes or packs per day	Yes/No (7)	0.30–0.95 (10)
Age started smoking	No (1)	0.57–0.93 (2)
Age stopped smoking	NR	0.53–0.87 (2)
Number of smokers at home in childhood	Yes (1)	0.79 (1)
Number of smokers at home as an adult	Yes (1)	0.67 (1)
Hours of tobacco smoke exposure at work	Yes (1)	0.46 (1)
Drinking	NR	0.34–1.00 (5)
Frequency or amount of alcohol drinking	Yes/No (6)	−0.12 to 0.86 (9)
Present or recent past intake of specific foods	No (4)	0.31–0.53 (4)
Dietary vitamin A intake	Yes/No (2)	0.11–0.37 (2)
Dietary vitamin C intake	No (1)	0.34–0.62 (1)

[a] Kolonel et al.1977; Blot et al.1978; Krueger et al.1980; Marshall et al.1980; Herrmann 1985a; Humble et al.1984; Rocca et al.1986; Cummings et al.1989; Metzner et al.1989; Hatch et al.1991; Boyle et al.1992; Halabi et al.1992; Lyon et al.1992; Graham and Jackson 1993; Gilpin et al.1994; Nelson et al.1994; Semchuk and Love 1995; Poulter et al.1996; Weiss et al.1996; Barnett et al.1997; Hyland et al.1997; Passaro et al.1997; Long et al.1998; Reed and Price 1998; Navarro 1999; MRC 2000; Colt et al. 2001; Demissie et al. 2001; Lien et al. 2001; Miller 2001.

[b] Refers to presence of difference between mean or median values for proxies and index subjects.

[c] Numbers in parentheses refer to numbers of studies on which assessment of bias or estimate of κ or r was based.

[d] κ, Cohen's κ or weighted κ; r, Pearson, Spearman, or intraclass correlation coefficient.

[e] NR, not reported.

Reliability of exposure data on death certificates

A number of studies have compared data derived from death certificates (provided most often by the next of kin) with data provided by the decedent during life. Two frequently quoted classic studies conducted in the USA in the middle of the twentieth century, which compared the occupations on death certificates to actual job history, observed a tendency to promote men with lower-status jobs into higher-status categories (Heasman *et al.* 1958, Kaplan *et al.* 1961). The levels of agreement between occupation on death certificates and some pre-mortem source of this information appear to have changed little over the years. For example, Steenland and Beaumont (1984) found agreement with respect to three-digit occupation codes in 51 per cent of cases for usual occupation and 70 per cent of cases for last occupation. Agreement was less for women and non-whites than it was for white males. Using five-digit codes, Shumacher (1986) found that occupation agreed in 67 per cent of individuals and industry agreed in 68 per cent.

Educational level, an alternative to occupation as a measure of socio-economic status, has likewise shown evidence of post-mortem promotion. In a study of death certificates in New York State and Utah, Shai and

Table 8.3 Summary of results of studies[a] in which data obtained from living index subjects were compared with data collected from proxy respondents after the index subjects had died

Measurement	Relative bias[b,c]	κ or r[c,d]
Height	Yes (1)	0.52 (1)
Weight	Yes (1)	0.48 (1)
Last or usual job	No (1)	0.48–0.78 (2)
Exposure to specific occupational hazards	No (1)	0.07–0.62 (1)
Cigarettes per day	No/Yes (3)	0.25–0.44 (2)
Age started smoking	No/Yes (1)[e]	0.48 (1)
Years of smoking	No (2)	0.91 (1)
Recent intake of specific foods	No (1)	0.14–0.24 (1)

[a] Todd (1966); Rogot and Reid (1975); Lerchen and Samet (1986); McLaughlin *et al.* (1987); Fryzek *et al.* (2000).

[b] Refers to presence of difference between mean or median values for proxies and index subjects.

[c] Numbers in parentheses refer to numbers of studies on which assessment of bias or estimate of κ or r was based.

[d] κ, Cohen's κ or weighted κ; r, Pearson, Spearman, or intraclass correlation coefficient.

[e] In the study by McLaughlin *et al.* (1987) proxies reported a higher average age at starting smoking in males only.

Rosenwaike (1989) found a high degree of error in recording of educational status in subjects who had either not started or not completed high school, in almost all instances in favour of a higher level of education.

Accuracy of recording of other socio-demographic variables on death certificates has also been investigated (Hambright 1969a,b). In US census records and death certificates for 1960, there was 69 per cent agreement on single year of age with up to 93 per cent agreement on 10-year age group depending on sex, age, and race. For marital status, agreement was good in single, married, and widowed categories, but poor in the divorced. Nativity was well reported (98 per cent agreement whether US or foreign born). Again, agreement on detail (actual country of birth) was less (93 per cent in those shown as foreign born on both records); there was least agreement on countries which had undergone substantial changes in political geography (e.g. Yugoslavia and Austria). There was very good overall agreement (99.6 per cent) on race (white, black, other non-white); other non-white were the least well identified. In another report, Native American race was misclassified for 9 per cent, mostly as white (Harwell *et al.* 2002).

Missing data in reports by proxy respondents

Missing data are a greater problem in information provided by proxies than by the subject, because the proxies may never have known the facts sought, or be more prone to forget them than the index subject because of the lower salience of the information for them.

Several studies have reported the prevalence of missing data (item non-response) in information provided by proxy respondents. Rogot and Reid (1975) found that the prevalence of non-response by proxy respondents varied from 17 per cent (for smoking) to 24 per cent (for age at migration) across seven variables. Rocca *et al.* (1986) obtained an appreciable proportion of 'don't know' responses from proxies only for history of general anesthesia (27 per cent), history of blood transfusion (10 per cent), history of antacid drug use (21 per cent), dementia in second-degree relatives (12 per cent), and age of mother and father at the subject's birth (27 per cent) among a wide range of variables covering socio-demographic characteristics, personal and family medical history, life habits, and animal contacts. McLaughlin *et al.* (1987) found that 35 per cent of proxies could not provide information on the age when the index subject began smoking, compared with 1 per cent of the subjects themselves. Nelson *et al.* (1994) found that, overall, non-response proportions were low (3 per cent or less) for demographic factors, body measures, cigarette and alcohol consumption, and physical activity, with increasing non-response as questions became more detailed. Non-response was considerably higher (6–25 per cent) for medical history and use of medication. Demissie *et al.* (2001) found that the lowest 'don't know' rates were for medical history, smoking, and alcohol use (1–9 per cent) and highest for oestrogen use (30 per cent) and medication history (18–24 per cent).

Several studies have examined the performance of particular types of proxies in providing complete information. While the prevalence of non-response was appreciably higher in the spouse than in the index subject for most questions, the prevalence of non-response was generally lower in the spouse than in other proxy respondents (Pickle *et al.* 1983; Nelson *et al.* 1994, MRC Cognitive Function and Ageing Study 2000; Demissie *et al.* 2001). These studies have shown the next least amount of missing data came from other relatives and the highest amount from non-related proxies. However in one study siblings had no more missing data than spouses and provided more complete data for country of birth and history of cancer in the parents and grandparents (Pickle *et al.* 1983). Similarly, Demissie *et al.* (2001) noted that when spouses were unavailable, siblings, especially sisters, provided the most complete data.

As noted above, the relationship between the amount of missing data and type of respondent may depend on the exposure of interest. With respect to age at uptake of smoking, McLaughlin *et al.* (1987) found that siblings and other proxies had the highest prevalence of non-response and parents of male subjects and spouses of female subjects had the lowest. This sex difference may relate to the ages at which smoking was taken up in people who are now old—teenage and early adult life in men and middle life in women.

Issues in the use of proxy respondents

Design of studies making use of proxy respondents

The design of studies which include proxy respondents should include proxies for some proportion of controls as well as for those requiring proxies (generally cases) (Nelson *et al.* 1990). This creates equivalent exposure assessment for cases and controls, but does not protect against differential exposure measurement error due to use of proxies. Ideally, where proxy respondents must be used for some subjects in a study, they should be used for all subjects in the study in addition to obtaining data direct from the index subjects who are able to provide it. This approach allows evaluation of the extent of error caused by the use of proxy respondents in both cases and controls (by comparison of responses obtained from proxies and index subjects when both provide data) and the potential for applying a correction for this error in the analysis (see Chapter 5).

Cost is probably the only disadvantage of obtaining proxy respondents for all subjects in a study in which they must be used. A suitable alternative approach, particularly in large studies, would be to obtain both proxy and subject data in samples of subjects sufficiently large to estimate the reliability of the proxy responses with reasonable precision (see Chapter 4).

Dead controls for dead cases?

Because the quality of response given by a proxy respondent may be different when the index subject has died, it is tempting to suggest that dead controls should be used for dead cases. This approach would also match proxy respondents for cases to proxy respondents for controls. However, Gordis (1982) pointed out that since death may have resulted from diseases caused by the exposure under study, the selection of dead controls may lead to biased estimates of the prevalence of the exposure in the source population and thus biased estimates of its effect. This phenomenon has been demonstrated empirically by McLaughlin et al. (1985a) with respect to smoking, drinking, and the use of medications.

The potential bias outlined above may be dealt with by either selecting living controls and obtaining proxy responses for them, or endeavouring to exclude from among the dead controls those who have died from diseases thought to be caused by any of the exposures of interest (McLaughlin et al. 1985b). We prefer the former approach, adequately supported by a comparison of the responses obtained from proxies and living subjects, because of the very highly selective nature of a control series made up of dead people and the uncertainty about whether deaths related to the exposures of interest can ever be adequately excluded. The evidence of McLaughlin et al. (1985b) is that they cannot, at least for smoking.

Selection of proxy respondents

Selection of the proxy respondents to be used should be based on consideration of which person within the subject's family would be most likely to know the facts required. Evidence reviewed above indicates that close relatives, particularly spouses, usually provide more complete data than other proxy respondents. The spouse or child will generally know more about the subject's adult life, while a parent or sibling will generally know more about his/her childhood, young adult life, and family history of diseases. Consideration should be given to obtaining the consensus view of more than one proxy respondent on the exposures of interest, especially when the whole of life is of interest.

Because the choice of proxy respondent is inevitably restricted by the availability of particular classes of relatives, there may be advantage in matching on proxy type or, at least, endeavouring to balance the distribution of proxy types among cases and controls so that this variable can be taken into consideration in the analysis.

Sample size

Use of proxy respondents will generally necessitate an increase in the sample size of a study over what would otherwise have been considered necessary. This is because of the probable greater degree of error in proxy responses, and the probable higher prevalence of item non-response (Nelson *et al.* 1990). Allowance for the effects of measurement error in sample size estimation is dealt with in Chapter 3. Assumptions about the likely prevalence of item non-response and the resulting reduction in effective sample size for each variable would be necessary to take this factor into account in estimating the required sample size.

Questionnaire design

Evidence reviewed above indicates that proxy respondents are more likely to be unable to reply or to be in error than index subjects themselves when detailed data are sought (e.g. age at starting smoking, and details of occupational history in someone who has had many jobs). Therefore it may be desirable, in the interests of reducing the burden on respondents, to seek rather simpler data from proxy respondents than from index subjects, or to simplify the questionnaire for both.

Pickle *et al.* (1983) have suggested that a question should be asked of proxy respondents regarding the closeness of their knowledge of the index subject. This variable may be used later in the evaluation of the reliability of proxy data and as a stratification variable in the analysis.

Analysis

The analysis of studies which make use of proxy respondents is beyond the scope of this book. It has been reviewed by Walker *et al.* (1988) and Nelson *et al.* (1990). It is enough to say here that where data are collected from both index subjects and proxy respondents among both cases and controls, as we have advocated above, the broadest range of analytical options is available. In addition, it should be noted that when this is done, rules should be set down in advance of the analysis as to which data will be used in each class of subjects for analyses involving each variable (Nelson *et al.* 1990). These rules will have regard to:

- prior perceptions as to the validity of each data source
- the likelihood of differential measurement error between cases and controls
- the likely consequences of a case series biased by the loss of dead subjects

◆ the effects of the reduction in sample size which would result from the exclusion of the deceased subjects.

Summary

There is substantial error in data provided by proxy respondents. This error is more likely to be present in measurements of variable and low-impact characteristics, and where detail is required, than in measurements of fixed and high-impact characteristics, and where the data required are comparatively simple. However, there are indications that the degree of error in the responses of proxy respondents may be only slightly greater than the error in responses from the subjects themselves. Of even greater importance is that responses obtained from proxies, for some variables at least, may be biased relative to those obtained from the index subjects. In particular, proxy respondents may over- or under-report certain exposures, so that this tendency would induce differential measurement error if proxies were only used for cases. Unfortunately, even if proxies are used for (some) cases and (some) controls, there is evidence that differential error would still occur because of the tendency for proxies to respond to questions differently based on whether they are reporting for a case or control.

Item non-response is more common in data provided by proxy respondents than by the index subjects. Close relations generally provide more complete data than proxy respondents who are more distantly related or not related at all.

In undertaking studies making use of proxy respondents, the following are recommended.

(a) The study design should include proxies for some (or all) controls as well as some (or all) cases, but dead controls should not be sought, preferentially, for dead cases.

(b) The sample size should be increased to allow for the greater error and prevalence of missing data that are likely.

(c) The proxy respondents selected should generally be close relatives and, as far as possible, those most likely to know the facts sought.

(d) Questionnaire design should make allowance for the reduced detail that may be available from proxy respondents so that respondent burden is not excessive.

References

Alanko, T. (1984). An overview of techniques and problems in the measurement of alcohol consumption. In *Research Advances in Alcohol and Drug Problems*, Vol. 8 (ed. R.G. Smart, F.B. Glaser, Y. Israel, H. Kalant, R.E. Popham, and W. Schmidt), pp. 209–26. Plenum Press, New York.

Allison, J.J., Wall, T.C., Spettell, C.M., *et al.* (2000). The art and science of chart review. *Joint Commission Journal on Quality Improvement*, **26**, 115–36.

Allor, K.M. and Pivarnik, J.M. (2001). Stability and convergent validity of three physical activity assessments. *Medicine and Science in Sports and Exercise*, **33**, 671–6.

Barnett, R., O'Loughlin, J., Paradis, G., and Renaud, L. (1997). Reliability of proxy reports of parental smoking by elementary schoolchildren. *Annals of Epidemiology*, **7**, 396–9.

Bassett, D.R., Ainsworth, B.E., Swartz, A.M., Strath, S.J., O'Brien, W.L., and King, G.A. (2000). Validity of four motion sensors in measuring moderate intensity physical activity. *Medicine and Science in Sports and Exercise*, **32**, S471–80.

Beaton, G.H., Milner, J., Corey, P., *et al.* (1979). Sources of variance in 24-hour dietary recall data: implications for nutrition study design and interpretation. *American Journal of Clinical Nutrition*, **32**, 2456–9.

Berg, J., Dunbar, J.J., and Rohay, J.M. (1998). Compliance with inhaled medications: the relationship between diary and electronic monitor. *Annals of Behavioral Medicine*, **20**, 36–8.

Black, A.E., Goldberg, G.R., Jebb, S.A., Livingston M.B.E., Cole, T.J., and Prentice A.M. (1991). Critical evaluation of energy intake data using fundamental principles of energy physiology. 2: Evaluation the results of published studies. *European Journal of Clinical Nutrition*, **45**, 583–99.

Blot, W.J. and McLaughlin, J.K. (1985). Practical issues in the design and conduct of case–control studies: use of next of kin interviews. In *Statistical Methods in Cancer Research* (ed. W.J. Blot, T. Hirayama, and D.G. Hoel), pp. 49–62. Radiation Effects Research Foundation, Hiroshima.

Blot, W.J., Harrington, J.M., Toledo, A., Hoover, R., Heath, C.W., and Fraumeni, J.F. (1978). Lung cancer after employment in shipyards during World War II. *New England Journal of Medicine*, **299**, 620–4.

Boyd, N.F., Pater, J.L., Ginsburg, A.D., and Myers, R.E. (1979). Observer variation in the classification of information from medical records. *Journal of Chronic Diseases*, **32**, 327–32.

Boyle, C.A., Brann, E.A., and Selected Cancers Cooperative Study Group. (1992). Proxy respondents and the validity of occupational and other exposure data. *American Journal of Epidemiology*, **136**, 712–21.

Brownson, R.C., Davis, J.R., Chang, J.C., DiLorenzo, T.M., Keefe, T.J., and Bagby, J.R., Jr (1989). A study of the accuracy of cancer risk factor information reported to a central registry compared to that obtained by interview. *American Journal of Epidemiology*, **129**, 616–24.

Buzzard, M. (1998). 24-hour dietary recall and food record methods. In *Nutritional Epidemiology* (2nd edn) (ed. W. Willett), pp. 101–47. Oxford University Press, New York.

Campbell, D.T. and Stanley, J.C. (1963). *Experimental and Quasi-Experimental Designs for Research*. Rand McNally, Chicago, IL.

Carney, M.A., Tennen, H., Affleck, G., del Boca, F.K., and Kranzler, H.R. (1998). Levels and patterns of alcohol consumption using timeline follow-back, daily diaries and real-time 'electronic interviews'. *Journal of Studies on Alcohol*, **59**, 447–54.

CDC (Centers for Disease Control) (1989). *Health Status of Vietnam Veterans. Supplement B: Medical and Psychological Data Quality*. US Department of Health and Human Services, Atlanta, GA.

Christensen, D.B., Williams, B., Goldberg, H.I., Martin, D.P., Engelberg, R., and LoGerfo, J.P. (1994). Comparison of prescription and medical records in reflecting patient antihypertensive drug therapy. *Annals of Pharmacotherapy*, **28**, 99–104.

Coleman, K.J., Saelens, B.E., Woedrich-Smith, M.D., Finn, J. D., and Epstein, L.H. (1997). Relationships between TriTrac-R3D vectors, heart rate, and self-report in obese children. *Medicine and Science in Sports and Exercise*, **29**, 1535–42.

Colt, J.S., Engel, L.S., Kiefer, M.C., Thompson, M.L., and Zahm, S.H. (2001). Comparability of data obtained from migrant farmworkers and their spouses on occupational history. *American Journal of Industrial Medicine*, **40**, 523–30.

Cummings, K.M., Markello, S.J., Mahoney, M.C., and Marshall, J.R. (1989). Measurement of lifetime exposure to passive smoke. *American Journal of Epidemiology*, **130**, 122–32.

Demissie, S., Green, R.C., Mucci, L., *et al.* (2001). Reliability of information collected by proxy in family studies of Alzheimer's disease. *Neuroepidemiology*, **20**, 105–11.

Dennis, B., Ernst, N., Hjurtland, M., Tillotson, J., and Grambsch, V. (1980). The NHLBI nutrition system. *Journal of the American Dietetic Association*, **77**, 641–7.

Dobie, S.A., Baldwin, L.M., Rosenblatt, R.A., Fordyce, M.A., Andrilla, C.H., and Hart, L.G. (1998). How well do birth certificates describe the pregnancies they report? The Washington State experience with low-risk pregnancies. *Maternal and Child Health Journal*, **2**, 145–54.

Dolecek, T.A., Stamler, J., Caggiula, A.W., Tillotson, J.L., and Buzzard, I.M. (1997). Methods of dietary and nutritional assessment and intervention and other methods in the Multiple Risk Factor Intervention Trial. *American Journal of Clinical Nutrition*, **65**, 196S–210S.

Feinstein, A.R., Pritchett, J.A., and Schimpff, C.R. (1969a). The epidemiology of cancer therapy. III: The management of imperfect data. *Archives of Internal Medicine*, **123**, 448–61.

Feinstein, A.R., Pritchett, J.A., and Schimpff, C.R. (1969b). The epidemiology of cancer therapy. IV: The extraction of data from medical records. *Archives of Internal Medicine*, **123**, 571–90.

Forster, J., Jeffery, R., Van Natta, M., and Pirie, P. (1990). Hypertension prevention trial. Do 24-h food records capture usual eating behavior in a dietary change study? *American Journal of Clinical Nutrition*, **51**, 253–7.

Fowles, J.B., Fowler, E.J., and Craft, C. (1998). Validation of claims diagnoses and self-reported conditions compared with medical records for selected chronic diseases. *Journal of Ambulatory Care Management*, **21**, 24–34.

Freudenheim, J.L., Johnson, N.E., and Smith, E.L. (1986). Relationships between usual nutrient intake and bone-mineral content of women 35–65 years of age: longitudinal and cross-sectional analysis. *American Journal of Clinical Nutrition*, **44**, 863–76.

Freudenheim, J.L., Johnson, N.E., and Wardrop, R.L. (1987). Misclassification of nutrient intake of individuals and groups using one-, two-, three-, and seven-day food records. *American Journal of Epidemiology*, **126**, 703–13.

Frost, F., Starzyk, P., George, S., and McLaughlin, J.F. (1984). Birth complication reporting: the effect of birth certificate design. *American Journal of Public Health*, **74**, 505–6.

Fryzek, J.P., Lipworth, L.L., Garabrant, D.H., and McLaughlin, J.K. (2000). Comparison of surrogate with self-respondents for occupational factors. *Journal of Occupational and Environmental Medicine*, **42**, 424–9.

Gerbert, B., Stone, G., Stulbarg, M., Gullion, D.S., and Greenfield, S. (1988). Agreement among physician assessment methods: searching for the truth among fallible methods. *Medical Care*, **26**, 519–35.

Gersovitz, M., Madden, J.P., and Smiciklas-Wright, H. (1978). Validity of the 24-hr dietary recall and seven-day record for group comparisons. *Journal of the American Dietetic Association*, **73**, 48–55.

Gibson, R.S. (1987). Sources of error and variability in dietary assessment methods: a review. *Journal of the Canadian Dietetic Association*, **48**, 150–5.

Gilliland, F.D., Larson, M., and Chao, A. (1997). Risk factor information found in medical records of lung and prostate cancer cases, New Mexico Tumor Registry (United States). *Cancer Causes and Control*, **8**, 598–604.

Gillmore, M.R., Gaylord, J., Hartway, J., *et al.* (2001). Daily data collection of sexual and other health-related behaviors. *Journal of Sex Research*, **38**, 35–42.

Gilpin, E.A., Pierce, J.P., Cavin, S.W., *et al.* (1994). Estimates of population smoking prevalence: self- versus proxy reports of smoking status. *American Journal of Public Health*, **84**, 1576–9.

Goodman, M.T., Nomura, A.M., Wilkens, L.R., and Kolonel, L.N. (1990). Agreement between interview information and physician records on history of menopausal estrogen use. *American Journal of Epidemiology*, **131**, 815–25.

Gordis, L. (1982). Should dead cases be matched to dead controls? *American Journal of Epidemiology*, **115**, 1–5.

Graham, P. and Jackson, R. (1993). Primary versus proxy respondents: comparability of questionnaire data on alcohol consumption. *American Journal of Epidemiology*, **138**, 443–52.

Greenberg, R.S., Liff, J.M., Gregory, H.M., and Brockman, E. (1986). The use of interviews of surrogate respondents in a case–control study of oral cancer. *Yale Journal of Biology and Medicine*, **59**, 497–504.

Halabi, S., Zurayk, H., Awaida, R., Darwish, M., and Saab, B. (1992). Reliability and validity of self and proxy reporting of morbidity data: a case study from Beirut, Lebanon. *International Journal of Epidemiology*, **21**, 607–12.

Hambright, T.Z. (1969a). Age on the death certificate and matching census record. United States—May–August 1960. *Vital and Health Statistics Series 2*, Vol. 29. US DHEW PHS Pub. No. 1000, Series 2, No. 29. US Department of Health, Education and Welfare, Washington, DC.

Hambright, T.Z. (1969b). Comparability of marital status, race, nativity, and country of origin on the death certificate and matching census record. United States—May–August 1960. *Vital and Health Statistics Series 2*, Vol. 34. US DHEW PHS Pub. No. 1000, Series 2, No. 34. US Department of Health, Education and Welfare, Washington, DC.

Harwell, T.S., Hansen, D., Moore, K.R., Jeanotte, D., Gohdes, D., Helgerson, S.D. (2002). Accuracy of race coding on American Indian death certificates, Montana 1996–1998. *Public Health Reports*, **117**, 44–9.

Hatch, M.C., Misra, D., Kabat, G.C., and Kartzmer, S. (1991). Proxy respondents in reproductive research: a comparison of self- and partner-reported data. *American Journal of Epidemiology*, **133**, 826–31.

Heasman, M.A., Liddell, F.D.K., and Reid, D.D. (1958). The accuracy of occupational vital statistics. *British Journal of Industrial Medicine*, **15**, 141–6.

Henry, H.J., Shepard, E.A., Woods, M., and Blethen, E. (1987). Quality control procedures to monitor the effects of coding four-day food records in the Women's Health Trial (Abstract). American Dietetic Association Meeting Abstracts, Atlanta, GA.

Herrmann, N. (1985a). Retrospective information from questionnaires. I: Comparability of primary respondents and their next-of-kin. *American Journal of Epidemiology*, **121**, 937–47.

Herrmann, N. (1985b). Retrospective information from questionnaires. II: Intrarater reliability and comparison of questionnaire types. *American Journal of Epidemiology*, **121**, 948–53.

Herrmann, N., Cayten, C.G., Senior, J., Staroscik, R., Walsh, S., and Woll, M. (1980). Interobserver and intraobserver reliability in the collection of emergency medical services data. *Health Services Research*, **15**, 127–43.

Hewson, D. and Bennett, A. (1987). Childbirth research data: medical records or women's reports? *American Journal of Epidemiology*, **125**, 484–91.

Hilsenbeck, S.G., Glaefke, G.S., Feigl, P., *et al.* (1985). *Quality Control for Cancer Registries*. US Department of Health and Human Services, Washington, DC.

Hilton, M.E. (1989). A comparison of a prospective diary and two summary recall techniques for recording alcohol consumption. *British Journal of Addiction*, **84**, 1085–92.

Hornsby, P.P. and Wilcox, A.J. (1989). Validity of questionnaire information on frequency of coitus. *American Journal of Epidemiology*, **130**, 94–9.

Horwitz, R.I. and Yu, E.C. (1984). Assessing the reliability of epidemiologic data obtained from medical records. *Journal of Chronic Diseases*, **37**, 825–31.

Horwitz, R.I., Feinstein, A.R., and Stremlau, J.R. (1980). Alternative data sources and discrepant results in case–control studies of estrogens and endometrial cancer. *American Journal of Epidemiology*, **111**, 389–94.

Humble, C.G., Samet, J.M., and Skipper, B.E. (1984). Comparison of self- and surrogate-reported dietary information. *American Journal of Epidemiology*, **119**, 86–98.

Hyland, A., Cummings, M., Lynn, W.R., Corle, D., and Giffen, C.A. (1997). Effect of proxy-reported smoking status on population estimates of smoking prevalence. *American Journal of Epidemiology*, **145**, 746–51.

Jamison, R.N., Raymond, S.A., Levine, J.G., Slawsby, E.A., Nedeljkovic, S.S., and Katz, N.P. (2001). Electronic diaries for monitoring chronic pain: 1-year validation study. *Pain*, **91**, 277–85.

Johnson, R.A., Mandel, J.S., Gibson, R.W., *et al.* (1993). Data on prior pesticide use collected from self- and proxy respondents. *Epidemiology*, **4**, 157–64.

Kaplan, D.L., Parkhurst, E., and Whelpton, P.K. (1961). *The Comparability of Reports on Occupation from Vital Records and the 1950 Census*. Vital Statistics Special Reports, Vol. 53, No. 1. US Public Health Service, Washington, DC.

Kolar, A.S., Patterson, R.E., White, E., *et al.* (2005). A practical method for collecting 3-day food records in a large cohort. *Epidemiology*, **16**, 579–83.

Kolonel, L.N., Hirohata, T., and Nomura, A.M.Y. (1977). Adequacy of survey data collected from substitute respondents. *American Journal of Epidemiology*, **106**, 476–84.

Kristensen, J., Langhoff-Roos, J., Skovgaard, L.T., and Kristensen, F.B. (1996). Validation of the Danish Birth Registration. *Journal of Clinical Epidemiology*, **49**, 893–7.

Krueger, D.E., Ellenberg, S.S., Bloom, S., *et al.* (1980). Fatal myocardial infarction and the role of oral contraceptives. *American Journal of Epidemiology*, **111**, 655–74.

Kubey, R., Larson, R., and Csikzentmihalyi, M. (1996). Experience sampling method applications to communication research questions. *Journal of Communication*, **46**, 99–120.

Kunin, C.M. and Ames, R.E. (1981). Methods for determining the frequency of sexual intercourse and activities of daily living in young women. *American Journal of Epidemiology*, **113**, 55–61.

La Porte, R.E., Kuller, E.H., Kupfer, D.J., *et al.* (1979). An objective measure of physical activity for epidemiologic research. *American Journal of Epidemiology*, **109**, 158–68.

Lerchen, M.L. and Samet, J.M. (1986). An assessment of the validity of questionnaire responses provided by a surviving spouse. *American Journal of Epidemiology*, **123**, 481–9.

Lien, N., Friestad, C., and Klepp, K.I. (2001). Adolescents' proxy reports of parents' socioeconomic status: how valid are they? *Journal of Epidemiology and Community Health*, **55**, 731–7.

Liu, K., Stamler, J., Dyer, A., McKeever, J., and McKeever, P. (1978). Statistical methods to assess and minimize the role of intraindividual variability in obscuring the relationship between dietary lipids and serum cholesterol. *Journal of Chronic Diseases*, **31**, 399–418.

Long, K., Sudha, S., and Mutran, E.J. (1998). Elder-proxy agreement concerning the functional status and medical history of the older person: impact of caregiver burden and depressive symptomatology. *Journal of the American Geriatrics Society*, **46**, 1103–11.

Lyon, J.L., Egger, M.J., Robison, L.M., French, T.K., and Gao, R. (1992). Misclassification of exposure in a case–control study: the effects of different types of exposure and different proxy respondents in a study of pancreatic cancer. *Epidemiology*, **3**, 223–31.

MacDiarmid, J. and Blundell, J.E. (1997). Dietary underreporting: what people say about recording their food intake. *European Journal of Clinical Nutrition*, **51**, 199–200.

McKeown, N.M., Day, N.E., Welch, A.A., *et al.* (2001). Use of biological markers to validate self-reported dietary intake in a random sample of the European Prospective Investigation into Cancer United Kingdom Norfolk cohort. *American Journal of Clinical Nutrition*, **74**, 188–96.

McLaughlin, J.K., Blot, W.J., Mehl, E.S., and Mandel, J.S. (1985a). Problems in the use of dead controls in case–control studies. I: General results. *American Journal of Epidemiology*, **121**, 131–9.

McLaughlin, J.K., Blot, W.J., Mehl, E.S., and Mandel, J.S. (1985b). Problems in the use of dead controls in case–control studies. II: Effect of excluding certain causes of death. *American Journal of Epidemiology*, **122**, 485–94.

McLaughlin, J.K., Dietz, M.S., Mehl, E.S., and Blot, W.J. (1987). Reliability of surrogate information on cigarette smoking by type of informant. *American Journal of Epidemiology*, **126**, 144–6.

Marr, J.W. (1971). Individual dietary surveys: purposes and methods. *World Review of Nutrition and Dietetics*, **13**, 105–64.

Marshall, J., Priore, R., Haughey, B., Rzepka, T., and Graham, S. (1980). Spouse–subject interviews and the reliability of diet studies. *American Journal of Epidemiology*, **112**, 675–83.

Martin, L.J., Su, W., Jones, P.J., Lockwood, G.A., Tritchler, D.L., and Boyd, N.F. (1996). Comparison of energy intakes determined by food records and doubly labeled water in women participating in a dietary-intervention trial. *American Journal of Clinical Nutrition*, **63**, 483–90.

Metzner, H.L., Lamphiear, D.E., Thompson, F.E., Oh, M.S., and Hawthorne, V.M. (1989). Comparison of surrogate and subject reports of dietary practices, smoking habits and weight among married couples in the Tecumseh diet methodology study. *Journal of Clinical Epidemiology*, **42**, 367–75.

Miller, J.E. (2001). Predictors of asthma in young children: does reporting source affect our conclusions? *American Journal of Epidemiology*, **154**, 245–50.

MRC (Medical Research Council) Cognitive Function and Ageing Study. (2000). Survey into health problems of elderly people: multivariate analysis of concordance between self-report and proxy information. *International Journal of Epidemiology*, **29**, 698–703.

Mundt, J.C. (1997). Interactive voice response systems in clinical research and treatment. *Psychiatry Service*, **48**, 611–2.

Navarro, A.M. (1999). Smoking status by proxy and self-report: rate of agreement in different ethnic groups. *Tobacco Control*, **8**, 182–5.

NCHS (National Center for Health Statistics) (1973). Net differences in interview data on chronic conditions and information derived from medical records. *Vital and Health Statistics*, Series 2, Vol. 57, 1–58. DHEW Publ. No. (HSM) 73–1331. US Department of Health, Education and Welfare, Washington, DC.

NCHS (National Center for Health Statistics) (2002a). National Vital Statistics System: Classification and Coding Instructions for Birth Records. Available online at: http://www.cdc.gov/nchs/data/3amanual.pdf

NCHS (National Center for Health Statistics) (2002b). National Vital Statistics System: Instruction Manuals. Available online at: http://www.cdc.gov/nchs/about/major/dvs/im.htm

Nelson, L.M., Longstreth, W.T., Jr, Koepsell, T.D., and van Belle, G. (1990). Proxy respondents in epidemiologic research. *Epidemiologic Reviews*, **12**, 71–86.

Nelson, L.M., Longstreth, W.T., Koepsell, T.D., Checkoway, H., and van Belle, G. (1994). Completeness and accuracy of interview data from proxy respondents: demographic, medical and lifestyle factors. *Epidemiology*, **5**, 204–17.

Paganini-Hill, A. and Ross, R. K. (1982). Reliability of recall of drug usage and other health-related information. *American Journal of Epidemiology*, **116**, 114–22.

Passaro, K.T., Noss, J., Savitz, D.A., Little, R.E., and Alspac Study Team. (1997). Agreement between self and partner reports of paternal drinking and smoking. *International Journal of Epidemiology*, **26**, 315–20.

Pickle, L.W., Brown, L.M., and Blot, W.J. (1983). Information available from surrogate respondents in case–control interview studies. *American Journal of Epidemiology*, **118**, 99–108.

Poulter, N.R., Chang, C.L., Farley, T.M.M., and Marmot, M.G. (1996). Reliability of data from proxy respondents in an international case study of cardiovascular disease and oral contraceptives. *Journal of Epidemiology and Community Health*, **50**, 674–80.

Raymond, S.A. and Ross, R.N. (2000). Electronic subject diaries in clinical trials. *Applications in Clinical Trials*, **9**, 48–58.

Rebro, S.M., Patterson, R.E., Kristal, A.R., and Cheney, C.L. (1998). The effect of keeping food records on eating patterns. *Journal of the American Dietetic Association*, **10**, 1163–5.

Reed, D.R. and Price, R.A. (1998). Estimates of the heights and weights of family members: accuracy of informant reports. *International Journal of Obesity*, **22**, 827–35.

Reisch, L.M., Fosse, J.S., Beverly, K., *et al.* (2003). Training, quality assurance, and assessment of medical record abstraction in a multisite study. *American Journal of Epidemiology*, **157**, 546–51.

Rocca, W.A., Fratiglioni, L., Bracco, L., Pedone, D., Groppi, C., and Schoenberg, B.S. (1986). The use of surrogate respondents to obtain questionnaire data in case–control studies of neurologic disease. *Journal of Chronic Diseases*, **39**, 907–12.

Roghmann, K.J. and Haggerty, R.J. (1972). The diary as a research instrument in the study of health and illness behavior. *Medical Care*, **10**, 143–63.

Rogot, E. and Reid, D.D. (1975). The validity of data from next-of-kin in studies of mortality among migrants. *International Journal of Epidemiology*, **4**, 51–4.

Savitz, D.A. and Grace, C. (1985). Determinants of medical record access for an epidemiologic study. *American Journal of Public Health*, **75**, 1425–6.

Searles, J.S., Perrine, M.W., Mundt, J.C., and Helzer, J.E. (1995). Self-report of drinking using touch-tone telephone: extending the limits of reliable daily contact. *Journal of Studies on Alcohol*, **56**, 375–82.

Semchuk, K.M. and Love, E.J. (1995). Effects of agricultural work and other proxy-derived case–control data on Parkinson's disease estimates. *American Journal of Epidemiology*, **141**, 747–54.

Sempos, C.T., Johnson, N.E., Smith, E.L., and Gilligan, C. (1985). Effects of intraindividual and interindividual variation in repeated dietary records. *American Journal of Epidemiology*, **121**, 120–30.

Shai, D. and Rosenwaike, I. (1989). Errors in reporting education on the death certificate: some findings for older male decedents from New York State and Utah. *American Journal of Epidemiology*, **130**, 188–92.

Shiffman, S. and Stone, A.A. (1998). Introduction to the special section: ecological momentary assessment in health psychology. *Health Psychology*, **17**, 3–5.

Shumacher, M.C. (1986). Comparison of occupation and industry information from death certificates and interviews. *American Journal of Public Health*, **76**, 635–7.

Stange, K.C., Zyzanski, S.J., Smith, T.F., *et al.* (1998). How valid are medical records and patient questionnaires for physician profiling and health services research? A comparison with direct observation of patients visits. *Medical Care*, **36**, 851–67.

Steenland, K. and Beaumont, J. (1984). The accuracy of occupation and industry data on death certificates. *Journal of Occupational Medicine*, **26**, 288–96.

Stergachis, A. (1989). Group Health Cooperative. In *Pharmacoepidemiology* (ed. B.L. Strom), pp. 149–160. Churchill Livingstone, Edinburgh.

Stolley, P.D., Tonascia, J.A., Sartwell, P.E., *et al.* (1978). Agreement rates between oral contraceptive users and prescribers in relation to drug histories. *American Journal of Epidemiology*, **107**, 226–35.

Tilley, B.C., Barnes, A.B., Bergstralh, E., *et al.* (1985). A comparison of pregnancy history recall and medical records: implications for retrospective studies. *American Journal of Epidemiology*, **121**, 269–81.

Todd, G.F. (1966). *Reliability of statements about smoking. Supplementary Report*, Research Paper 2A, pp. 25–7. Tobacco Research Council, London.

Verbrugge, L.M. (1980). Health diaries. *Medical Care*, **18**, 73–95.

Verbrugge, L.M. (1984). Health diaries: problems and solutions in study design. In *Health Survey Research Methods* (ed. C.F. Cannell and R.M. Groves), pp. 171–92. Research Proceedings Series, DHHS Pub. No. PHS 84–3346. National Center for Health Services Research, Rockville, MD.

Walker, A.M., Velema, J.P., and Robins, J.M. (1988). Analysis of case–control data derived in part from proxy respondents. *American Journal of Epidemiology*, **127**, 905–14.

Walter, S.D., Clarke, E.A., Hatcher, J., and Stitt, L.W. (1988). A comparison of physician and patient reports of Pap smear histories. *Journal of Clinical Epidemiology*, **41**, 401–10.

Weiss, A., Fletcher, A.E., Palmer, A.J., Nicholl, C.G., and Bulpitt, C.J. (1996). Use of surrogate respondents in studies of stroke and dementia. *Journal of Clinical Epidemiology*, **49**, 1187–94.

Willett, W. (1998). *Nutritional Epidemiology* (2nd edn). Oxford University Press, New York.

Willett, W.C., Sampson, L., Stampfer, M.J., *et al.* (1985). Reproducibility and validity of a semiquantitative food frequency questionnaire. *American Journal of Epidemiology*, **122**, 51–65.

Youland, D.M. and Engle, A. (1976). Practices and problems in HANES. *Journal of the American Dietetic Association*, **68**, 22–5.

9

Measurements in the human body or its products

Ideally in an epidemiological study [subjects] should be classified into exposure groups according to their concentration of bioactive chemical at the biological receptor.
(Droz et al. 1991)

Introduction

Exposures can often be measured directly in the subject's internal environment—in cells, body fluids, or body products. These measurements are commonly described as 'biological measurements' or measurements of 'biological markers' (biomarkers), although in most cases the measurement procedures do not make use of biological properties but, rather, are chemical or physical in nature.

Three types of biological measurements can be used to measure exposure.

(a) The presence or concentration of the agent of interest itself in various biological media, such as blood, urine, expired air, hair, adipose tissue, saliva, etc.

(b) The concentration of products of biotransformation of the agent in the same media.

(c) The biological effects which result from contact of the agent with the human body.

The agents measured are, in some instances, *endobiotic*, i.e. body constituents which are normally present and necessary for healthy bodily function; they range from polymorphic variants of a gene to levels of circulating hormones. In others, they are *xenobiotic*, i.e. agents that are foreign to the human body such as drugs, cosmetics, and environmental contaminants absorbed through the skin, lungs, or gastrointestinal tract.

The biological effects of these agents may be harmless, harmful, or helpful; reversible or irreversible after cessation of exposure; and may appear early or late after exposure begins. Logically, those effects measured to evaluate exposure should not be the disease under study itself, or any of its direct effects. The inhibition of serum pseudocholinesterase by exposure to organophosphorus pesticides (Lauwerys 1984) is an example of a reversible and substantially harmless effect, at least at low levels of exposure. On the other hand, effects such as chloracne after exposure to chlorinated organic compounds, skin erythema after irradiation, and the very early radiological manifestations of pneumoconioses are indicators of harmful exposure, although some may be reversible.

In general, biological effects are measured when there is no possibility of measuring the agent or its biotransformation products in the body; this is the case for physical agents like sound or electromagnetic waves. Thus, for example, changes in the skin due to degeneration of dermal collagen have been used as indicators of total accumulated exposure to sunlight (Holman and Armstrong 1984). In addition, biological effects, when they can be measured accurately, may provide a more error-free measure of the actual exposure of interest (e.g. total accumulated exposure to the sun) than an alternative subjective measurement (e.g. a personal interview).

The epidemiological application of measurements of exposure in the human body and its products, together with increasingly refined measurements of biological effects for exposure, individual susceptibility, and outcome determination, characterize what has come to be called molecular epidemiology (Hulka *et al.* 1990; Schulte and Perera 1993).

The detailed rationale, development, application, and technical interpretation of biological measurements belong largely to experts in disciplines other than epidemiology. This chapter deals particularly with those aspects of these measurements which demand most directly attention or personal action from the epidemiologist during the course of a study, such as sampling, storage of biological specimens, and quality control procedures. Following a general account of the characteristics, value, and limitations of biological measurements, particular aspects of the measurement of exposure to xenobiotic and endobiotic compounds will be considered separately and exemplified, respectively, with reference to measurement of exposure to carcinogens and measurement of genetic exposures and diet. Quality control and the establishment of 'banks' of biological specimens will be given special attention.

The value and limitations of measurements in the human organism

Measuring exposure biomarkers

In principle, measuring an exposure directly in the human body or its products can make an exposure assessment:

+ *objective*, i.e. independent of the observed person's perceptions and substantially independent of the observer if instrumental or laboratory methods are used

+ *individualized*, i.e. exactly targeted on each subject at times relevant to causation of the disease under study

+ *analytically specific* and *sensitive* to the exposure of interest.

Here '*analytical specificity*' denotes the ability of a method to respond only to the agent of interest with or without minimal response to other agents, and '*analytical sensitivity*' denotes the ability to respond in a quantitative way to the agent down to a very low limit of detection. For practical purposes, 'very low' means a level well below the minimum concentration likely to induce a detectable biological effect.

Because of these favourable characteristics, biological measurements of exposure may be regarded in principle as optimal, at least for present exposure.

In practice, biological measurements are *objective* to the extent that they are automated and that the technicians in charge of the procedure are ignorant of the status (exposed or not exposed, case or control) of the subjects. Subjectivity on the part of the subjects of the study is introduced when they must participate cooperatively in the collection of specimens (e.g. when the collection of urine specimens is required; a complete 24-hour collection may be difficult to achieve). Similarly, subjectivity may affect instrumental measurements when, for example, the subject must exhale air into instruments which detect and measure volatile compounds (e.g. carbon monoxide and alcohol).

Individualization of the measurements is absolute with biological measurements, apart from errors of identification of specimens and readings. Individualization of the measurement is a prime strength of biological measurements. However, if the wrong compartment within a person's body is sampled, or samples are taken at the wrong time, an exposure may be missed completely when it might have been correctly identified by a cruder measurement in the environment or by answers to a questionnaire.

The possibility of achieving a high degree of analytical specificity for single substances or biologically relevant fractions (e.g. the active site of a hormonally active molecule) represents the other major strength of biological measurements.

Developments, particularly in the area of immunoassays using monoclonal antibodies, have provided some highly specific methods of measurement of both endobiotic and xenobiotic substances. However, many methods still fall short of optimal specificity. For example, in radio-immunoassays of cotinine, non-specific cross-reactivity with other substances in the urine may reduce specificity if volumes of urine larger than 20 μl are used. These cross-reacting substances prevent the use of large volumes of urine to increase the sensitivity of the assay when the concentration of cotinine is low, and call for a more complex process of prior extraction and concentration (Van Vunakis *et al.* 1987).

A common problem affecting specificity, particularly in biological measurements of metals, is incomplete 'speciation'. Measurements of metals in biological specimens are still based mainly on tests for the elementary metal, while biological properties such as kinetics and toxicity are usually specific to a particular chemical form of the metal. For example, trivalent chromium salts are less water soluble than hexavalent chromium salts, are less capable of crossing biological membranes, and have different tissue and organ affinities; they also exhibit different toxicities. Occupational exposure to hexavalent chromate causes lung cancer in man, and hexavalent chromic acid is capable of producing skin ulcers and perforation of the nasal septum (IARC 1990). These effects have not been observed with trivalent chromium compounds.

Biological measurements have the potential to be more specific for relevant exposure than measurements in the environment (see Chapter 10). Measurements in the environment estimate the *available* dose of an agent or, at best, the *administered* or external dose (intake), while biological measurements estimate the *absorbed* or internal dose (uptake) (see Chapter 1, Figure 1.2). Thus, for example, biological measurements of exposure to an airborne agent occurring in the workplace, unlike measurements of its concentration in the air, will reflect individual variations in factors such as the use of respirators, personal hygiene, and metabolism. They will also usually measure the presence of an agent in the body whatever its external sources and route of entry. Depending on the object of the investigation, this may be an advantage or a disadvantage. For example, as noted in Chapter 1, in an investigation of the possible role of aluminium in the aetiology of Alzheimer's disease, all sources of intake, and not just that from, say, antacid drugs, would need to be taken into account. In this case, a biological measurement reflecting the total body uptake of aluminium would be appropriate. On the other hand, in a study of the relationship between pollution from car engine exhaust gases and myocardial infarction, the use of blood carboxyhaemoglobin concentration, an accurate measure of recent exposure to carbon monoxide, would be inappropriate, at least by itself, because it measures exposure to carbon monoxide from all sources including tobacco smoke. In this case, a measurement in the environment or by way of interview might be more pertinent.

In some circumstances, biological measurements may also permit estimation of the *active* or biologically effective dose, namely the dose at the level of the structures (organs, cells, subcellular, and molecular constituents) which are targets of the action of the agent.

Specificity, combined with absolute individualization and objectivity, allows the possibility that biological measurements will be able to measure 'the right thing in the right person in the right way'. These characteristics are even more important for epidemiological purposes than high analytical sensitivity, an asset which biological methods of measurement also posses, often to a high degree. Pursuit of sensitivity has often been spectacularly successful. For example, the most sensitive technique for detecting adducts of carcinogens with DNA (^{32}P post-labelling) needs as little as 10 mg of tissue, a quantity orders of magnitude smaller than that required by other analytical methods (Randerath *et al.* 1988).

Whether or not biological measurements also allow measurement 'at the right time', i.e. at a time relevant aetiologically to the disease under study, depends on the natural history of the disease, the characteristics of the biological marker, and the study design. In case–control studies biological measurements are suitable only if there is evidence that they can measure exposure at the relevant times in the past and that they are not altered by the occurrence of disease. These limitations do not apply to measurements in prospective cohort studies, although in these studies measurements at a single point, or even several points, in time may not be able to capture the long-term pattern of exposure.

Problems in the timing of biological measurement, added to error in the assay procedure and short-term physiological variability, may produce appreciable misclassification of subjects with respect to the relevant exposure and reduce or eliminate the gains in accuracy of exposure measure that might otherwise have been anticipated. These possibilities underline the need for validity and/or reliability studies comparing alternative methods of biological measurements of exposures, and comparing biological with other kinds of measurements (e.g. interview-based measurements or measurements in the environment), before biological measurements can be confidently adopted for widespread use in epidemiological studies.

In addition to the above considerations, the practical usefulness of biological measurements depends on their feasibility and cost. Both will be influenced by the nature of the specimens required, the logistic difficulties in collecting them, and the technology required to make the actual measurements. Feasibility will also be influenced by the adverse effects that inclusion of some biological measurements may have on the willingness of subjects to participate. Costs may be substantially reduced in prospective studies by storage of specimens and analysis only of those from subjects who develop disease and a sample of those who do not. Issues related to storage ('banking') of specimens for later use are discussed in the last section of this chapter.

Exposure biomarkers as reference or supportive measurements

Measurements of exposure biomarkers may be employed as *comparison measurements* for other measurements, obtained by questionnaire for example, to determine the validity and reliability of the latter under conditions closely similar to those of planned studies (e.g. on papilloma virus and cervical cancer). To qualify as reference for another measurement instrument a biomarker should either represent itself as the 'true' variable of interest (the presence of virus in target cells) or have known validity and reliability with respect to it, as a serological marker of the virus may have. In some circumstances, extrapolating from the conditions of the validity and reliability study to a set of different conditions might have some justification but it implies reasoning by analogy. For example, in the short term, of the order of a week or less, exposure to environmental tobacco smoke (ETS) reported by questionnaire in non-smoking women correlates well with urinary cotinine levels, which measure the bodily uptake of ETS (Riboli *et al.* 1990). This offers support, by analogy, to the contention that in the long term, over years, self-reported exposure to ETS reflects actual exposure to ETS.

Within epidemiological studies biomarkers are used not only as primary exposure measurements but occasionally as *supportive measurements*. Typically this arises when only crude measurements are available of past exposures, spanning back decades, acquired through some highly indirect procedure of reconstruction. For example, an association may have been found between length of occupational employment as a sprayer of pesticides likely to be contaminated in the past with dioxin (TCDD) and soft tissue sarcomas, but the causal nature of the association may be in doubt mainly because of the uncertainty about the actual exposures. Finding that that the levels of TCDD in the few and sparse samples of fat tissue available from pesticide sprayers are on average higher than in the general population offers some supportive independent evidence for a causal association, even if the properties of the biomarker itself (TCDD in fat tissue) may not be fully known.

Measurement of xenobiotic compounds

Principles of sampling

The principal matters to be specified in a sampling scheme are the body sites (tissues and products) from which the samples will be taken, and the times and numbers of the samples. They are determined substantially by the kinetics of absorption, distribution, storage, metabolism, and elimination of the xenobiotic substances in question.

Knowledge of the distribution of a substance and of the products of its biotransformation or its early effects within the body, and the time course of these processes, is essential for correct sampling. Plasma or, more exactly, plasma water is most often the central compartment in which an agent becomes distributed after absorption. From this compartment it may be transferred into a number of other compartments (e.g. blood cells, liver, fat, cerebrospinal fluid, and urine). Some of these compartments are of particular importance because they may lend themselves to easy sampling (e.g. urine, saliva, and hair). In general, the distribution of a substance involves more than a single compartment, with some organs or tissues concentrating it either because they are targets of the action or because they act as storage sites.

Biological measurements on the substance itself, on metabolites, or on markers of effect can be made either during exposure or after exposure has ended. When past exposure is being measured, the time since exposure began and/or ended must be taken into consideration. In the simplest case, the substance itself is measured in plasma in the post-exposure period with the body behaving as a single homogeneous compartment and with the disapperance of the substance from plasma governed by first-order (single exponential) kinetics. In this case a constant proportion R of the substance present at a time t is lost in the subsequent very small time interval Δt. If the plasma concentration values are plotted on the natural logarithmic ordinate of a graph with time on the arithmetic abscissa, the value of the fractional constant of elimination R is given by the slope of the straight line going through the points (Figure 9.1). The biological half-life $t_{1/2}$, i.e. the time required for the concentration of the substance to be reduced by half, can also be read directly from the graph as the time interval between any two concentrations, the second of which is half the first. Alternatively, it can be obtained as $t_{1/2} = \ln 0.5/R = 0.693/R$, a relationship from which R can be derived reciprocally once the value of $t_{1/2}$ has been obtained graphically.

If the body behaves as a system of several compartments, exchanging reversibly or irreversibly at different rates with the central plasma compartment, the curve of the concentration of the substance in plasma will be composed of

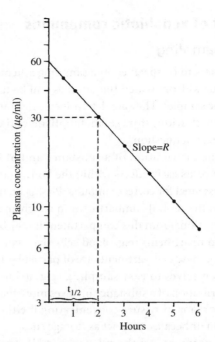

Figure 9.1 Fall in plasma concentration of a xenobiotic compound for which the body behaves as a single homogeneous compartment obeying first-order kinetics. (Reproduced with permission from C.D. Klaassen (1980). Absorption, distribution, and excretion of toxicants. In *Casarett and Doull's Toxicology* (2nd edn) (ed. J. Doull, C.D. Klaassen, and M.O Amdur), pp. 28–55. MacMillan, New York.)

as many single exponentials as there are compartments. A two-compartment model is represented in Figure 9.2 in which lines A and B represent the two single exponentials. The exponential with the shallower slope (B) on this semilogarithmic plot corresponds to the compartment from which the elimination of the substance is the slowest. This may often be a storage site such as a plasma protein (e.g. albumin for many xenobiotics), liver, kidney, fat (for all lipophilic substances), bone, etc. The substance in these storage sites is always in equilibrium with the free substance, and as the free substance is metabolized or excreted more is released from storage. The disappearance of substances from the storage compartment(s), as expressed by the rate of elimination, may be very slow, of the order of years (e.g. lead from bone).

Measurements will frequently be taken during continuous or intermittent exposure rather than in the post-exposure phase. The former can be regarded as a particular case of the latter, with very short pulse exposures separated by very short intervals. Figure 9.3 shows the concentration curve of nicotine in

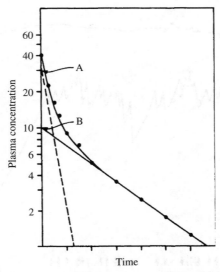

Figure 9.2 Fall in plasma concentration of a xenobiotic compound for which there are two compartments of distribution in the body, each obeying first-order kinetics, as represented by lines A and B. (Reproduced with permission from C.D. Klaassen (1980). Absorption, distribution, and excretion of toxicants. In *Casarett and Doull's Toxicology* (2nd edn) (ed. J. Doull, C.D. Klaassen, and M.O Amdur), pp. 28–55. MacMillan, New York.)

the plasma of a smoker; each cigarette produces a pulse exposure. After about five cigarettes a plateau level of nicotine is reached which fluctuates with and between each cigarette smoked subsequently (Teeuwen 1988). The plateau is reached asymptotically at $t = \infty$, but 90–95 per cent of the plateau level is reached in a time equal to three to four half-lives, whatever the frequency of the repeated exposure. However, the level of the plateau depends, for a given half-life, on the frequency of the repeated exposure (Rowland and Tozer 1980). The plateau occurs when the concentration lost in the interval T between two exposures exactly equals the rise in concentration given by a new absorbed dose.

Samples can be taken directly from secondary compartments rather than from the central one, plasma water. If this is done the relevant items of information become the concentration versus time curve in the secondary compartment sampled and its relationship to the absorbed dose and the amount of the exposure. Secondary compartments in which elimination occurs, such as urine and expired air, may simply reflect, *moment by moment* and in accordance with fixed proportionality factors, the concentration curve

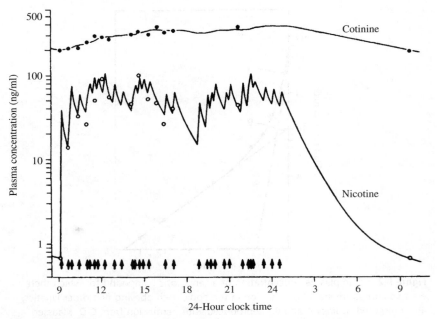

Figure 9.3 Concentration curves of nicotine and cotinine in the plasma of a smoker where each arrow (↑) represents the smoking of one cigarette delivering 1.1 mg of nicotine. (Reproduced with permission from H.W.A. Teeuwen (1988). Clinical pharmacokinetics of nicotine, caffeine, and quinine. PhD Thesis, University of Nijmegen. CiP-DATA, Koninklijke Bibliotheek, Den Haag.)

of the substance in plasma water. Therefore they may not only be particularly convenient and easy to sample but also be capable of providing as much information as would be derived from the analysis of plasma. Other secondary compartments may accumulate and store substances circulating in plasma. For example, fat accumulates lipophilic substances such as PCBs (used industrially, for example, as insulators in electrical capacitors and found both in workplace and general environments) and the insecticide DDT. The concentration of a substance in such storage compartments, when measured at a particular time, will reflect the cumulative exposure to it up to that time.

For secondary compartments containing metabolites of the parent substance (and even more so for markers of biological effect), the relationship of the concentration versus time curve to absorbed dose and to exposure is less direct. Indeed, it may be quite complex, requiring both extensive empirical data and complex formal modelling for an exact description. For example, a few empirical data exist on the times of appearance and disappearance, in relation to exposure, of the micronucleus marker (a non-specific indicator of exposure to DNA-damaging agents) in erythrocytes, lymphocytes, and exfoliated buccal mucosa cells (Vine 1990). In these cases, the micronucleus marker appears almost immediately after exposure in circulating lymphocytes, after about 3–4 days in red cells (the time from exposure to the appearance of new red cells in the blood) and after about 5–7 days in epithelial cells (the time it takes for a cell to migrate from the basal layer to the surface of the epithelium and then to be exfoliated).

In summary, knowledge of the kinetics of the measured substance in the central plasma compartment, in elimination compartments, especially urine, and in accessible storage compartments, like plasma proteins, fat, nails, and hair, is essential to establishing the correct *site* and *time* for sampling and the number of samples that should be taken. Time is especially critical if, as is often the case in epidemiological studies, only one sample per subject can be taken on a given occasion or even in the course of the whole study, and if the exposure is of brief duration or highly variable in time. Chronic near-constant exposures pose fewer problems. While this knowledge of kinetics does not need to go as far as complete characterization of the kinetic model, it needs to be detailed enough to define what differences in the time of sampling for the different study subjects can be tolerated without introducing appreciable non-comparability in the measurements of their exposure. For example, if plasma concentrations of a substance with a plasma half-life of 3 hours were to be measured after exposure during a night work shift, four- to eightfold differences in concentrations could be found if the workers were examined sequentially throughout the day, without there being any appreciable differences in exposure.

Two other matters arising from knowledge of the kinetics of xenobiotic compounds should be noted.

(a) This knowledge not only allows the establishment of the conditions for valid measurements but may also permit back-calculation of the initial absorbed dose from the observed concentration in the body and knowledge of the time since exposure.

(b) Kinetic parameters are not narrowly fixed biological constants, but vary as a function of age, previous exposure to the same substance, or concurrent exposures to other substances which may modify rates of metabolism (e.g. by way of enzyme induction or inhibition). There is widespread exposure to substances, such as alcohol and tobacco, capable of inducing P-450-dependent microsomal monoxygenases which metabolize many lipid-soluble xenobiotics (Berlin *et al.* 1984; Bartsch *et al.* 1988). Therefore the potential for the introduction of further variability in biological measurements of exposure (Saracci 1984*)* as a result of other exposures must be carefully considered in the light of available knowledge on the metabolism of the xenobiotic under study. Where this potential exists, collection of information on these other exposures is essential for a correct interpretation of the study.

Assays for xenobiotic compounds

A number of analytical procedures for biological measurement of xenobiotic compounds to suit the medium-to large-scale needs of epidemiological research have become available in the last decades. These procedures are also suitable for routine 'biological monitoring' of working or general populations, which shares a number of practical requirements with epidemiology.

In 1985 a review put at 53 the number of compounds which could be validly measured in specimens of blood, plasma or serum, urine, breast milk, placenta, hair and nails, expired air, and faeces. Included in the 53 were 12 metals (elements and their inorganic or organic compounds), five organochlorine pesticides, four polyhalogenated hydrocarbons of low volatility, six volatile halogenated hydrocarbons, five aromatic and aliphatic hydrocarbons, 19 other organic compounds, and three internal asphyxiants (Zielhuis 1985). A tabulation in the year 2000 of biomonitoring levels requiring action as formulated by occupational health organizations in four countries (USA, UK, Germany, Finland) includes 71 substances for which standard methods of analysis are available (Aitio 2000).

To be usefully applied, analytical methods need to be complemented, as outlined above, by information on the distribution and kinetics in the body of the substance to be measured. For example, carbon monoxide can be measured either to assess exposure to the compound itself or to methylene chloride, a volatile solvent widely used as an aerosol propellant, paint stripper, degreasing agent, and fat extractant. The measurements can be made in blood, by measuring carboxyhaemoglobin, or on carbon monoxide levels in expired air; the half-life of carbon monoxide is the same in both compartments. However, if the measurement is to assess external exposure to carbon monoxide, the half-life is 5 hours, while if the agent is present in the environment as methylene chloride, the half-life is about 10 hours. In this case carbon monoxide derives from the biological transformation of methylene chloride, which continues after exposure has ceased (Zielhuis 1985).

Similarly, as shown in Figure 9.3 (Teeuwen 1988), the plasma concentration of nicotine after daytime exposure to tobacco smoke, which has a half-life of only about 2 hours, rapidly reverts to a low baseline level when smoking is stopped overnight. However, its main metabolite, cotinine, has a longer half-life of 24 hours. As a consequence, not only are its fluctuations around the plateau concentration smaller, but its concentration remains high so that it can still be assayed even in the post-exposure phase (say, next day).

Some metals and asbestos have very long half-lives. For example, lead remains in the blood for several weeks, and cadmium remains for years. In some circumstances, measurement of their concentrations at one point in time may reflect reasonably accurately cumulative exposure up to that point. However, care must be exercised. Figure 9.4 shows a considerable difference between tremolite (a variety of amphibole asbestos) and chrysotile asbestos when cumulative exposure (measured here in millions of particles per cubic foot years), assessed by work history and environmental measurement, is plotted against the concentration of fibres in the lungs of deceased miners (Sébastien *et al.* 1986). The amphibole concentration in the lung increases linearly with cumulative exposure; but the chrysotile concentration levels off, indicating an equilibrium between rates of deposition and clearance. While the reasons for this difference are poorly understood (the data available on the deposition and clearance of the two types of asbestos are not so different as to explain the observed effect), the difference highlights the danger of simply taking, without qualification, fibre concentration in the lungs at a single point in time as reflecting cumulative exposure.

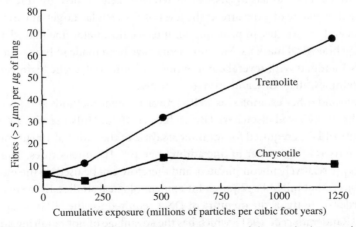

Figure 9.4 Concentration of asbestos fibres in the lungs of deceased miners and millers of chrysotile asbestos contaminated with tremolite. (Reproduced with permission from P. Sébastien *et al.* (1986). Inhalation of chrysotile dust. In *The Biological Effects of Chrysotile. Accomplishments in Oncology*, Vol. 1, No. 2 (ed. J.C. Wagner), pp. 19–29. J.B. Lippincott, Philadelphia, PA.)

Assays for carcinogens

There has been a great expansion in methods of biological measurement of xenobiotic carcinogens over the last decades. Carcinogens aptly illustrate the whole spectrum of possible biological measurements of exposure. For convenience in this discussion, they will be grouped into measurements of carcinogens and other metabolites, and measurements of the biological effects of carcinogens.

Measurements of carcinogens and their metabolites

Measurements of carcinogens and their metabolites may be specific or non-specific. Mutagenic activity in urine reflecting exposure to mutagens or pro-mutagens, and urinary thioethers reflecting exposure to electrophilic substances, are the most popular non-specific markers of exposure to carcinogens. Because of their non-specificity they are, for example, appreciably influenced by substances in tobacco smoke. However, they may be of use in directing attention to unsuspected exposure to mutagens or electrophilic substances during the last 1–3 days, rather than for the quantitative assay of a single substance. More specific measurements of exposure to carcinogens include measurement of free carcinogens and their metabolites, and of chemical adducts of carcinogens with macromolecules in cells and body fluids.

Adducts are 'addition products' resulting from covalent binding of the reactive form of a carcinogen to macromolecules like nucleic acids and proteins. Measurement of adducts to DNA extracted from cells is the most direct measurement available of exposure at the level of the cellular target of carcinogen action, and constitutes, in principle, an internal dosimeter unequalled among existing biological markers. Measurements have been made in human subjects of DNA adducts with several compounds including polycyclic hydrocarbons, nitrosamines, aflatoxins, and aromatic amines.

These and other examples, as well as measurement methods and problems, have been reviewed elsewhere (Bartsch et al. 1988; Hulka et al. 1990). The quantity of DNA required for immunoassays is of the order of 100 μg, and the sensitivity is of the order of one adduct per 10^6–10^8 nucleotides. The techniques are relatively uncomplicated, and therefore can be used on the numbers of subjects that might be required for epidemiological studies. Even smaller, of the order of 10 μg, is the quantity of DNA required for the ^{32}P post-labelling assay (Randerath et al. 1981), which has the advantage of not requiring advance knowledge of which adducts to look for, as it can detect the presence of any adduct with a high sensitivity of one to two adducts per 10^{10} nucleotides. However, the method is technically elaborate, particularly if the often necessary step of identifying the specific chemical producing the adduct is pursued.

The usefulness of DNA adducts as measures of exposure to carcinogens and mutagens is limited by a number of factors which may affect the measured concentrations. These factors include:

+ production of several different adducts by a single compound
+ rates of removal of adducts which depend on DNA repair and cell turnover, and vary according to adduct, organ, and tissue
+ inter-individual variation in formation of adducts
+ background presence of certain adducts
+ stability in storage
+ intra-laboratory and inter-laboratory variability in assay.

A critical issue for the application of measurements of adducts in epidemiology is their persistence in target tissues, including blood cells and tissues like intestinal or respiratory mucosa, which, under certain conditions, can be sampled through biopsy or surgery. Lymphocytes are widely used for the measurement of adducts. They can themselves be possible target cells, although non-proliferating lymphocytes contain low concentrations of activating enzymes and are less capable of adduct formation than other cells (Lucier and Thompson 1987), or they can take up reactive carcinogens from the variety of tissues with which they come into contact. As the lifespan of different lymphocyte subpopulations may vary from a few days to several years, and this and the size of these populations can be influenced by a variety of immunological stimuli, the persistence of DNA adducts in lymphocytes and the period of time over which they measure exposure cannot be estimated in general. Some human data indicate the possibility of persistence for several weeks (Haugen *et al.* 1986).

Since some adducts are removed from cellular DNA and RNA by repair enzymes and excreted in urine, measurement of nucleic acid adducts in urine can be used to reflect recent exposure. However,its accuracy for this purpose is influenced by variability in the capability for repair of DNA.

Protein adducts may also be useful in measuring exposure to carcinogens, although they have no role in the carcinogenic process. To date, most investigations have been of adducts with haemoglobin. Their use is analogous to the use of glycosylated haemoglobin to monitor exposure of diabetic patients to blood glucose which provides a picture of exposure to excess glucose integrated over time. Carcinogens of diverse structure have been shown to bind to haemoglobin *in vivo*, either directly, as with alkylating agents, or after metabolic activation. Adducts of haemoglobin with ethylene and propylene oxides, 4-aminobiphenyl, benzo(a)pyrene, and some *N*-nitroso compounds, have been measured in human samples. These adducts appear to be stable over the lifespan of the average erythrocyte (120 days) and therefore offer a measure of cumulative exposure over a period of several months.

Adducts of albumin, for example with aflatoxin B1 (Wild and Turner 2001), have been investigated and may also prove useful as markers of recent exposure, given that most xenobiotics are metabolized in the liver, where albumin is synthesized, and that the half-life of albumin is not too short (20 days).

Measurement of the biological effect of carcinogens

Several indicators of early biological effects of carcinogens are measurable in somatic cells or germ line cells. They include gene mutations, chromosomal aberrations, sister chromatid exchanges, micronuclei, and unscheduled DNA synthesis. Some of these early markers have been measured in groups exposed to ionizing radiation or chemical agents. Indicators arising later in the process of carcinogenesis, such as measurement of tumour markers or abnormalities in exfoliative cytology, may not measure exposure in any direct way but simply indicate the presence of malignant cells.

As measurements of exposure to carcinogens, all measurements of biological effects are non-specific. This restricts their usefulness for exposure measurement, particularly as quantitative measures, except in certain cases. One such exception is the quantitative indication of cumulative exposure to ionizing radiation given by structural chromosomal aberrations in lymphocytes. This exception occurs because ionizing radiation can induce aberrations at all stages of the cell cycle. However, structural chromosomal aberrations in lymphocytes are not useful for measuring exposure to most chemical carcinogens. This is because these carcinogens usually require metabolic activation and the cell must be in the S-phase (i.e. during the period of DNA synthesis) when exposure occurs, or pass an S-phase between exposure and observation, if aberrations are to be observed. Most circulating lymphocytes are in the resting phase (Bloom 1981) and can only go into the S-phase after mitogen stimulation *in vitro*, by which time a substantial and variable proportion of lesions will have been eliminated by repair processes. In principle, exposure-specific mutations as measurable in the minute amounts of free DNA circulating in plasma, a handy material for analyses, could be specific dosimeters. An example is the ser[249] mutation in codon 249 of the P53 gene in subjects exposed to aflatoxin B1; however, it is not clear whether the presence of the mutation in detectable concentrations reflects the clonal expansion of a cell which has acquired the mutation or, instead, a substantial exposure to the carcinogen (Kirk *et al.* 2000).

Measurement of endobiotic compounds

Introduction

Endobiotic compounds include not only substances that are produced endogenously but also exogenous compounds that are of importance to normal body function (e.g. nutrients). It may be possible to infer nutrient intake from biological measurements of nutrients or their effects. These measurements are being undertaken increasingly, both because analytical methods have improved and because the error associated with other methods of measuring nutrient intake is often substantial. Measurement of other endobiotic compounds has been used more to elucidate the pathogenesis and role of host factors in disease, rather than to measure exposure to external causes of disease. However, where such measurements are known to be influenced by external agents they may assist in drawing inferences about exposure to these agents.

Principles of sampling

Sampling to measure physiological compounds demands knowledge of their distribution in tissues and over time which, unlike that of xenobiotic compounds, is substantially influenced by homeostatic mechanisms. The concentrations of endobiotic compounds depend on time in various systematic ways. They vary with age, as instanced by the falling plasma concentration of calcitonin and the rising concentration of parathyroid hormone with increasing age, and in response to external stimuli, like the response of gastrointestinal and pancreatic hormones to food intake. Major hormonal variations take place during the menstrual cycle. A diurnal variation of as much as 30–50 per cent is found in the plasma concentrations of corticosteroids, catecholamines, and oestriol. The concentrations of nutrients are also subject to diurnal variation in relation to eating and homeostatic mechanisms, and to sizable fluctuations from day to day caused by variations in diet.

These within-person variations have an important effect on the use of endobiotic compounds as markers of exposure to external agents. For example, when plasma total cholesterol concentration, a non-specific marker of lipid intake, was measured twice at an interval of 2 years, it showed a ratio of within-person to between-person variance of 0.54 (Shekelle *et al.* 1981), i.e. an intraclass correlation coefficient R of 0.65. As explained in Chapter 3, this implies that if one random measurement of plasma total cholesterol concentration is taken for a number of subjects, a true relative risk of, say, 2.00 between two classes of subjects with different average values of plasma cholesterol would be attenuated, because of the intra-individual variability over time, to an observable relative risk of 1.57. For beta-carotene concentration, a ratio of within-person to between person variances of 0.62 ($R = 0.62$) has been reported for a four-week interval between measurements (Tangney *et al.* 1987). This implies that a single measurement would reduce a true relative risk from 2.00 to an observed relative risk of 1.53. For 24-hour urinary sodium, a marker of sodium intake, a ratio of within-person to between-person variances as high as 3.20 has been reported ($R = 0.24$), which would imply a reduction of a true relative risk from 2.00 to an observed relative risk of 1.18 (Liu *et al.* 1979).

To reduce the effect of some of these variations, the time of specimen sampling can be standardized. For example, blood could be drawn for all subjects in the morning, after fasting for 10–12 hours, or at a fixed time in a woman's menstural cycle. In addition, when practical, the use of the average of multiple measures over the appropriate time period improves the precision of the exposure measurement and lessens the attenuation of the relative risk (see Chapter 5).

Measurements of genetic exposures

Before the advent of contemporary methods of molecular biology, the possibility of determining the genotype of an individual, regarded as an (internal) exposure with biological effects, was essentially limited to those traits for which the unmeasurables underlying gene variants (alleles) are expressed one to one into measurable phenotypes, as in the ABO blood group system, or to gross chromosomal alterations with health effects, as in Down syndrome.

Exposure to potentially pathological gene variants could be measured indirectly by the degree of relatedness of subjects to persons affected by a disease. Typically, first-degree relatives of, for example, breast cancer cases would be regarded as genetically exposed and their incidence of breast cancer compared with the incidence in the general population. However, this approach leads to a strong attenuation, even of one or two orders of magnitude, of the risk ratio between genetically 'susceptible' and 'non-susceptible' subjects (Peto 1980). The attenuation derives from the fact that the general population contains, unidentifiable to the observer, both susceptible and non-susceptible subjects, as well as from the fact that not all cancer patients are susceptible, and even fewer of their relatives are (again, susceptible and non-susceptible remaining unidentifiable to the observer).

In sharp contrast genotypes are today accessible to measurements by a large array of techniques which are evolving at a fast pace with the objective of permitting rapid exploration of many genes in large numbers of subjects.

In broad terms, measurements of genetic exposures can be performed at the two levels of genotype and phenotype.

Genotype measurements are performed on DNA. The DNA macromolecule is normally constituted by two complementary chains of nucleotides, each composed of a pentose sugar, a phosphate group, and a nitrogenous base paired by a hydrogen bond to a corresponding base on the opposite chain. The total amount of DNA in the haploid human genome is about 3.3×10^9 base pairs long, and for the greatest (about 99 per cent) is common to all humans; however, the remaining 1 per cent roughly corresponds to 3×10^7 base pairs, providing substantial room for variation between individuals. Variations involve sequences of different length along a chromosome, ranging from an entire chromosomal region to a single nucleotide, and may have different phenotypic effects, from a lethal disease to a neutral effect. Conventionally the term *polymorphism* is reserved for those variants, or alleles, which occur at given DNA locations (loci), are present in at least 1 per cent of individuals, and do not have markedly deleterious effects (highly deleterious and less frequent variants are usually referred to as mutations). Chromosomes contain a large amount of 'tandem repeats', namely repeated sequences of base pairs which can occur in chromosomal regions both coding and non-coding for proteins. In 'minisatellites', the repeated unit is of the order of 10–25 nucleotides; in 'microsatellites', the repeated unit includes one to four nucleotides, a frequent unit being the two-nucleotide sequence 'citosine–adenine' repeated n times. Minisatellites and, even more, microsatellites are widely distributed in loci over all chromosomes; each of them may vary in the number of repeat units, and hence in length, between individuals, thus representing different allelic forms of a polymorphic marker. These are recognizable by measuring methods like gel electrophoresis which separates DNA fragments of different lengths. Most, but by no means all, satellite markers have loci in non-coding regions. They are essential for linkage studies investigating the intrafamilial coheritance of a polymorphic marker whose chromosomal location is already known and a disease. The inference could then be drawn that a hypothetical susceptibility gene should also be coherited with the marker and be linked to it on the same chromosome. While these linkage studies in families contribute to ascertaining the existence and mapping the approximate location of hypo- thetical susceptibility genes, the actual identification of such genes can be directly pursued via classical epidemiological studies (case–control or prospec- tive) in which allele–disease associations are investigated. Single-nucleotide polymorphisms (SNPs), i.e. base changes occurring in a single nucleotide (and in its corresponding nucleotide on the complementary strand), are exten- sively used for these studies. When an SNP occurs in a coding region of an aetiological 'candidate gene', it can be classified as synonymous (silent) or non-synonymous; the former does not lead to a change in the amino acid sequence of the coded protein, while the latter does. It is obviously the latter type of SNP which is functionally of interest. Often alleles positioned close to each other along a chromosome are inherited together (instead of being dissociated by meiotic recombination) as a complex called a haplotype. This presents the opportunity of identifying and measuring in association studies only those few SNPs which are essential, as they capture the haplotypes present in a chromosomal region while omitting the redundant ones ('haplotype tagging') (Johnson *et al.* 2001). If an association with one haplotype emerges, a second-stage finer analysis can be conducted to identify the specific allele variant(s) responsible for it. Such multiple stage investigations are becoming more common: the most recent technologies allow testing for half a million or a million SNP's making feasible genome-wide first stage explorations ('genome-wide association' or GWA studies).

A host of methods exist for SNP measurements, some of which are suited for high-throughput analyses in epidemiological studies (Syvänen 2001). These have tended to supplant the traditional method of restriction site analysis which permitted the first successes in identifying polymorphisms relevant to disease causation, for example the polymorphisms of apolipoprotein E (de Andrade *et al.* 1995). Restriction sites are short specific sequences of DNA which are recognized by restriction enzymes which cut the DNA at these sites. If a nucleotide change occurs within a restriction site, creating a different allele sequence, the enzyme will be unable to cut it and an enzymatic digestion of DNA will result in fragments of different length from the original ones (restriction fragment length polymorphism (RFLP)). The main determinants of the choice of a method are the quantity of DNA available, the number of SNPs to be measured, the measurement plan (whether all SNPs are measured in all subjects or whether some SNPs are measured only in a subset of subjects identified by the results of the initial measurement of other SNPs), and the time required for the analyses. The common issues of method sensitivity and specificity are also considered. As new techniques are continuously developed and modifications to existing techniques are introduced, consultation with experienced scientists working in the molecular genetics laboratory is mandatory at the planning stage of an epidemiological study.

DNA for measurements of minisatellite, microsatellite, and single-nucleotide polymorphisms can be obtained from nucleated cells in the body, most commonly from white blood cells. In epidemiology, DNA is often extracted from the cells after a period of storage. In this procedure centrifugation of the collected blood with an anticoagulant (e.g. sodium citrate) separates three strata: the lowest is composed of erythrocytes, the intermediate thin layer is composed of white cells (the '*buffy coat*'), and the top stratum is composed of plasma. The buffy coat can be pipetted and stored in a biobank for future DNA extraction. In the international European Prospective Investigation into Cancer and Nutrition (EPIC) (Riboli *et al.* 2002), involving the collection of blood from several hundred thousand subjects, in most centres buffy coats were stored in plastic straws of 500 µl capacity kept at −196°C. The content of a straw, which, depending on the accuracy of the manual pipetting, includes white cells mixed with minor and variable amounts of erythrocytes and plasma, derives from approximately 5 ml of blood. On average 50 µg of DNA could be extracted from the content of a straw, with extremes ranging from 5 to 100 µg (M. Friesen 2004, personal communication). As the most efficient techniques require 2 ng for an SNP determination, about 25 000 different SNPs could be measured; however, less efficient but current techniques would require up to 10 ng for an SNP determination, bringing down to 5 000 the number of possible determinations. Materially higher yields of DNA (up to 50 µg/ml blood), can be obtained if storage is avoided and DNA is extracted from blood immediately after collection. Tests of the purity of the extracted DNA need to be carried out in any case, particularly as most measurements use a preliminary step of DNA amplification in order to minimize the amount of DNA required for a single determination. This is carried out through several cycles of the polymerase chain reaction (PCR), which amplifies the segment of DNA of interest for a given SNP measurement a million or a billion times. However, non-specific products can be generated in this process. DNA measurement and related techniques are not only used to measure various kinds of polymorphism but are also increasingly being adapted to investigating how a series of genes in DNA are actually transcribed into RNA, producing expression profiles in normal and pathological tissues. These profiles may have potential aetiological significance when measured in normal tissues and prognostic significance when measured in pathological tissues (e.g. in a neoplasm). The need to introduce sound methodological principles to evaluate these measured profiles has recently been stressed (Simon *et al.* 2003; Ransohoff 2004). Specimens other than blood, such as buccal cells, can be used under appropriate conditions for DNA banking in epidemiological studies (Steinberg *et al.* 1997; King *et al.* 2002).

Phenotype measurements can be used as an indirect way of determining genotype.They have the added advantage that they address not the structure of the gene but the functional results of it, which is what matters most for health and disease investigations. However, they have the major disadvantage that the chain of events from gene to a functional phenotype, for example the activity of an enzyme metabolizing a xenobiotic, is very often influenced by other factors (endogenous and external) which not only make the measurement an unreliable indicator of the underlying genotype but may themselves be predictors of the disease. An obvious example is case–control studies in which the presence of the disease as well as possible treatments may influence the measurements among cases but not controls. As a consequence, inferring a relation between genotype and a disease from an observed association between phenotype and disease may be distorted by 'metabolic confounding' (Saracci 1997). In investigations of the role of genotype difference in cancer causation, considerable attention has been given over the last two decades to metabolic phenotypes genetically controlled and involved in the activation of environmental pre-carcinogens or in the detoxification of carcinogens (Vineis *et al.* 1999). Commonly employed measurements are the activity levels (basal or after challenge with a test drug) of genetically controlled metabolizing enzymes in cancer cases and in control subjects. In these studies great care is required in ascertaining potential confounders, such as physiological rhythms, recent diet, and chronic and recent use of substances such as alcohol, tobacco, and medications, in order to control for them. In the case of strong known effects (e.g. of a medication), it may be preferable to exclude the subjects taking it from the study (which may introduce another kind of bias). When a challenge with a test drug is planned, the possible adverse effects (at the dose employed) in some subjects must be taken into consideration and the appropriate remedial action incorporated in the measurement protocol.

Biological measurements of diet

Dietary factors were the most common main exposure in the 311 papers from the *American Journal of Epidemiology* reviewed in Chapter 1 (see Table 1.1); these are often measured by nutrient concentrations in body fluids. The use of these measurements, and of measurements of nutrient effects, is increasing and so it considered important to pay some specific attention here to biological measurements of diet. They are treated in much more detail in Willett (1998).

A biological measurement suitable for an epidemiological investigation of diet should be specific and sensitive for the dietary component (nutrient, group of related nutrients, or food item) of which the uptake is to be measured. Unfortunately, even the best available biological measurements do not represent purely the effect of dietary uptake, and the boundary between measurements of exposure and measurements of biological effect, i.e. nutritional status, is not well defined. Specificity can be improved if variables other than dietary intake which influence the values of measurements can be identified and controlled. For example, lipid-soluble vitamin E is carried by plasma lipoproteins, and its level in serum or plasma is influenced by the concentration of cholesterol in the blood. Adjusting for cholesterol concentraton can improve the ability of the vitamin E concentration to reflect vitamin E intake and uptake.

Many physiological variables can be measured and may be of interest *per se*, but they may not be sensitive to the uptake of dietary components. For instance, experiments in metabolic wards demonstrate that dietary intake of cholesterol affects plasma cholesterol concentration. However, large changes in cholesterol intake produce small changes in its plasma concentration, so that in any cross-sectional study, given the presence of other factors affecting cholesterol concentration, the correlation between intake and blood concentration is bound to be weak (Willett 1987). Similarly, the plasma concentration of retinol reflects vitamin A intake poorly, except in severe nutritional deficiency, as it is mostly controlled by strict homeostatic mechanisms (Peto 1983).

It is plausible that the cumulative effect of diet over some prolonged period of time (months or years) is more relevant to the aetiology of diet-related disease than diet over shorter spells. Thus good measurements of diet ought preferably to reflect the integrated uptake over prolonged timespans.

Although the range of feasible biological measurements bearing some kind of relationship to diet is broad, there are few good measurements of dietary uptake. In this respect it is useful to distingush two major types of dietary biomarker (Kaaks *et al.* 1997). The first type are *recovery markers* based on physiological knowledge about the balance between intake and excretion of specific compounds, i.e. the percentage recovery of a compound or its metabolites in excretion products such as urine and breath. These markers are time related; they reflect the balance between intake and output over a representative time period, usually 24 hours, and can be translated into estimates of absolute intake level over 24 hours. Probably the best known example is the 24-hour urinary excretion of nitrogen as a marker of average 24-hour protein intake. After allowing for extra-urinary losses, 24-hour urinary nitrogen excretion correlates well with intake of protein during the preceding 24 hours. However, repeated measurements are necessary for the accurate assessment of *usual* protein intake which varies from day to day. The results of some long-term studies indicate that measurements of urinary nitrogen over 6–8 days allow a valid estimate of the usual protein intake of an individual.

A further problem that the measurement of urinary nitrogen shares with other measurements is the need for a complete 24-hour collection of urine. Prolonged collection of urine is always difficult, and may be a source of major error when attempted on a large population rather than in the more tightly controlled conditions possible in a small-scale study. Measurement of urinary creatinine with expression of the results of other measurements as units of the substance excreted per unit of creatinine excreted has been the tool usually employed to take into account possible losses in the collection of urine. However, this adjustment may not work well because of intra-individual variation in creatinine excretion. A method of evaluating the completeness of collection of urine, based on the administration of 250 mg of para-aminobenzoic acid, has been proposed (Bingham and Cummings 1983). Para-aminobenzoic acid is completely recoverable in the urine over the 24 hours following administration and thus appears to be a good check for completeness of collection.

Urinary excretion of potassium as a measurement of potassium intake and average energy expenditure (measured through the 'doubly labelled water' method) as a measurement of average energy intake are two other examples of reasonably well-established recovery markers. Satisfactory measurements of the recovery type are not available for key macronutrients such as fats, fibres, and sucrose.

The second type of dietary biomarker, *concentration markers*, is measured as concentrations of specific substances in biological fluids or cells. The vast majority of biomarkers of dietary intake are of this type; they are not time related and they cannot be translated into absolute measurements of intake.

A summary of the measurements of dietary uptake available for use in epidemiological studies is presented in Table 9.1. This table was prepared with particular reference to studies of the aetiology of cancer, and this orientation has been particularly reflected in the assessment of acceptability to the subjects; for example, it is not usually feasible to approach cancer patients repeatedly to assess their past diet. The paper from which this table is adapted (Riboli *et al.* 1987) presents a detailed discussion of biochemical markers of nutritional intake. A similar discussion with a description of the essentials of assay procedures can be found in Hunter (1998) and an updated discussion of these biomarkers is presented in a series of articles in the *Journal of Nutrition* (volume 133, supplement 3, 2003).

Quality control in biological measurements

Many of the general quality control procedures descitbed in Chapter 5 and listed in Table 5.3 can be applied to meaures in the human body. These include the need for clear written protocols for both field and laboratory procedures, pre-testing and resolving problems with the protocol, and good training and supervision of study personnel. In addition, monitoring the laboratory results by comparing the distribution between laboratory technicians (to test for technician effects) and over time (to test for laboratory 'drift') will improve the quality of the data. Also, procedures to deal with outliers and failures should be applied to reduce the amount of spurious or missing data.

In terms of specific quality control procedures for biological meaures, 'quality control ... begins before the sample is collected ...' (Pickard 1989) and extends from a systematic scrutiny, in consultation with specialists in laboratory methods, of the materials and procedures for specimen collection, storage, and analysis, through their implementation to the review of results before they are accepted and incorporated into a study database.

Collection of specimens

Epidemiological studies make use of biological specimens specially collected for the purpose of the study or make secondary use of materials, or portions of materials, collected for other reasons, usually for diagnostic or therapeutic purposes. Clinical activities may be an easy source of biological materials but the specimens may be inadequate for an epidemiological investigation, particularly if collected by a number of different people only remotely connected with the study. For example:

- 'leftovers' of blood and tissues may be insufficient in volume or quality (e.g. fragments of normal tissues mixed with adjacent pathological tissue, when only the former was required for the study)

- specimens may have remained too long in less than optimal conditions of preservation

- contamination with extraneous materials may also have occurred.

If, for ethical or practical reasons, certain specimens can only be obtained as by-products of clinical procedures (typically surgical or diagnostic specimens), it is advisable that a representative from the epidemiological study team, who is thoroughly familiar with the collection protocol, is present in the biopsy room or operating theatre. This was done, for example, in a study of carcinogen activation which used lung tissue specimens from lung cancer cases and controls (Petruzzelli et al. 1988).

Members of the epidemiological study team should also be directly responsible for the collection, initial processing, and storage of specimens collected expressly for an epidemiological study. At these stages, a number of variables should be controlled by standard procedures and any departure from these procedures immediately recorded in a log book indicating the specimens affected. These records will permit departures from accepted collection procedures to be addressed during analysis of the data.

As an illustration of what should be addressed in developing the measurement procedures, the following are variables that should be controlled during the collection of blood (Young and Bermes 1986; Pickard 1989).

Table 9.1 Summary of biological measurements of dietary uptake available for use in epidemiological studies[a]

Measurement	Value as an indicator of dietary intake	Useful for: Short- or long-term diet[b]	Prospective or retrospective studies	Number of measurements required	Acceptability To researcher[c]	To subject
Protein						
24 h urinary nitrogen	Very high	Short	Prospective	2+	Medium	Low
24 h urinary 3-methylhistidine	Very high	Short	Prospective	2+	Medium	Low
Fat						
Fatty acids in adipose tissue	Very high	Long	Both	1	High	Medium
Fatty acids in red cell membranes	High	Long	Both	1	Very high	Very high
Fatty acids in other cell membranes	High	Long	Both	1	Low	Very high
Fatty acids in plasma lipids	Very high	Short	Prospective	2+	Very high	Very high
Vitamins						
Vitamin A in plasma	Low	Uncertain	Uncertain	Uncertain	High	Very high
Carotenoids in plasma	High	Both	Both	1	High	Very high
Ascorbic acid in:						
Plasma	Medium	Short	Prospective	2+	Very high	Very high
Leucocytes	Medium	Both	Both	1	High	Very high
Lingual ascorbic acid test	Low	Uncertain	Uncertain	Uncertain	High	Very high
Saliva	Low	Uncertain	Uncertain	Uncertain	High	Very high
α-Tocopherol in plasma	Medium	Both	Prospective	1	High	Very high

Trace minerals

Selenium in:						
Plasma	Low (?)	Short (?)	Prospective	2+ (?)	High	Very high
Red cells or whole blood	High (?)	Both	Both	1	High	Very high
Nails or hair	High (?)	Long	Both	1	High	Very high
24 h urine	Medium (?)	Short (?)	Uncertain	2+	Medium	Low
Glutathione peroxidase activity	Medium (?)	Long	Uncertain	1	Low	Very high

Zinc in:						
Plasma	Low	Uncertain	Prospective	Uncertain	High (?)	Very high
Saliva	Low	Uncertain	Prospective	Uncertain	High (?)	Very high
24 h urine	Medium (?)	Short	Uncertain	2+	Medium	Low
Hair	High	Long	Both	1	High	Very high
Tolerance test	Low	Uncertain	Uncertain	Uncertain	Medium	Low

[a] Adapted and updated from Riboli et al (1987).

[b] Short = days; long = weeks to months or more.

[c] Acceptability taking into account complexity and cost of analysis.

Contamination of collection tubes

A large variety of collection and storage tubes are now commercially available. Especially for measurement of substances that are at low concentration in blood and common in the environment, such as trace metals, it is necessary to ensure that all materials (needles, tubes, pipettes, stoppers, additives (if any), etc.) do not release the substance and that manipulations are conducted in such a way that no contamination from the ambient environment occurs.

Types of additive

Serum, requiring no additive, and plasma, collected with added heparin, are the most commonly used 'all-purpose' materials. Other additives may be needed depending on the desired analytical determinations (e.g. citrate or EDTA for coagulation and fibrinolysis measurements). The comments above clearly apply in the choice and control of additives.

Order of collection tubes

When several tubes are filled, one should first fill those with no additive, then those with additives (say, heparin), leaving to the last those with the chelating agent EDTA. This procedure is designed to avoid carry-over of additives from tubes with additives to tubes without additives.

Time of venepuncture

The importance of the timing of blood collection, with reference to the time of the external exposure and the time of day, has been discussed above. Time factors which may affect the value of exposure measurements (e.g. time since exposure to a xenobiotic agent, time within the menstrual cycle, time since the last meal) should preferably be controlled by the protocol and/or be recorded and accounted for in the analysis of the data.

Subject posture

Posture has been shown to influence the plasma concentrations of several physiological compounds (e.g. total protein, iron, total cholesterol and its fractions) which can be increased by as much as 5–15 per cent in the standing position compared with the supine position because of orthostatic reduction in plasma volume.

Use of tourniquet

Tourniquets should be applied only very briefly, as a stasis of more than a couple of minutes may alter the concentration of many blood components, particularly proteins and protein-bound compounds.

Haemolysis

Smooth gentle manipulations are required to avoid visible or occult, and therefore uncontrollable, haemolysis which alters the concentrations of many compounds. Haemolysis may also occur during transport of tubes if they are incompletely filled.

Transport and storage conditions

The optimal transport and storage conditions vary according to the substances to be measured. The prevention of oxidation caused by contact with air or the action of light is a prime requirement. Under normal circumstances, cells should be separated from serum or plasma within 2 hours after venepuncture. During this period, the specimens can be left at room temperature, but preferably held at 4°C. Immediate treatment with an appropriate additive, centrifugation, and deep freezing are necessary for some substances, for example vitamin C (Galan *et al.* 1988).

Similar guiding principles apply to the collection, initial processing, and storage of specimens other than blood. Particular care is necessary in instructing study subjects, and in checking that instructions have been followed, when specimen collection depends on them (e.g. urine collection).

Sending samples by batch to the laboratory

The researcher should specify the protocol for sending specimens to the laboratory for analysis. First, specimens should be sent to the laboratory *blinded*, i.e. without information on case/control or exposure status (including the way that subject ID numbers are assigned). Secondly, for case–control and nested case–control studies, the effects of variations between laboratory batches (e.g. because of differences in chemicals or drift in calibration of instruments over time) can be reduced by including both cases and controls within each batch (in the same ratio of cases to controls as in the biomarker study) (Tworoger and Hankinson 2006). This automatically leads to a proper balance of cases and controls by the laboratory technician, which is also important if there is a technician effect on the laboratory measure. To control further for other variations which might affect the accuracy of the measurement (e.g. the length of storage time in the freezer or the number of freeze–thaw cycles), cases and control might be individually or group matched on these factors, and the matched set(s) included in a batch. For intervention trials, where the goal is to look for within-person *change* over time, samples from the same participant should be assayed in the same batch. When multiple specimens per subject are analysed to reduce measurement error by creating an *average*, inclusion of the multiple samples per person in the same batch is less important. Finally, some of these sources of variation can be controlled at the time of data analysis; for example, one can statistically control for laboratory technician or length of specimen storage.

Laboratory quality control

Laboratory quality control (Westgard and Klee 1986; Copeland 1989) is the responsibility of the laboratory staff and is substantially beyond the scope of this book. However, an epidemiologist depending on laboratory-based measurements of exposure should be familiar with laboratory control procedures and be assured that they are being applied in the laboratory being used.

The following are essential for the purpose of an epidemiological study.

(a) If any specimen is rejected by the laboratory as 'unacceptable' for analysis, the reasons should be stated, as they may point to faults in collection, initial processing, storage, or transport which may be amenable to correction.

(b) Time from collection of the specimen to analysis should be known and as a rule controlled, either at the stage of allocating specimens to days of analysis or during statistical analysis of the study. As specimens generally accrue over long periods of time and a laboratory can only process a limited number of specimens each day, it is neither correct nor feasible to have all specimens analysed on a single occasion. The interval between collection and analysis should be kept to a minimum unless a long-term storage approach, with its additional requirements (see below), is adopted.

(c) The imprecision and bias of the measurements of interest due to variations in the laboratory procedure should be known and monitored at regular intervals (as a rule, daily), and maintained within the laboratory's acceptable limits.

These limits can be quite narrow for the best methods of analysis. For example, measurements of electrolytes (sodium, potassium, and calcium) may have day-to-day coefficients of variation of less than 2 per cent (Copeland 1989). For plasma total cholesterol concentration, most current assays have a day-to-day coefficient of variation of 3–6 per cent (Naito 1989). Even higher values (5–10 per cent or more) may apply to other measurements, for example, measurements of oestriol (Kaplan 1989) or of other hormones in serum. Imprecision leads to random misclassification of subjects, and variable accuracy over time has the same effect. Moreover, bias, if unknown, prevents comparison of absolute values of biological measurements made in different places or at different times.

Imprecision is monitored through control measurements on replicate samples from a standard specimen or reference material made without the analyst being aware of their identity as replicates. Bias can also be assessed if the reference material contains a known concentration of the substance of interest. For example, frozen aliquots from a pool of sera can be used for reference. The reference concentration is determined under optimal conditions using the best available reference method, and the sera can be stored and used for up to about a year. If a reference material is not available, accuracy (intermethod reliability) can be monitored by double assaying some specimens with the current method and with a reference method. It may also be possible to carry some specimens over for some time and assay them repeatedly. A sufficient number of control measurements should be taken to provide sufficient statistical power to promptly detect increasing imprecision or trends in bias over time (Saracci 1974).

It is the epidemiologist's responsibility to ensure that statistical quality control procedures are being applied by the responsible laboratory scientists to biological measurements of exposure. Usually there will be no difficulties with well-established methods of measurement, for which good laboratories routinely apply intra-laboratory quality control, often supplemented by inter-laboratory controls. However, problems may arise with methods still in development, as is the case for many of those used for measuring exposure, because requirements for a regular quality control may be difficult to meet: the assay may be time-consuming and cumbersome, an accepted reference method may not exist, reference materials may not be available, etc. Compromise approaches may then be necessary, varying from mere 'spot checking' for inaccuracy and imprecision to a systematic quality control programme. As a rule, however, no large series of biological measurements should be started until regular quality control procedures are applicable.

A final requirement, more in the nature of a safety precaution than a quality control procedure, is to ensure that study staff and subjects are protected against the risk of infection from microbiological contamination of specimens, notably with HIV and hepatitis viruses. The 'universal precautions' recommended by the US Centers for Disease Control are relevant to all persons dealing with human biological specimens (US DHHS 1987) (available online at: http://www.cdc.gov/ncidod/dhqp/bp_universal_precautions.html).

Banks of biological specimens

Epidemiological investigations of exposure–disease relationships can make use of banks of biological specimens collected from large groups of identifiable subjects. For example, the relationship between breast cancer and selenium intake could be studied by comparing subjects with breast cancer and control subjects from a population from which blood, hair, or toenail specimens had been collected in the past. Obviously, the investigation would be much more informative and its results more clearly interpretable if, in addition to the collection of biological specimens, other information had been gathered, such as food habits, reproductive history, etc.

The banking approach has three main advantages.

(a) It avoids having to perform the biological measurements of exposure after a disease has been diagnosed. Measurement after onset of disease may be useless if the aetiologically relevant period of exposure goes back decades and the exposure level has changed with time. In addition, it may result in a misleading measurement of exposure if the presence of the disease has altered the metabolism of the substance to be measured or has made the subjects change their exposure (e.g. their food habits).

(b) By restricting the number of biological determinations to, say, a few hundred cases and controls rather than to the tens of thousands of subjects in the source population it can make an investigation feasible that would otherwise be impracticable.

(c) As new analytical techniques are developed they may be applied to specimens in existing banks and thus greatly shorten the time needed to obtain results relating outcome to newly measurable exposures.

Against these advantages must be weighed the disadvantage of the cost of establishing and maintaining a large bank of specimens and the potential problems arising from the fact that the analytical procedures have to be applied to stored rather than fresh materials.

Long-term preservation of biological specimens is made possible by freezing or freeze-drying; the former method is more generally applicable to samples of blood, serum, plasma, urine, cells, and tissues. For long-term preservation, temperatures of at least −70°C to −80°C (in an electrically operated deep freezer) or, better, −130°C to −160°C (nitrogen vapour) or −196°C (liquid nitrogen) are currently used. The results, in terms of maintaining all the properties of the fresh sample qualitatively and quantitatively, usually vary inversely with the biological complexity of the stored material. For example, urine is an easier material to preserve than tissue.

While −70°C may be adequate for many purposes, several biological degradation processes still continue at that temperature and, indeed, some enzymatic activity is even present at −196°C. Degradation is also influenced by the frequency with which a specimen has been left to withstand temperatures above the nominal storage temperature (say, −70°C), whether this is through a failure of the freezing system or because the specimen was thawed and refrozen when part of it was used in the past. In fact, some of the changes resulting from storage at low temperatures only come about during thawing. If thawing is not rapid (as it is when the specimen is transferred directly from the freezer to a 37°C bath), micronuclei of ice formed within cells during freezing act as starting points for crystal growth which is capable of seriously damaging biological structures.

These general considerations point to four requirements.

(a) Any freezing system must incorporate back-up facilities, adequate in size and performance, to overcome the effects of failure of the main system. In this respect liquid nitrogen, which does not depend on an electrical power supply, has a definite advantage.

(b) Specimens should be stored in aliquots so that sub-specimens can be easily and correctly identified and retrieved with minimal change in the temperature of the other specimens and without the need for thawing and refreezing of the whole material from the subjects to be studied.

(c) A 'history' or chart of the storage conditions should be kept for all specimens. This chart should include, in particular, the speed of freezing, the speed of thawing, and the temperature of storage, which may vary in different positions within a freezer.

(d) Several specimens containing different concentrations of a number of substances of interest should each be stored in multiple small aliquots and then analysed at regular intervals (say, every 3 months initially and then every year) to monitor time-related changes in concentrations.

It is also common, if there is more than one specimen per participant, to store the specimens in different freezers in case there is a catastrophic failure affecting one freezer.

Experience in dealing with the technical and logistic problems of biological specimen banks set up specifically for epidemiological purposes has been described (Fondation Marcel Mérieux 1987; Jellum *et al.* 1987). The feasibility of setting up very large banks for the purpose of long-term prospective studies on diet and health carried out in different national contexts has been proved in the last decade (Riboli *et al.* 2002). When developing a bank project, direct contact and consultation not only with laboratory specialists, but also with professionals in charge of banks maintained for medical care purposes (blood, bone marrow, organs, semen, etc.), is advisable.

Biological specimen banks can be used for measuring exposure at both the individual level and the group level. At the group level, it has been proposed that specimens from various subjects are mixed together and the measurements made on the pool of blood instead of on each specimen individually, particularly when a large number of different measurements (say, of a variety of vitamins in blood) are to be made (Peto 1983). The groups for which the pooling is done could be defined by sex or age, or geographically, or might be the cases and controls in a case–control study. The former would be a special case of the 'ecological' approach to the investigation of exposure–disease relationships, which has both advantages and disadvantages.

In a case–control study the pooling approach might be used to screen a large number of variables for differences between cases and controls, with advantages in terms of both cost and amount of blood used. It would then be necessary to proceed to measurements in individuals for the variables found to differ between cases and controls so that a full statistical analysis of the study, including consideration of confounding variables, could be undertaken.

At the individual level, biological measurements are increasinly being made in case–control studies nested within cohort studies. This is an efficient way of processing specimens and analysing data from large cohorts of subjects followed up prospectively (Breslow and Day 1987). Samples are formed consisting of the cases of the disease under study and random samples of controls from each 'risk set' of subjects under observation at the same age and calendar period in which a case occurs. Biological measurements are then made on specimens from the cases and the selected controls. A loss of statistical power compared with the results which would have been obtained if the measurements and statistical analysis had been carried out on the whole cohort rather than on the cases and selected controls is unavoidable. To make this loss negligible, particularly for categories of exposures within which few cases are observed (e.g. those with extreme exposure levels), as many as 10 controls per case may have to be selected. However, this approach still usually produces a large saving in cost and other resources in comparison with making measurements on specimens from every individual in the cohort.

Summary

Measurements made directly in the human body or on its products represent, in principle, the ideal approach to measuring exposure. They can be:

- objective, i.e. independent of the observed person's perceptions and of the observer, if instrumental or laboratory methods are used
- individualized, i.e. exactly targeted on each subject at times relevant to causation of the disease under study
- quantitatively specific and sensitive to the exposure of interest.

In practice, these valuable characteristics are realized to a variable extent depending on the exposure to be measured and the methods employed.

It is essential to sample the correct site within the body (or the correct body product) at the appropriate time, lest an exposure goes undetected which could have been correctly identified by a cruder measurement in the environment or even by a simple answer to a questionnaire.

For xenobiotic compounds, correct sampling implies a knowledge of the kinetics of absorption, distribution, transformation, and elimination (or storage) of the compound of interest. For endobiotic substances (e.g. hormones), the distribution in tissues and in time is substantially influenced by homeostatic mechanisms as well as by important day-to-day variations reflecting changes in diet. This within-person variation, which is often the same size as or larger than the between-person variation, causes substantial misclassification of subjects with respect to the exposure when only a single measurement of exposure is made. Multiple measurements can reduce this source of variation.

The materials used for sampling, the sampling procedures, and the storage and analysis of biological specimens require systematic quality control. Even though many methods for measuring exposure in the human body or its products are currently still at a developmental stage, no large series of biological measurements should be embarked upon until a regular quality control programme can be set up.

The realization that it is becoming possible to expand the range of exposures, particularly individual genotypes, accessible to measurement in biological materials is one of the reasons behind the establishment of banks of biological specimens from large groups of subjects from whom other information has also been gathered (personal characteristics, habits, etc.). Typically, the stored specimens can be analysed for selected exposures when new cases of a disease of interest occur and compared with similar measurements on a sample of the specimens from the whole population.

The development of methods of measurement of exposures in biological materials is a rapidly advancing front. The epidemiologist can contribute, in collaboration with laboratory scientists, to ensure that these methods acquire properties of objectivity, individualization, specificity, sensitivity, and technical and economic practicability to a sufficient degree to make them usable and to have an advantage over other methods in epidemiological studies.

References

Aitio, A. (2000). Biological monitoring in the occupational environment. In *General and Applied Toxicology* (ed. B. Ballantyne, T.C. Marrs, and T.Syversen), pp.1899–914. MacMillan, London.

Bartsch, H., Hemminki, K., and O'Neill, I.K. (1988). *DNA Damaging Agents in Humans: Applications in Cancer Epidemiology and Prevention*. IARC Scientific Publication No. 89. International Agency for Research on Cancer, Lyon.

Berlin, A., Draper, M., Hemminki, K., and Vainio, H. (1984). *Monitoring Human Exposure to Carcinogenic and Mutagenic Agents*. IARC Scientific Publication No. 59. International Agency for Research on Cancer, Lyon.

Bingham, S. and Cummings, J.H. (1983). The use of 4-aminobenzoic acid as a marker to validate the completeness of 24h urine collections in man. *Clinical Science*, **64**, 629–35.

Bloom, A.D. (1981). *Guidelines for Studies of Human Populations Exposed to Mutagenic and Reproductive Hazards*. March of Dimes Birth Defects Foundation, White Plains, NY.

Breslow, N.E. and Day, N.E. (1987). *Statistical Methods in Cancer Research*. Vol. 2, *The Design and Analysis of Cohort Studies*. IARC Scientific Publication No. 82. International Agency for Research on Cancer, Lyon.

Copeland, B. (1989). Quality control. In *Clinical Chemistry: Theory, Analysis and Correlation* (2nd edn) (ed. L.A. Kaplan and A.J. Pesce), pp. 270–89. C.V. Mosby, St Louis, MO.

de Andrade, M.,Thandi, I., Brown, S., Gotto, A., Jr, Patsch, W., and Boerwinkle, E. (1995). Relationship of the apolipoprotein E polymorphism with carotid artery atherosclerosis. *American Journal of Human Genetics*, **56**, 1379–90.

Droz, P.O., Berode, M., and Wu, M.M. (1991). Evaluation of concomitant biological and air monitoring. *Applied Occupational and Environmental Hygiene*, **6**, 465–74.

Fondation Marcel Mérieux (1987). *Sérothèque Rhône-Alpes. 9ème Séminaire Y. Biraud*. Fondation Marcel Mérieux, Lyon.

Galan, P., Hercberg, S., Keller, H.E., Bellio, J.P., Bourgeois, C.F., and Fourlon, C.H. (1988). Plasma ascorbic acid determination: is it necessary to centrifuge and to stabilize the blood sample immediately in the field? *International Journal of Vitaminology and Nutritional Research*, **58**, 473–4.

Haugen, A., Becher, G., Benestad, C., *et al.* (1986). Determination of polycyclic aromatic hydrocarbons in the urine, benzo(a)pyrene diolepoxide-DNA adducts in sera from coke oven workers exposed to measured amounts of polycyclic aromatic hydrocarbons in the work atmosphere. *Cancer Research*, **46**, 4178–83.

Holman, C.D.J. and Armstrong, B.K. (1984). Cutaneous malignant melanoma and indicators of total accumulated exposure to the sun: an analysis separating histogenetic types. *Journal of the National Cancer Institute*, **73**, 75–82.

Hulka, B.S., Wilcosky, T.C., and Griffith, I.D. (1990). *Biological Markers in Epidemiology*. Oxford University Press, New York.

Hunter, D. (1998). Biochemical indicators of dietary intake. In *Nutritional Epidemiology* (2nd edn) (ed. W. Willett), pp. 174–243. Oxford University Press, New York.

IARC (International Agency for Research on Cancer) (1990). *Chromium, Nickel and Welding. Monographs on the Evaluation of Carcinogenic Risks to Humans*, Vol. 49. International Agency for Research on Cancer, Lyon.

Jellum, E., Andersen, A., Orjasaeter, H., Foss, O. P., Theodorsen, L., and Lund-Larsen, P. (1987). The JANUS serum bank and early detection of cancer. *Biochimica Clinica*, **11**, 191–5.

Johnson,G.C., Esposito, L., Barratt, B.J., *et al* (2001). Haplotype tagging for the identification of common disease genes. *Nature Genetics*, **29**, 233–7.

Kaaks, R., Riboli, E., and Sinha, R. (1997). Biochemical markers of dietary intake. In *Application of Biomarkers in Cancer Epidemiology* (ed. P. Toniolo, P. Boffetta, D.E.G. Shuker, N. Rothman, B. Hulka, and N. Pearce), pp. 103–26. IARC Scientific Publication no. 142. International Agency for Research on Cancer, Lyon.

Kaplan, L.A. (1989). Estriol. In *Clinical Chemistry: Theory, Analysis and Correlation* (2nd edn) (ed. L.A. Kaplan and A.J. Pesce), pp. 944–50. Mosby, St Louis, MO.

King, I.B., Satia-Abouta, J.S., Thornquist, M.D., *et al.* (2002). Buccal cell DNA yield, quality and collection costs: comparison of methods for large scale studies. *Cancer Epidemiology Biomarkers and Prevention*, **11**, 1130–33.

Kirk,G.D., Camus-Randon, A.M., Mendy, M., *et al.* (2000). Ser-249 mutations in plasma DNA of patients with hepatocellular carcinoma from the Gambia. *Journal of the National Cancer Institute*, **92**, 148–53.

Klaassen, C.D. (1980). Absorption, distribution, and excretion of toxicants. In *Casarett and Doull's Toxicology* (2nd edn) (ed. J. Doull, C.D. Klaassen, and M.O Amdur), pp. 28–55. MacMillan, New York.

Lauwerys, R. (1984). Basic concepts of monitoring human exposure. In *Monitoring Human Exposure to Carcinogenic and Mutagenic Agents* (ed. A. Berlin, M. Draper, K. Hemminki, and H. Vainio), pp. 31–6. IARC Scientific Publication No.59. International Agency for Research on Cancer, Lyon.

Liu, K., Cooper, R., McKeever, J., *et al.* (1979). Assessment of the association between habitual salt intake and high blood pressure: methodological problems. *American Journal of Epidemiology*, **110**, 219–26.

Lucier, G.W. and Thompson, C.L. (1987). Issues in biochemical applications to risk assessment: when can lymphocytes be used as surrogate markers? *Environmental Health Perspectives*, **76**, 187–91.

Naito, H.K. (1989). Cholesterol. In *Clinical Chemistry: Theory, Analysis and Correlation* (2nd edn) (ed. L.A. Kaplan and A.J. Pesce), pp.974–83. Mosby, St Louis, MO.

Peto, J. (1980). Genetic predisposition to cancer. In *Cancer Incidence in Defined Populations* (ed. J.Cairns, J.L. Lyon, and R.Skolnick), p. 203. Banbury Report No.4, Cold Spring Harbor Laboratory, Cold Spring Harbor, NY.

Peto, R. (1983). The marked differences between carotenoids and retinoids: methodological implications for biochemical epidemiology. *Cancer Surveys*, **2**, 327–40.

Petruzzelli, S., Camus, A. M., Carrozzi, L., *et al.* (1988). Long-lasting effects of tobacco smoking on pulmonary drug-metabolizing enzymes: a case–control study on lung cancer patients. *Cancer Research*, **48**, 4695–700.

Pickard, N.A. (1989). Collection and handling of patients specimens. In *Clinical Chemistry: Theory, Analysis and Correlation* (2nd edn) (ed. L.A. Kaplan and A.J. Pesce), pp. 40–8. Mosby, St Louis, MO.

Ransohoff, D.F. (2004). Rules of evidence for cancer molecular-marker discovery and validation.*Nature Reviews: Cancer*, **4**, 309–14.

Randerath, K., Reddy, M.J., and Gupta, R.C. (1981). ^{32}P-labelling test for DNA damage. *Proceedings of the National Academy of Sciences of the USA*, **78**, 6126–9.

Randerath, K., Miller, R.H., Mittal, D., and Randerath, E. (1988). Monitoring human exposure to carcinogens by ultrasensitive post-labelling assays: application to unidentified genotoxicants. In *DNA Damaging Agents in Humans: Applications in Cancer Epidemiology and Prevention* (ed. H. Bartsch, K. Hemminki, and I. K. O'Neill), pp. 361–7. IARC Scientific Publication No. 89. International Agency for Research on Cancer, Lyon.

Riboli, E., Rönnholm, H., and Saracci, R. (1987). Biological markers of diet. *Cancer Surveys*, **6**, 685–718.

Riboli, E., Preston-Martin, S., Saracci, R.,Haley, N.J.,Trichopoulos, D.,and Becher, H. (1990). Exposure of non-smoking women to environmental tobacco smoke: a 10-country collaborative study.*Cancer Causes and Control*, **1**, 243–42.

Riboli, E., Hunt, K.J., Slimani, N., *et al.*(2002) European Prospective Investigation into Cancer and Nutrition (EPIC): study populations and data collection. *Public Health Nutrition*, **5**, 1113–24.

Rowland, M. and Tozer, T.N. (1980). *Clinical Pharmacokinetics*. Lea & Febiger, Philadelphia, PA.

Saracci, R. (1974). The power (sensitivity) of quality control plans in clinical chemistry. *American Journal of Clinical Pathology*, **62**, 398–406.

Saracci, R. (1984). Assessing exposure of individuals in the identification of disease determinants. In *Monitoring Human Exposure to Carcinogenic and Mutagenic Agents* (ed. A. Berlin, M. Draper, K. Hemminki, and H. Vainio), pp. 135–42. IARC Scientific Publication No. 59. International Agency for Research on Cancer, Lyon.

Saracci, R. (1997). Comparing measurements of biomarkers with other measurements of exposure. In *Application of Biomarkers in Cancer Epidemiology* (ed. P. Toniolo, P. Boffetta, D.E.G. Shuker, N. Rothman, B. Hulka, and N. Pearce), pp. 303–312. IARC Scientific Publication No.142. International Agency for Research on Cancer, Lyon.

Sébastien, P., Bégin, R., Case, B.W., and McDonald, J.C. (1986). Inhalation of chrysotile dust. In *The Biological Effects of Chrysotile. Accomplishments in Oncology*, Vol. 1, No. 2 (ed. J.C. Wagner), pp. 19–29. J.B. Lippincott, Philadelphia, PA.

Shekelle, R. B., Shryock, A. M., Paul, O., *et al.* (1981). Diet, serum cholesterol and death from coronary heart disease. *New England Journal Medicine*, **304**, 65–70.

Schulte, P.A. and Perera, F.P. (ed.) (1993). *Molecular Epidemiology*. Academic Press, San Diego, CA.

Simon, R., Radmacher, M.D., Dobbin, K., and McShane, L.M. (2003). Pitfalls in the use of DNA microarray data for diagnostic and prognostic classification. *Journal of the National Cancer Institute*, **95**, 14–18.

Steinberg, K.K., Sanderlin, K.C., Ou, C.Y., Hannon, W.H., McQuillan, G.M., and Sampson, E.J. (1997). DNA banking in epidemiologic studies. *Epidemiologic Reviews*, **19**, 156–62.

Syvänen, A.C. (2001). Accessing genetic variation: genotyping single nucleotide polymorphisms. *Nature Reviews: Genetics*, **2**, 930–942.

Tangney, C.C., Shekelle, R.B., Raynor, W., Gale, M., and Betz, E.P. (1987). Intra- and inter-individual variation in measurements of β-carotene, retinol and tocopherols in diet and plasma. *American Journal of Clinical Nutrition*, **45**, 764–9.

Teeuwen, H.W.A. (1988). Clinical pharmacokinetics of nicotine, caffeine, and quinine. PhD Thesis, University of Nijmegen. CiP-DATA, Koninklijke Bibliotheek, Den Haag.

Tworoger, S.S., and Hankinson, S.E. (2006). Use of biomarkers in epidemiologic studies: minimizing the influence of measurement error in the study design and analysis. *Cancer Causes and Control*, **17**, 889–899.

US DHHS (US Department of Health and Human Services) (1987). Recommendations for prevention of HIV transmission in health care settings. *Morbidity and Mortality Weekly Report*, **36**, 1S–18S.

Van Vunakis, H.,Gjika, H.B., and Langone, J.J. (1987). Radioimmunoassay for nicotine and cotinine. In *Environmental Carcinogens: Methods of Analysis and Exposure Measurement.* Vol. 9, *Passive Smoking* (ed. I.K. O'Neill, K.D. Brunnemann, B. Dodet, and D. Hoffmann), pp. 317–330. IARC Scientific Publication No. 81. International Agency for Research on Cancer, Lyon.

Vine, M.F. (1990). Micronuclei. In *Biological Markers in Epidemiology* (ed. B.S. Hulka, T.C. Wilcosky, and J.D. Griffith), pp. 125–46. Oxford University Press, New York.

Vineis, P., Malats, N., Lang, M., *et al.* (ed.) (1999). *Metabolic Polymorphisms and Susceptibility to Cancer.* IARC Scientific Publication No.148. International Agency for Research on Cancer, Lyon.

Westgard, J.O. and Klee, G.G. (1986). Quality assurance. In *Textbook of Clinical Chemistry* (ed. N.W. Tietz), pp. 424–58. W.B. Saunders, Philadelphia, PA.

Wild, C. and Turner, P.C. (2001). Exposure biomarkers in chemoprevention studies of liver cancer. In *Biomarkers in Cancer Chemoprevention* (ed. A.B. Miller, H. Bartsch, P. Boffetta, L. Dragsted, and H. Vainio), pp.215–22. IARC Scientific Publication No. 154. International Agency for Research on Cancer, Lyon.

Willett, W. (1987). Nutritional epidemiology: issues and challenges. *International Journal of Epidemiology*, **16**, 312–17.

Willett, W. (1998). *Nutritional Epidemiology.* Oxford University Press, New York.

Young, D.S. and Bermes, E.W. (1986). Specimen collection and processing: sources of biological variation. In *Textbook of Clinical Chemistry* (ed. N.W. Tietz), pp. 478–518. W.B. Saunders, Philadelphia, PA.

Zielhuis, R.L. (1985). Biological monitoring studies in occupational and environmental health. In *Epidemiology and Quantitation of Environmental Risk in Humans from Radiation and Other Agents* (ed. A. Castellani), pp. 291–306. Plenum Press, New York.

10

Measurements in the environment

In the last decade, recognition of the complexity of the determinants of individual exposure to air pollutants and the impact of misclassification has led to the need for a new conceptual framework for exposure assessment.
(National Research Council 1985)

Introduction

Environmental agents include physical, chemical, and biological components or contaminants of the general environment (soil, air, water), the local environment (home, workplace, recreational sites), or the personal environment (food, drinks, cosmetics, drugs). Frequently, exposure to these agents is unknown or unsensed by the exposed individual. Under these circumstances, the exposure as such cannot be recalled or recorded by the study subject, and so it can only be documented through measurements in the environment. In other circumstances, measurements in the environment represent an alternative or complementary approach to questioning the subject.

Methods of making measurements in the environment vary in sophistication from rating by skilled observers (e.g. the dustiness of air in the workplace) through measurements made in the field by simple or complex instruments (e.g. concentration of dust in the atmosphere measured by nephelometry) to measurements in the laboratory of the concentration of substances in samples taken from the environment (e.g. counting specific mineral fibres in air samples by electron microscopy). The choice of method depends on the environment to be sampled, the agent to be measured, the availability of the appropriate technology, and the cost.

This choice, together with the development and application of the relevant technical methods, belongs mainly to the disciplines of industrial and environmental hygiene and other technical disciplines rather than to epidemiology. For this reason, the emphasis of this chapter, like that of the last, is on those aspects of these methods of measurement which most demand the epidemiologist's attention and action.

In this chapter, we outline the characteristics, value, and limitations of measurements in the environment, and address issues of measuring both present and past exposure by way of examples taken mainly from the occupational environment. For present exposure, the selection of exposures to be measured and the places and substances to be sampled, the extent of sampling, and some analytical aspects are discussed. Reconstruction of measurements of past exposure are considered in circumstances in which complete, incomplete, or no actual measurements of the relevant past environment are available. The use of conversion tables, together with data derived from questionnaires, as a substitute for direct measurements in the environment is also considered.

The value and limitations of environmental measurements

Measuring an exposure in the external environment by instrumental and laboratory methods may render exposure assessment objective, individualized, and quantitatively specific and sensitive. Because of these desirable characteristics, the use of these methods for measuring environmental exposure in epidemiological studies is becoming more common. However, the increasingly popular belief that they are intrinsically superior to questionnaires and related subjective approaches on every occasion that they can be applied has no general validity in practice. The extent to which the potential superiority of instrumental and laboratory methods can be achieved depends on circumstances particular to each epidemiological study.

Also particular to the design and conduct of each study are the consequences of deficiencies in objectivity, individualization, sensitivity, and specificity of environmental measurements. The two types of error that can occur are (see Chapter 3):

- error variance (lack of precision) in the measure whereby individual levels of exposure are over- or underestimated but the mean exposure of a group (e.g. cases and controls) is correct
- systematically incorrect estimation of exposure levels, whereby the mean exposure level for a group is over or under-estimated.

The first type of error leads to attenuation of the observed relationship (e.g. the risk ratio) of the exposure to disease, such that the risk per unit increase of exposure is less than the true risk per unit of exposure. The latter error may lead to over- or underestimation of the risk at a fixed level of exposure, which is a major problem in public health terms, especially when control limits for exposure to an environmental agent must be established. This kind of error had, for example, been found for the earlier estimates of radiation exposure following the atomic bombing in Hiroshima and Nagasaki (Preston and Pierce 1987). Most measurements have both types of error to varying degrees.

The *objectivity* of a measurement in the environment depends on two steps: first, the sampling of the environment, and, secondly, the measurement procedure proper. Both steps can be highly objective such as, for example, when a personal sampler is used to take a sample of air during a working shift for subsequent automated measurement of the concentration of a gaseous pollutant. Often, however, only the second step can be objective, while identification and selection of the sample involves substantial subjectivity. Typically, reliance must be placed on information provided by the study subject to identify environmental materials to be sampled. For example, the subject must identify recently consumed food and drinks to be tested in the laboratory for chemical and microbiological contaminants when investigating an outbreak of diarrhoea. Similarly, when studying lung cancer in relation to inhaled carcinogens (other than those from active tobacco smoking), the work and residential histories gathered from the subjects, sometimes corroborated by pre-existing records, identify which part of the environment should be searched for records of past measurements of airborne contaminants. Subjectivity also enters into the second step, the analytical procedure, to the extent that it is not totally automated but demands the intervention of human operators in the form of manipulation of samples, taking readings, and recognition of objects to be measured or counted (e.g. asbestos fibres in a microscopic field).

Individualized measurement can be achieved fully only when personal sampling is practicable over repeated and extended periods of time. In many circumstances it can only be approximated by average measurements over time or groups of persons (or personal space), for example when an area sample of air is taken with a static sampler in the workplace. The approximation is even more distant when only a few haphazardly collected spot samples of the environment are available. Measurements on such samples, however accurate analytically, may be only rough guides to the amount of exposure and cannot be regarded as unbiased estimates of individual values. Error in obtaining the original specimens from the environment and in sub-sampling for laboratory analysis may be the main source of error in environmental measurements. For example, in measures of food contamination, random samples of kernels are drawn from commercial lots of shelled peanuts and comminuted in a mill to produce sub-samples. These sub-samples are then tested for aflatoxin, a highly hepatotoxic and carcinogenic mycotoxin. In one investigation, it was found that, at a concentration of 20 parts per billion of aflatoxin, 66 per cent of the random measurement error could be attributed to the initial sampling of kernels, 21 per cent to sub-sampling, and only 13 per cent to the analytical method (Whitaker and Dickens 1974). This example emphasizes the importance of an adequate sampling strategy when aiming at accurate measurements of individual exposures, especially when the concentration of the agent of interest varies widely. This is the case for aflatoxin in batches of peanuts, where a few peanuts account for most of the contamination.

Analytic specificity and sensitivity (see Chapter 9), which jointly describe the accuracy of a method, also deserve careful consideration before choosing instrumental or laboratory-based measurements of the environment in preference to some alternative method of exposure measurement. If the exposure relevant to the epidemiological study is a mixture of chemicals (e.g. air pollutants), measurements specific for a single chemical may be inappropriate if that chemical is not the one responsible for the biological effect under study (or is not responsible on its own), and its concentration is not highly correlated with that of the active agent(s) or with the total activity in the mixture. For example, in attempting to evaluate the possible carcinogenicity of chlorination by-products in water, a number of epidemiological studies have used measurements of concentrations of particular trihalomethanes (e.g. chloroform) to indicate the exposure. However, the chemical(s) measured may not be the only potentially carcinogenic by-products of chlorination of water. High analytic sensitivity (the ability to detect low levels of exposure) is never a disadvantage, but there is little point, at least for epidemiological purposes, in pursuing it to concentrations of the agent much below those likely to produce epidemiologically detectable effects.

Whether or not measurements in the environment will be useful in practice also depends on their cost and the feasibility of their use on a large scale, as is commonly required in epidemiology. Neither cost nor logistic feasibility will usually present insurmountable difficulties if the number of measurements can be restricted to the range of hundreds rather than thousands or tens of thousands. This restriction may be achieved by limitation of the collection and analysis of environmental specimens to a sample of all subjects in the study for the purpose, for example, of validating some less expensive measure of exposure. Alternatively, if the cost of obtaining and storing the samples compares favourably with the cost of the analysis, one or more environmental specimens may be collected and preserved for each study subject while only a proportion are later analysed, or specimens from subgroups of subjects may be pooled so that the exposure of the subgroup can be characterized by measurements in the 'pool'. The application of these 'banking' and 'pooling' approaches has been discussed in Chapter 9.

Whatever the part of the environment to be studied, the exposure to be assessed, and the properties (chemical, physical, or biological) by which it is measured, several issues require detailed consideration. They include sampling of and measurements in present and past environments, and the use of records or questionnaires in place of actual measurements to estimate environmental exposures. These issues are considered below, mainly focusing, by way of example, on measurement of exposure to an airborne agent in the working environment. However, the principles outlined are general. They can be applied, with modification, to measurements of different kinds of agents in a variety of general, local, or personal environments. Several issues of quality control of measurements have been considered already, particularly in Chapters 5 and 9. Their specific application to measurements in the environment should be developed in collaboration with environmental hygienists, and will not be dealt with here.

Sampling and measuring present exposures

In epidemiology, measurements of present environmental exposures are made for two main purposes:

(a) to be used as such in prospective cohort studies aimed at relating present exposure to future disease occurrence

(b) to be entered as one element in the process of estimating past exposure within cross-sectional, retrospective cohort, or case–control studies.

In principle, use can be made in epidemiology of measurements of present exposure gathered for other purposes, such as measurements of workplace contaminants carried out for checking compliance with regulatory standards or monitoring process leakages, the effect of process changes, or the success of technical control measures. However, such measurements cannot usually be used to define the exposure of individual subjects. An *ad hoc* environmental survey is desirable, especially in a prospective cohort study. Even such a survey cannot possibly characterize *all* the environmental exposures of every member of a population, and it is necessary to determine how the scope of an environmental survey can be focused and restricted with respect to both the number of agents to be measured and the number of measurements to be made of each agent.

Selecting the exposures to be measured

Taking airborne agents in the workplace as an example, the first step is to make an inventory of all airborne agents present. It is not uncommon, in moderate-sized production plants (500 workers or so), for the total inventory to include 500–1000 chemicals (Corn 1981). A full inventory requires first the listing of all incoming materials, which is best undertaken by systematic review of the purchase records for the last 1–2 years. Sole reliance on data provided informally by key informants (managers, engineers, other staff) is best avoided, because important items may be missed. If records are not available then, at the very least, data from key informants should be elicited by means of a standard questionnaire. Next, a department-by-department review of the plant is made to list all the products, both intermediate and final, derived from the incoming materials. The exposures to be measured are then selected from the lists of incoming materials and their transformation products. In a less structured situation, for example when the environment to be measured is a water supply rather than workplace air and a complete inventory of chemical or biological inputs and transformation products cannot be prepared, a complete list of probable constituents and contaminants should still be prepared with reference to relevant empirical data and theory.

Which variables are selected for measurements depends critically on the objectives of the study being undertaken. For example, in a cohort study of lung cancer in relation to exposure to ceramic fibres, a decision would have to be made whether to limit the measurement to ceramic fibres, or to include established and suspected carcinogens for the human lung, which may also be present as potential confounders, and biologically plausible effect modifiers, should any be present. The selection of the agents to be measured may need to be more extensive if several endpoints are to be investigated, such as cancer at several sites, as each may call for measurement of some additional confounding variables.

Methods of environmental sampling

As the purpose of sampling is to measure the exposure of individuals, a sampling strategy, centred on individuals rather than on broad sections of a plant, for example, should be adopted. There are two broad approaches to sampling an environment:

(a) measurement at fixed points (static sampling) within the environment and inferring individual exposure from the concentration of contaminants measured in the parts of the environment covered by each sampler

(b) measurement of the immediate and continually changing environment of individual subjects by some form of personal sampling.

The latter is the preferred approach because it takes into account the subject's position in the environment, the concentrations of the environmental agent there, and behaviours which may modify exposure in particular circumstances (e.g. avoidance of sudden increases in emissions at particular points, use of protective devices, etc.)

In the case of sampling for airborne contaminants in the workplace, a personal sampler is worn by each worker whose environment is to be sampled. The sampler consists of a power source and a pump connected to an aspirating head containing, for example, a filter membrane onto which the substance to be tested is deposited. The aspirating head is placed anywhere within the breathing zone, i.e. a zone of air extending to 30 cm from the head of the subject. Unless the pump is of a self-correcting type, the flow of air is checked regularly during sampling periods extending over several hours, lest the quantity of air captured and filtered should vary and cause error in measurement of the concentration of the substance under study. Wearing a pump and a battery for hours may be considered a nuisance, and a high participation rate in measuring sessions may be difficult to maintain. 'Passive' samplers (Thain 1980), based on the diffusion or permeation of gases and vapours into some chemical trap, have been developed and used, for example, to measure the level of NO_2 as a component of traffic-related air pollution in relation to atopy in children (Krämer et al. 2000). Passive samplers minimize the weight and eliminate the noise of the sampler and can be worn for long periods, as may be necessary when the concentration of the substance to be measured is very low, which is not a rare circumstance for pollutants in the general environment. Passive samplers may not match the accuracy and precision of aspiration samplers, and may need to be compared and validated against the latter before actual field use.

The measurement of dietary intake of nutrients and other components of food by sampling and analysis of the diet provides a very different example of personal sampling. Three techniques may be used.

(a) In the *duplicate portion technique*, portions of all foods and beverages (except for water) identical to those consumed by the individuals are collected and analysed chemically.

(b) In the *aliquot sampling technique*, all foods and beverages (except for water) consumed by an individual during the survey period are weighed, and aliquot samples (e.g. one-tenth of all foods and beverages consumed) are collected daily for chemical analysis.

(c) In the *equivalent composition technique*, the weights of all foods and beverages (except for water) consumed by an individual are recorded during the whole survey period. Afterwards, a sample of raw foods equivalent to the foods eaten by the individual during the survey period is analysed chemically.

The highly intrusive nature of these methods may discourage participation and is likely to alter normal eating patterns. These problems, together with the cost of direct chemical analyses, limit the use of these methods to small-scale studies.

Selecting subjects for environmental sampling

At one extreme, measurement of the environment could entail continuous sampling of the environment of each subject throughout all periods of exposure relevant to the study. While in some circumstances this is comparatively simple (e.g. film-badge monitoring of exposure to ionizing radiation), in most cases it is neither practicable nor necessary. To make the measurements logistically and economically feasible and to ensure that quality is not sacrificed to quantity, sampling of both subjects and exposure time is usually undertaken.

Two main approaches have been used for the sampling of subjects in the workplace:

(a) random selection of subjects and then grouping those appearing to share common levels of exposure to the environmental agent (Woitowitz *et al.* 1970)

(b) pre-definition of strata presumptively homogenous with respect to the exposure and sampling randomly within the strata.

Measurements of environmental exposures in these samples are then used to estimate the exposure of *all* subjects in the classes into which the sampled subjects were grouped or from which they were taken. The first approach requires definitions of statistical criteria to separate *a posteriori* groups of measurements into classes, and it may result in very few measurements being available for classes at the low and high extremes of the exposure, which are more informative when relating exposure levels to biological effects. The second approach stands on the assumption that strata can be *a priori* identified, with exposure(s) levels relatively homogenous within strata while different between strata. These strata have been defined as 'exposure zones' (Corn and Esmen 1979; Corn 1985), and their definition is a valuable approach to the sampling of subjects for environmental measurements. In the analysis of exposure–disease relationships (linear or logistic regressions) individual measurements averaged within zones have been shown, using actual sets of data from a variety of occupational environments and simulation exercises (Tielemans *et al.*1998), to provide nearly unbiased estimates of the relative risk, while individual measurements produced appreciably attenuated estimates.

In the occupational environment, an exposure zone is defined with reference to knowledge of the production or other process, work tasks, sources of contaminants, and devices used for their removal. The procedure for selecting zones involves an examination of all processes, job classifications, material inventories, and ventilation and exhaust facilities in the plant. The definition of exposure zones should rely purely on these *a priori* criteria. Any measurements that may be available should not be used for definition of the zones because they will rarely, if ever, have been derived from a previous random sampling survey. For example, knowledge of high concentrations of a contaminant found at some of the few sites in a plant checked during a compliance control survey may lead to their grouping together to form a zone, removing them from the zones to which they would have been assigned on the basis of the *a priori* criteria used to classify all other sites. A zone can be, but it is not necessarily, a definable area or volume of the physical plant space that might be suitable for static sampling. Indeed, it is commonly found that a proportion of the workers in a given plant area belong to a zone which they share with a proportion of the workers in another area, for example workers undertaking the same tasks but on another production line which is differently located. Conversely, some workers sharing physical space may not belong to the same zone because of different tasks, and different positions with respect to sources of pollutants and exhaust and ventilation devices.

Each zone should meet four basic criteria (Corn 1981, 1985).

(a) *Work similarity*. Employees in the zone must perform similar tasks, so that similar mechanisms generating environmental contaminants exist.

(b) *Similarity with respect to hazardous agents*. Zone members must use the same agents (chemicals, heat, electricity), and the potential for exposure to the agents under investigation must be similar. Where multiple agents are present, the potential for exposure to all of them must be similar for all persons included in the zone.

(c) *Environmental similarity*. Process equipment and ventilation must be similar for all zone members.

(d) *Identifiability*. The same employee must not be classifiable to more than one zone. This requirement is important for the subsequent random selection of workers from a zone. Employees classified to a zone must be identifiable in company records as belonging to that zone by, for example, job title and plant department. It is not uncommon to find that in some departments there is no distinct job classification and all workers may be involved in the different phases of the operation on a non-specific schedule, i.e. while tasks can be distinguished, workers cannot be readily identified with them. In this situation, the number of different zones will be small, the heterogeneity of exposure within them potentially great, and error in individual measurement more likely.

Once employees have been preliminarily assigned to zones they are observed individually to see whether changes in zone assignments are needed.

The zoning process characterizes the work with respect to exposure in such a way that any person with any job title identified as belonging to a given zone can be expected to experience the exposure value representative of that zone. This marks the limit of the degree of individualization possible in the zoning approach. Such a limit reflects the trade-off between direct measurement of the environment of every exposed person and feasibility, cost, and the assurance of quality.

The definition of zones requires close cooperation with the industrial hygienist primarily responsible for making the measurements on workers, plant engineers, and other staff. It is also highly desirable that the epidemiologist who is going to use the exposure measurements in the analysis of health effects is present at some time during the assessment of exposure in zones to become familiar with the source of the exposure data and the errors which may affect it, such as biased selection of subjects, poor response rate among those selected, failure to follow instructions, etc.

The concepts of exposure zones and personal sampling, intuitively straightforward and developed for sampling the occupational environment, can be extended and adapted to sampling current exposure to a variety of agents in other parts of the environment. The essential elements for defining zones, prior to any measurements, are similarity of the subjects' activities, the hazards present and the environmental conditions, and unique identifiability, i.e. assignment of each subject to one zone only. These criteria can be readily applied when sampling indoor environments as well as some features of the general environment. For example, a proportional sampler can be used to sample tap water in the home (5 per cent of water flowing through the tap) so that measurements of the constituents of water can be made and related to individuals' or, at least, household consumption of water for different purposes. The households to be sampled would be selected according to 'zoning criteria'.

It may be problematic to employ the exposure zone approach when sampling the general environment over a relatively large area because only scanty information may be available to characterize a large non-captive population according to the zoning criteria. In these circumstances, a topographical approach to sampling may be of help (Gilbert 1987). In the case of general air pollution, for example, a grid would be superimposed on the area to be studied, and cells of the grid selected by simple random, multi-stage random, or stratified random sampling. It may be desirable, for example, to stratify by topographical orientation, dominant wind direction, and proximity to a particular point source of pollution, and more generally to ensure that a correct representation is obtained of the temporal and spatial distribution specific for each pollutant emanating from a source, for example atmospheric arsenic from coal burning in a power station (Colvile *et al* 2001). Systematic sampling may also be considered, as it is usually easier to implement under field conditions, although it may lead to substantial bias to the extent that the surveyed population is not randomly distributed in space. Within each cell selected for the sample, measurements would be carried out by choosing, at random, a number of subjects to wear personal samplers, or by use of fixed area samplers, or both. Other approaches may be used to define zones in the general environment. For example, with respect to contamination of water, zones may be defined by characteristics such as town area, socio-economic status, and features of housing, water supply, and plumbing, which may be readily ascertainable through a simple questionnaire.

Special sampling schemes have been suggested for cases in which, prior to any consideration of zones in the general environment, a pollution source or 'hot spot' must be located, for example buried waste or a point source contaminating a water distribution network (Gilbert 1987).

Extent of sampling

The extent of sampling within each exposure zone is defined in terms of the number of measurements to be made, the duration of collection (or size) of each sample, the period during which the measurements are taken, and the distribution of the measurements over this survey period. As the survey will extend over several days or weeks, the selection of zones for measurement, and of subjects within zones, should be random with respect to time.

The number of measurements often corresponds to the number of subjects whose environment is to be sampled, but may be larger if more than one measurement per subject is done. Subjects are chosen at random from all members of each exposure zone, their number being determined following different approaches. First, if the number of subjects in most zones happens to be small (say one or two), there may be no other sensible choice than to take all of them plus only a proportion, as practically convenient, of the subjects in the few zones with more individuals. Secondly, when the numbers of subjects in each zone permit, one may aim at achieving a predetermined level of precision, constant or variable from zone to zone, in the estimation of the average concentration of the substance of interest in each zone. In the case of airborne contaminants, a reasonable assumption is that the measurements will be lognormally distributed and, if no preliminary measurements are available, a geometric standard deviation between 2 and 3 can be assumed (Corn 1985) (the geometric or multiplicative standard deviation is the antilogarithm of the standard deviation of the logarithms of the measurements). Table 10.1, which has been derived by standard methods of sample size calculation (Mace 1964; Hale 1972), shows the approximate number of measurements required to estimate their median value or geometric mean (assuming a log-normal distribution) with a given precision, i.e. with a 90 per cent confidence interval of given width. Thus, for example, with 10–20 measurements (one per subject) in each zone, the true median will be included in an interval ranging from 50 to 150 per cent of the observed median in 90 per cent of the zones. A similar precision will be achieved for the estimate of the arithmetic mean (and taking 10–20 measurements will also give 90 per cent confidence that the sample range covers 75–80 per cent of the possible values of individual measurements in a zone).

While this criterion may be appropriate when the interest centres on the substance concentration itself, as may be the case for descriptive or control purposes, in an epidemiological context another approach aimed at obtaining an unbiased and as precise as possible estimate of the relative risk expressing the exposure–disease association is more relevant. Even the best methods of measurement are affected, at the very least, by some random error with respect to an ideal perfect method capable of providing 'true' values; hence the observable relative risk will be attenuated towards the null value 1, as described in Chapter 3. Tielemans *et al.* (1998) provide equations to evaluate different

Table 10.1 Approximate number of measurements required to estimate the median with given precision

90% confidence limits around the median (expressed as % of median)	Number of measurements	
	GSD[a] = 2	GSD = 3
±10%	145	360
±20%	40	100
±30%	20	50
±40%	15	30
±50%	10	20

[a] GSD, geometric standard deviation of individual measurements.

strategies of group-based exposure assessment to help guide the choice of number of measurements within each zone. Also, Equation 5.6 in Chapter 5, which gives the number of repeated measures needed to yield a given level of validity for the average measure, may provide some guidance. For this use of that equation, an estimate of the reliability coefficient within zone (rather than within person) would need to be assessed.

The duration of sampling is first determined by the need to obtain enough material for accurate analysis; this entails consideration of the probable concentration of the contaminant, the efficiency of its collection, and the sensitivity of the analytical method. Secondly, the nature of the biological effect expected and its relationship to onset of exposure and the amount of agent absorbed and retained in the body must be considered. The latter depends, in turn, on the airborne concentration of the substance, the time a given concentration is maintained, and the biological half-life of the agent. For irritants, asphyxiants, sensitizers, and allergenic agents, i.e. agents which produce rapid biological responses, short-term sampling of, say, 15 minutes or less may be used. In general, the sampling time should be in proportion to the biological half-life of the substance. It has been proposed (Roach 1966) that an optimum duration is about one-tenth of the half-life. This turns out to be neither so short as to miss fluctuations in airborne concentration capable of being reflected in important variations in body burden, nor so long as to dampen and mask such variations. When the objective is to study late effects of exposures, such as pneumoconiosis or cancer, sampling over a full working shift (8 hours) is usually adopted, as variations in exposure which may occur within this interval are regarded as being of negligible relevance.

The choice of the period of the year in which to perform the measurements must take into account the fact that concentrations of environmental agents may vary not only within a day (e.g. between shifts) but also from season to season. While the variability from hour to hour and between shifts can be accommodated in a single survey lasting from several days to a few weeks, documentation of seasonal or yearly variation may necessitate repetition of the survey. If resources are limited it is better to target the survey on periods when the highest concentrations can be found (e.g. winter, when there is less ventilation of the workplace, in the case of an airborne contaminant). Repetition might then be limited to sub-samples, to ascertain the stability or variability of the concentration established in the survey.

The exact programme of sampling adopted depends on the objectives and type of the epidemiological study proposed. For any kind of study of a disease or other biological effect with a short induction period (i.e. a short interval from commencement of exposure to onset of the effect) it is desirable to sample close in time to the period during which occurrence of the effect is being determined. In the case of a prospective cohort study, or a case–control study within a cohort study, repetition of sampling at intervals within the period over which cases are determined is desirable. The frequency of repetition should be determined by the length of the induction period and the day-to-day, week-to-week, or month-to-month variability of the exposure. At one extreme, if the induction period is very short (e.g. of the order of a few hours), variability is high, and there is little discrimination between exposure zones, useful measurements may only be obtained by very frequent sampling. At the other extreme, if the exposure varies little with time or there are substantial and stable differences in level of exposure between zones, a single survey of exposure may suffice.

For cohort studies of an effect with a long interval (years or decades) between first exposure and effect (like most cancers), an initial complete survey should be supplemented by at least partial repetition periodically over the period of follow-up.

Analytical aspects

Repetition of a survey means that the collection of specimens and the analytical procedures are carried out at intervals of months or years. To ensure uniformity of the whole measurement process, strict attention to quality control is essential. At the very least, this requires that all procedures are carried out according to a written protocol and that reference samples are included in all batches of analyses. When measurements are done at different laboratories, there is a need for inter-laboratory, as well as intra-laboratory, comparisons to monitor and maintain accuracy and precision within fixed limits.

Some methods of measurement involve substantial subjectivity and analyst fatigue, for example, counting fibres by optical microscopy, for which the advice is that no operator should do more than six counts a day. These methods may have coefficients of variation for repeated measurements of the same sample of 20 per cent or more (Rajhans and Sullivan 1981). For chemical methods, substantially lower coefficients, below 10 per cent and down to 2–3 per cent or less, may be found (Horwitz 1977). However, beside the analytical errors, a variability between parallel replicates of some 5 per cent, for example in obtaining an air sample by pump and filter, has to be taken into account. This brings the total error (coefficient of variation) for repeated measurements of the same part of the environment to near 10 per cent. Further non-negligible variability is introduced if several different laboratories are used.

Whereas the size of the total error and its components are of direct interest to the epidemiologist who is going to use the environmental measurements, technical aspects relevant to its minimization are the province of the environmental hygienist and the analyst.

These aspects include choice of equipment and procedures for collecting, handling, and storing specimens (by definition, if an agent is present in the environment it has the potential for contaminating containers, equipment, hands, and clothes), analytical methods, and quality control procedures.

A point worth noting is that, depending on the concentration of the agent to be measured and the concurrent presence of other agents, different methods of measurement may need to be used, even for the same medium (e.g. air or water). For example, the number of fibres >5 μm long counted on membrane filters by phase contrast microscopy has been in use as a measure of exposure to asbestos in the occupational environment (Rajhans and Sullivan 1981), although these fibres form only a small proportion of the total number of fibres present and the method is not specific for asbestos fibres. This lack of sensitivity and specificity has not represented a measurement problem at the level of contamination subject to control in occupational environments where asbestos has been the predominant fibre present. However, measurements in the general environment are complicated by the low concentration of asbestos and the predominance of other mineral particulates. Under these circumstances it has proved necessary to resort to examination of the sampled material by electron microscopy which permits both sensitive and specific identification of asbestos fibres at the level found in urban air, although it produces measurements that are not directly comparable with those derived by optical microscopy from the higher concentrations present in the occupational environment (Dupré *et al.* 1984; Nicholson 1989).

The specific sampling strategies and analytical methods for different agents in different environments will be chosen, in the context and for the purposes of an epidemiological study, by the environmental hygienist.

Sampling and measuring past exposures

Measurements of present exposure to agents in the environment are applicable to cross-sectional, case–control, and retrospective cohort studies only when it can be reasonably assumed that measurements of concentrations of agents in the present environment are highly correlated with the concentration as present at aetiologically relevant periods in the recent or remote past. As an alternative to making this often unrealistic assumption, records of past measurements of relevant exposures may be sought. These can be used, alone or in combination with results from surveys of present exposures, to infer 'best estimates' of past exposure for each subject in an epidemiological study.

While usually useful to some degree, the records and the measurements they document are frequently far less than ideal for epidemiological purposes. Therefore their use requires the utmost care.

The reconstruction of measurements of past exposure in the environment can be conveniently divided according to whether past records are complete, incomplete, or unavailable. The epidemiologist is confronted today, and will continue to be confronted in the future, with all three situations, as it is practically impossible to adequately monitor *all* agents present in the environment, including those which may one day turn out to be worthy of epidemiological investigation.

Complete past measurements

When a complete set of measurements in exposure zones or similar strata are available, carried out in the past for epidemiological purposes by methods still judged as acceptable, they are as good as measurements obtained in contemporary surveys. However, the position is different when the measurements were collected for purposes other than an epidemiological investigation. Commonly, the measurements available were collected to check compliance with regulatory standards. Care is required in the use of such data. It is important to ascertain the purpose of the measurements and the frame within which they were collected, as these two factors determine the way in which the samples were selected and the way they reflect the pattern of exposure of the study subjects. For example, compliance may have been monitored by measurement of some readily measurable substance, which may have represented only a fraction (e.g. the water-soluble part) of the mixture of interest. Compliance control may also have concentrated on measurements in 'maximum risk employees', i.e. the employees judged to have had the highest potential for exposure at a given time. Attributing their levels of exposure to everyone would be likely to introduce substantial errors.

Incomplete past measurements

Past measurements may be incomplete because they were made only in selected exposure zones, or by methods that are sub-optimal according to present-day knowledge, or they were only some correlate of the exposure of interest (e.g. total dust concentration when only the concentration of mineral fibres is of interest).

In principle, incomplete past measurements may be used in the same way as complete past measurements or present measurements to reconstruct past exposure to environmental agents. Detailed estimates are made of the exposure levels in each exposure zone, or like stratum, at a single point or at different points in time in the past. Individual subjects are then assigned to zones in the usual way, i.e. in the case of an occupational exposure by matching job histories (by job titles and plant department) to jobs and areas included in a zone.

This approach was adopted by Stewart *et al.*(1986) to estimate past exposure to formaldehyde in a retrospective cohort study of the mortality of approximately 30 000 workers employed by 10 companies. The procedure consisted of estimating the concentration of formaldehyde in inhaled air in each exposure zone as belonging to one of six 8-hour time-weighted average levels:

- *trace* (it was assumed that regardless of where a person worked in a formaldehyde plant, his/her exposure would be greater than that of a person not working in such plant)
- *<0.1 ppm* (e.g. an employee who occasionally went into the production area)
- *0.1–0.5 ppm* (odour occasionally noticeable in each 8-hour day)
- *0.5–2.0 ppm* (odour consistently present throughout the 8-hour day)
- *>2.0 ppm* (eye irritation or lacrimation and odour occurring throughout the 8-hour day)
- unknown.

These categories were developed before the estimation process was carried out.

The estimation process involved several steps. First, personnel records were abstracted to list, standardize, and aggregate the job titles held by cohort members and the areas in which they worked (the components of allocation to exposure zones). Next, other plants were walked through to gather historical and current production, control, and air-monitoring data. From these data a matrix of exposures by job and time was developed, which took detailed account of the tasks performed within each job at each time and the effects of engineering controls and production or process changes. Exposure estimates made by industrial hygienists belonging to the plant were then reviewed, and the present-day operation monitored to a total of about 2000 measurements of formaldehyde concentrations in air.

In addition to supplementing historical monitoring data, this procedure allowed standardization of measurements across the different plants. Finally, the information from these sources was integrated to produce the estimates of historical exposure levels by job and area used for the study. These estimates fully characterized past exposures at particular points in time, and were matched to the workers' job history files to provide individual estimates of exposure.

A more general approach to the estimation of past exposure was proposed by Esmen (1979). In essence, he broke down each job or occupational title into component elementary tasks called 'uniform tasks' which, unlike job titles, applied to the whole of an industry in a relatively uniform way, independently of plant. A set of uniform task units, adaptable to several kinds of production industries, is shown in Table 10.2. The major objective of this breakdown was the reduction of variability in exposure within these units.

Estimates of exposure levels were then made for each uniform task category at appropriate times in the past. If only current measurements were available, possibly supplemented by a few measurements in the past, they were extrapolated back, correcting for four factors:

◆ changes in the process
◆ changes in the physical characteristics of the agent
◆ periodic use of personal protective devices
◆ rate of output of the product.

If, instead, there were only current measurements for the agent of primary interest, but current and past data existed for some other agent, the two sets of current measurements were correlated, always within uniform task units, to permit estimation of past exposure to the agent of primary interest. Once estimates of exposure had been made for the uniform tasks, exposures for each job in each plant were estimated as weighted averages of exposure levels in uniform tasks, with the time each task contributed to a job used as its weight.

The work of both Stewart et al. (1986) and Esmen (1979) indicates that estimation of levels of exposure, whether in exposure zones or similar strata, is a painstaking endeavour, requiring a combination of search of documents, interviews with key informants, inspection of plants, and current measurements. The person-time required to make the exposure estimates for the study by Stewart et al.(1986) is summarized in Table 10.3 and gives an idea of the amount of work involved. It is a safe general rule that a feasibility investigation should be carried out as a first step to find out what type of information can be obtained at what cost, and what this may yield in terms of validity and precision of risk estimates.

Estimation of past exposures is apparently simpler when a set of measurements is available which is incomplete only in that it was obtained by methods different from those now regarded as acceptable or optimum. In principle, the establishment of some form of equivalence between measurements taken with different methods is all that is required. However, that objective may prove to be difficult to achieve.

Table 10.2 Uniform task categories in which separate estimates of exposure can be made[a]

Making A
Tasks which involve direct contact with the agent or precursors of the agent in operations that 'make' or 'get' the product, i.e. direct mining, mixing ingredients, loading raw material to processor

Making B
Tasks which involve direct contact with the agent or precursors of the agent in operations that 'make' or 'get' the product, e.g. indirect mining, joy loader operating, controlling mixers, kettles, or process ovens

Production A
Tasks which involve direct contact with the agent as the material is produced to be formed by a manufacturing process or formed to be shipped as is, e.g. moulding operations, process helping, mill operations, and process machine operations

Production B
Tasks which involve direct or indirect contact with the agent through the manufacture of a finished product from the material containing the agent by the use of cutting or abrasive tools, e.g. trimming, sawing, weaving, and sending operations

Production C
Tasks which involve direct or indirect contact with the agent through the manufacture of a finished product from the material containing the agent using heated tools, e.g. welding, hot joining, soldering, heat treating, and drying operations

Production D
Tasks which involve general manufacturing operations where exposure to the agent is less likely than in tasks A, B or C, e.g. painting finished product, handling packaged material, packaging finished product (foremen and floor supervisors).

Clean up A
Tasks which involve general cleaning of non-production areas

Clean up B
Tasks which involve cleaning production machinery and production areas, e.g. sweeping floor in production areas, cleaning particulate control devices

Maintenance
Tasks which involve the repair and upkeep of production machinery

Quality control
Tasks which involve sampling the product and performing tests to ascertain product quality

Shipping
Tasks which involve transportation of packaged material, forklift truck operations, and shipping yard operations

Isolated tasks
Tasks which are isolated from production areas and do not involve contact with the agent except for general plant exposure, e.g. boiler operations, tool crib, and shipping yard supervision

---

[a] From Esmen (1979).

Table 10.3 Time taken to estimate exposure to formaldehyde from an incomplete set of past exposure measurements in a cohort of approximately 30 000 workers employed by 10 companies[a]

Activity	Participants	Time (person-months)
Abstracting 30 000 personnel records	Abstracting team	45
Development of protocol and form	Industrial hygienists	5
Standardization of job titles	Industrial hygienists	9
Walk-throughs	Industrial hygienists	3
Estimation of exposures	Industrial hygienists	15
Monitoring	Industrial hygienists	9
Review of jobs	Company personnel	7
Integration to make final estimates	Industrial hygienists	2

[a] From Stewart *et al.* (1986).

Measurements of exposure to asbestos (Doll and Peto 1985) illustrate the difficulty of establishing equivalence of measurement methods. Table 10.4 shows the main changes which took place in the methods of measuring asbestos dust in one British asbestos textile factory over a 30-year period. They reflect the evolution of measurement technology over that period. There were several changes in the approach to measurement, instrumentation, and sensor devices, and in different periods different components of the dust were measured. In addition, personal sampling gradually replaced area sampling after 1975, thus introducing a further difference. That the measurements obtained with different techniques are not directly comparable is obvious, but is it possible to find valid factors for conversion from one method to another? The key conversion is from measurements in the form of particles per unit volume made by the older particle counting methods (the midget impinger, used in North America, and the thermal precipitator used, for example, in the UK) to measurements in terms of 'regulated' fibres (i.e. particles longer than 5 μm and with a length-to-diameter ratio of at least 3) counted by optical microscopy. Unfortunately, no simple conversion is possible. Fibre counts ranging from 3 per cent to more than 50 per cent of the particle counts have been obtained in different processes (mining and milling and manufacture of textiles, friction materials, and asbestos cement) and a similar range of variation has been found among areas within a single plant. No comparable measurements of particles and fibres are available at all for exposure during the use of asbestos insulation. Moreover, when measurements have been made simultaneously by different methods in the same environment, the correlations

Table 10.4 Methods used to measure asbestos dust concentrations in a British asbestos textile factory in different time periods [a]

Period	Instrument	Method of evaluation	Object measured	Unit [b]
1951–1960	Casella thermal precipitator (CTP)	Incinerated × 1000 dark field	Particles (including fibres)	particles/ml
1961–1964	Ottway long-running thermal precipitator (LRTP)	Not incinerated × 500 dark field	Fibres >5 μm long Length:diameter ratio >3:1	f/ml
1965–1974	Membrane filter sampler	× 500 phase contrast, full field	Fibres >5 μm long Length:diameter ratio >3:1	f/ml
	or			
	Royco automatic particle counter (RPC)	Automatic	Fibres >5 μm long Length:diameter ratio >3:1	f/ml
1975 and later	Membrane filter sampler	× 600 phase contrast, graticule grid count	Fibres >5 μm long Length:diameter ratio >3:1	f/ml

[a] From Doll and Peto (1985).

[b] Particles counted down to a diameter of 0.5 μm; 35 particles/ml is equivalent to 1 million particles/cubic foot (mppcf); f/ml, fibres (as defined by regulations) per millilitre.

obtained have invariably been weak (correlation coefficients of 0.3–0.6), and the relationship between particles and regulated fibres has not always been linear on an arithmetic scale.

The difficulty in finding a valid conversion factor is clearly shown by data from the Quebec mines and mills, where a large series of parallel measurements of particles counted by the midget impinger and fibres collected on membrane filters and counted by use of an optical microscope are available. A logarithmic transformation of both sets of measurements was chosen and a linear relationship sought between them. Estimates of the arithmetic conversion factor were derived from the regression line. Three selected values corresponding to typical counts (0.1, 1 and 10 million particles per cubic foot) are shown in Table 10.5.

As expected from a linear relationship, on a log–log scale the arithmetic conversion factor systematically decreases with increasing values of particle concentrations. Also, the arithmetic 95 per cent confidence intervals about the conversion factors were very wide because of the large scatter of the points from which the regression line was calculated.

Table 10.5 Values of multiplying factor to convert measurements of asbestos particle concentrations into asbestos fibre concentrations (f/ml)[a]

Particle concentration (mppcf)[b]	Multiplying factor to convert to f/ml	95% confidence interval about factor
0.1	23	1.2–116
1.0	11	0.6–58
10.0	5	0.3–27

[a] From Dagbert (1976).

[b] mppcf, millions of particles per cubic foot.

The regression line summarized in Table 10.5 can be regarded as correctly predicting the fibre concentrations from the particle concentrations under the conditions in which this limited series of parallel measurements was obtained. However, the very reason for deriving a conversion factor is to use it outside these strict circumstances, and this requires estimating a regression line corrected for the biasing effect or the measurement error in the 'independent' variable (particle concentration). This error has the effect of flattening the slope and increasing the intercept, with the consequence that at low concentrations the fibre concentrations would be overestimated from the particle concentrations, while at high concentrations they would be underestimated. One possible way of correcting for this bias is to force the regression line through the origin. If, in addition, a logarithmic model is not assumed, and instead the assumption is made that the variance of the estimated fibre counts increases in proportion to the values of the particle counts on an arithmetic scale, the estimator of the regression coefficient reduces to the simple ratio of the two mean values (Snedecor and Cochran 1980). This estimator, which is relatively insensitive to large random errors and outliers, has been used (Doll and Peto 1985) to derive a single conversion factor from a series of British measurements made with the Casella thermal precipitator (particles) and a membrane filter and optical microscopy (fibres). The value of the factor turned out to be 35.

Equivalence approaches, which use single conversion factors or regression equations, are virtually unavoidable if maximum use of available exposure measurements, obtained with different methods and under different conditions, is to be made for quantitative risk assessment. However, it is clear that they are subject to substantial error. Similar approaches are used when one agent is measured as a surrogate for another or for a mixture.

A particular case is the use of routinely collected measurements of variable degree of completeness, for instance measurements of air pollutants in the outdoor environment as recorded in fixed monitoring stations; these have been used as surrogates for individual exposures in epidemiological studies relating exposure differences between areas (Dockery *et al* 1993) or between days (Zanobetti *et al* 2003) to mortality.

No past measurements

When no past measurements of the environment are available, any characterization of subjects according to their likely past exposure to environmental contaminants will of necessity be crude and at the level of broad groups of subjects rather than individuals. A simple solution, often adopted in retrospective cohort studies of occupational exposures, is to group subjects according to their dates of first employment or, better, first exposure after employment (the two do not necessarily coincide). This calendar classification should reflect trends in exposure levels: decreasing because of new exposure being added to the environment, or, perhaps, increasing because of new exposures being added to the environment or more activity being carried out within the same factory area. The dates defining different levels of exposure can be selected according to whatever knowledge is available on secular trends affecting the exposure of interest. The more extensive and specific this information, the more detailed will be the chronological criterion.

This approach can be illustrated from a retrospective cohort study of workers in the synthetic mineral fibre industry in 13 production plants located in seven European countries (Saracci *et al*. 1984). Once it became clear that the data obtained in an *ad hoc* survey of present concentrations of airborne fibres (Cherrie *et al*. 1986) were not representative of past conditions, a reconstruction of past exposure was attempted (Dodgson *et al*. 1987). Since no past measurement was available, information about the technical history of each factory was obtained by means of self-administered questionnaire first introduced at a meeting with staff of the plant, completed by the staff, and then discussed at an interview with the research team. Great care was taken with the design of the questionnaire so that experienced plant managers could provide the best possible information on factors likely to affect exposure to fibres or other potential risk factors. Table 10.6 lists the major factors relevant to changes in fibre concentrations in the air. Reduction in nominal fibre size (i.e. length-weighted average fibre diameter in the bulk product) could produce an increase in emission of respirable fibres by up to a factor of 10. On the other hand, addition of oil to the fibrous material reduced the concentration of airborne fibres by a factor of about 10, by causing them to form larger conglomerates which are non-respirable and settle rapidly. Change from a discontinuous manually intensive process to a continuous process was also

Table 10.6 Factors considered to influence airborne fibre concentrations when estimating airborne fibre concentrations of synthetic mineral fibres in 13 plants in Europe for which no past measurements were available[a]

◆ Fibre size in the bulk product

◆ Binder and oil content

◆ Type of process

◆ Size of building

◆ Production rate

◆ Ventilation

◆ Use of respirators

◆ Cleaning of workplace

◆ Secondary production processes

[a] From Dodgson *et al.* (1987).

judged to reduce dust levels, by a factor of somewhat less than 10. Each of the other listed factors, some of which are interrelated (size of factory building, production rate, and ventilation), were judged not to contribute more than twofold variation to concentrations.

By use of this information on the presence and probable size of the effects of the main factor affecting fibre concentrations, it was possible to subdivide the production history of *each* plant into three technological phases:

(a) *early phase*, when a discontinuous production system was in use and/or no oil was added to the fibres during production

(b) *late phase* when continuous modern techniques were used to manufacture the fibres and oil was added

(c) *intermediate phase* in which a mixture of these techniques operated.

Critical dates were established separately for each of the 13 plants so that workers could be classified and grouped according to the phase in which they were first employed. Although seemingly crude, this classification was employed to relate exposure to health outcomes (Simonato *et al.* 1987), and was regarded as being able to rank workers according to their exposure to fibres more accurately than the much more refined, but much less relevant, measurements of airborne fibres under present-day conditions. A small-scale simulation experiment of an early production process was also performed to gauge the airborne fibre concentrations more directly (Cherrie *et al.* 1987). This experiment provided data broadly supportive of the ranking classification. In some of the same plants a further study was later conducted to reconstruct past exposure to fibres, as well as to other agents present in the working environment, at the level of the individual worker (lung cancer cases and control workers were studied). The reconstruction method, which may be of use in general when no past measurements are available, used descriptive information on jobs and processes in a structured subjective assessment based on a model of the exposure situation (Cherrie *et al* 1996; Cherrie and Schneider 1999). It involved four steps, two of which ((b) and (c)) are the core of the method.

(a) Expert panels formed at each plant by foremen and experienced workers reconstructed the work history of each worker in the study with information on job titles, dates of employment, work areas, and tasks.

(b) The panels, assisted by local industrial hygienists, characterized the different job titles in different periods using a standard form to identify details about how tasks within jobs were carried out, which materials were used and how they were handled, the local environment, and pollutants.

(c) For each plant, task, and period the information so collected was independently used by three industrial hygienists (trained blindly on scenarios in which the actual levels of fibre concentrations were known) to estimate exposure levels to each task and, taking a time-weighted summation over the tasks, to each job in each time period within each plant.

(d) The job estimates of the three hygienists were averaged and could then be used jointly with the information on job history in (a) to characterize the exposure of each individual over time.

Use of conversion tables with data derived from questionnaires

In the absence of actual measurement of the concentration of agents in the present or past environments, an attempt may be made to quantitate exposure by the use of conversion tables constructed from data bases external to the population under study and linked to data derived from records or questionnaires.

Some points on the use of conversion tables can be illustrated with reference to 'job-exposure' matrices used in studies of occupational epidemiology, and food tables used in studies of nutritional epidemiology.

The term *job-exposure matrix* has been loosely used to cover any method for converting job titles into exposures. More precisely and restrictively, an *a priori* job-exposure matrix (JEM) is a generic instrument (hence also the label of 'generic JEM') prepared prior to or separately from any data collection for the study in which it is used, and consisting of a typical two-entry conversion table with job classification along one axis, a list of potential exposures along the other axis, and an indication in the cells of the matrix of whether the particular exposure occurs or occurred in the particular job. Thus knowledge of the occupations of subjects allows an automatic coding of their possible exposures. The exposure classifications for each job all build on what is generally known about exposures associated with particular tasks in particular industries in particular time periods. This approach is necessarily limited by the fact that, even within narrowly defined occupational groups, exposure may vary from worker to worker according to their specific tasks, from country to country, from plant to plant, and from period to period. Exposures are assigned at the group level, i.e. at the level of occupation, industry, or a combination of the two, without reference to the particular exposure circumstances of individual workers. The *a priori* JEM could be particularly useful when only minimal information on occupation is available to the epidemiologist, although its use in these circumstances makes it correspondingly prone to error. In fact the performance of generic JEM has not lived up to the hopes placed initially in this method; for example, it was found (Siemiatycki 1996) that, for 160 substances, comparing the exposure derived from the JEM with exposure as assessed by experts, taken as the gold standard, the mean sensitivity of the JEM was 57% and the mean specificity 95%. Some performance improvement may ensue if the matrix does not simply declare an exposure present or absent for a given job but if it roughly specifies the probability of its occurrence (present/likely/unlikely/absent) for the job in a particular period of time.

A related but different and better performing method of assigning exposure is the subject-by-subject approach (sometimes, and confusingly, called the *a posteriori* matrix approach) involving the examination of each subject's work history by a team of trained experts who use their expertise and other sources of information to infer the exposures for each subject (Gérin *et al.* 1985). This approach is similar to what we have described above for reconstruction of exposures in workplaces when past measurements are incomplete or absent. However, here it is applied to individual workers in different industries rather than groups of workers in one industry. In fact both the subject-by-subject method and the *a priori* JEM have been developed mainly for reconstructing past exposures in case–control studies.

Food composition tables have been in use for many decades. In essence, they are two-entry conversion tables with food items on one axis, nutrients on the other axis, and the amounts of given nutrients per unit weight of each food item in the cells of the table. The tables are used to convert estimates of amounts of food items eaten by a subject during a specified time into estimates of intake of water, nutrients, and nutrient-derived energy. They are based on analyses of samples of foods obtained in particular countries at particular times, but are commonly applied to the equivalent foods eaten in other countries and at other times.

There are number of problems in the use of food tables. First, they rarely cover exactly the same list of food items as the dietary questionnaire, and so some pooling and averaging of the values from different foods may be needed. This process increases the measurement error for the subjects under study (i.e. reduces the degree of individualization of the measurements of nutrients) and reduces the power of the study to detect differences between groups.

A second important approximation in the use of food tables derives from the way the nutrient concentrations are estimated. The concentrations are derived from either review of the literature on composition of foods or *ad hoc* analyses. The tables available today are compiled from a mixture of these two sources. Unfortunately, one food item may vary substantially in its chemical composition. For example, composition may depend on the geographical origin (soil conditions, climate, fertilizer, method of husbandry and slaughter, etc.), the sampling procedure (time of collection, whether the sample was fresh, frozen, raw, cooked, etc.), and the treatment of samples before analysis (Paul and Southgate 1988). Composition may also change over time, making periodical revision necessary. The variability in nutrient composition of one food item is inadequately captured by the fixed conversion values of the table.

A third problem with food tables is lack of standardization of their methods of analysis and expression of concentrations of nutrients. For example, concentrations of nutrients may be expressed per unit weight of 'food as purchased', 'edible matter', or 'dry matter'. This lack of standardization can lead to both incorrect application of the tables (e.g. estimation of intake based on 'edible' quantities of food when the table refers to food 'as purchased') and artefactual differences in the results of studies based on different food tables. A further source of variability between food tables results from the factors used to convert nitrogen into protein, when nitrogen content of an item has been determined to estimate protein content, and to convert carbohydrate, fats, and proteins into energy values.

Even though they are affected by a number of limitations ('Anyone, who uses a table of food composition as an oracle is misleading himself' (Paul and Southgate (1978)), food tables are employed as an almost universal tool in studies of nutritional epidemiology. The tables to be used should be examined with the same detailed and critical attention as would be given to methods of direct chemical determination for which they are substitutes; numerous particularly delicate problems arise in epidemiological studies involving different countries as no internationally standardized food tables are yet available even within an area like Western Europe (Deharveng *et al* 1999).

With reference to the use of conversion tables, Kaldor (1991) noted that whereas the exposure variables measured directly in a study may be crude, they have the advantage that they can be interpreted unambiguously. They are independent of the conversion table, and do not contain the additional error arising from use of the tables which, in some cases, could overwhelm the reduction in error obtainable through more specific identification of the exposure of interest. Thus analyses, based on derived variables (e.g. nutrients) should not be carried out to the exclusion of analyses based on the measured variables (e.g. foods or food groups). This may be of particular importance in exploratory studies aimed at finding aetiological clues.

Summary

Components of the external environment which may be measured include physical, chemical, and biological constituents or contaminants of soil, air, water, food, drinks, cosmetics, and drugs occurring specifically in homes, workplaces, or recreational sites, or in the general environment. The exposed individual may not sense these exposures, or even be aware of their existence, and in these circumstances the exposures can only be documented by measurements in the environment.

Objectivity and individualization of measurements in the environment are best achieved by personal sampling and measuring devices. Most often, however, reliance must be placed on sampled collected over relatively short periods of time, following subjective advice from the person exposed on where to sample, and analysed by methods which are not fully automated. The result may be substantial error in the measurement of exposure.

The sensitivity of environmental measurements can be very high when modern methods are used, and this is never a disadvantage. However, for epidemiological purposes, there is a little point in pushing it to concentrations of the agent much below those likely to produce epidemiologically detectable effects. The specificity characteristics of an environmental measurement may be more difficult to determine. For example, where the biologically relevant exposure is a complex mixture, it may be more appropriate to base measurements on a biologically relevant characteristic of the whole mixture than to measure a specific chemical.

The measurement of present exposures and the reconstruction of past exposures require quite different approaches. Sampling strategies for current exposures have to take into account the nature of exposure and its expected effect, whether immediate or delayed in time. The extent of sampling in space and time must also be determined and requires knowledge, not often available in adequate detail, of exposure variability, for example between and within groups of workers exposed to a pollutant in a working environment.

Actual measurements taken in the past may occasionally be available for measurement of past exposure. These measurements will usually have been taken for purposes other than an epidemiological study, typically environment control, and may not be representative of the actual distribution of the exposure. Most often, few or no past measurements will be available for the reconstruction of past exposure.

Substantial experience has been gained in recent years in the reconstruction of past occupational exposures. Job titles, as they appear in work histories, are broken down into elementary task components. An estimate is made, for each of these components, of exposure levels at appropriate times in the past by use of whatever measurements are available and knowledge of factors likely to have affected exposure, such as the production processes in use, the physical characteristics of the agent, use of protective devices, etc.

When some past measurements are available, it may be necessary to convert measurements obtained by one method to estimates of those that would have been obtained by another, usually more recent and more accurate, method. The 'conversion factors' used may be subject to substantial uncertainty.

When no direct measurements are feasible for either past or present environments, an attempt may be made to measure exposure by use of conversion tables, such as job-exposure matrices and food tables linked to data derived from records or questionnaires. However, additional error may be introduced because of the errors inherent in the conversion tables themselves.

References

Cherrie, J. and Schneider,T. (1999).Validation of a new method for structured subjective assessment of past concentrations. *Annals of Occupational Hygiene*, **43**, 235–45.

Cherrie, J., Dodgson, J., Groat, S., and McLaren, W. (1986). Environmental surveys in the European man-made fiber production industry. *Scandinavian Journal of Work Environment and Health*, **12** (Suppl.1), 18–25.

Cherrie, J., Krantz, S., Schneider, T., Öhbert, I., Kamstrup, O., and Linander, W., (1987). An experimental simulation of an early rock wool/slag wool production process. *Annals of Occupational Hygiene*, **31**, 583–93.

Cherrie, J., Schneider, T., Spankie, S., and Quinn, M. (1996). A new method for structured, subjective assessment of past concentrations. *Occupational Hygiene*, **3**, 75–83.

Colvile, R.N., Stevens, E.S., Keegan,T., and Nieuwenhuijsen, M.J. (2001). Atmospheric dispersion modelling for assessment of exposure to arsenic in the Nitra Valley, Slovakia. *Journal of Geophysical Research: Atmospheres*, **106**, 17421–32.

Corn, M. (1981). Strategies of air sampling. In *Recent Advances in Occupational Health*, Vol. 1 (ed. J.C. McDonald), pp. 199–210. Churchill Livingstone, Edinburgh.

Corn, M. (1985). Strategies of air sampling. *Scandinavian Journal of Work Environment and Health*, **11**, 173–80.

Corn, M. and Esmen, N.A. (1979). Workplace exposure zones for classification of employee exposures to physical and chemical agents. *American Industrial Hygiene Association Journal*, **40**, 47–57.

Dagbert, M. (1976). *Études de Correlation de Mesures d'Empoussierage dans l'Industrie de l'amiante, Document 5 (Beaudry Report)*. Québec Comité d'étude sur la Salubrité dans l'Industrie de l'Amiante, Montreal.

Deharveng, G., Charrondière,U.R., Slimani, N., Southgate, D.A.T., and Riboli, E.(1999). Comparison of nutrients in the food composition tables available in the nine European countries participating in EPIC. *European Journal of Clinical Nutrition*, **53**, 60–79.

Dockery, D.W., Pope, A., III, Xu, X., *et al.* (1993) An association between air pollution and mortality in six US cities. *New England Journal of Medicine*, **329**, 1753–9.

Dodgson, J., Cherrie, J., and Groat, S. (1987). Estimates of past exposure to respirable man-made mineral fibres in the European insulation wool industry. *Annals of Occupational Hygiene*, **31**, 567–82.

Doll, R. and Peto, J. (1985). *Asbestos: Effects on Health of Exposure to Asbestos*, pp. 19–22. HMSO, London.

Dupré, J.C., Mustard, J.F., Uffen, R.J., Dewees, D.N., Laskin, J.I., and Kahn, L.B. (1984). *Report of the Royal Commission on Matters of Health and Safety Arising from the Use of Asbestos in Ontario*, Vol. 2, pp. 659–70. Ontario Ministry of the Attorney General, Toronto.

Esmen, N. (1979). Retrospective industrial hygiene surveys. *American Industrial Hygiene Association Journal*, **40**, 58–65.

Gérin, M., Semiatycki, J., Kemper, H., and Bégin, D. (1985). Obtaining occupational exposure histories in epidemiological case–control studies. *Journal of Occupational Medicine*, **27**, 420–6.

Gilbert, R.O. (1987). *Statistical Methods for Environmental Pollution Monitoring*. Van Nostrand Reinhold, New York.

Hale, W.E. (1972). Sample size determination for the log-normal distribution. *Atmospheric Environment*, **6**, 419–22.

Horwitz, W. (1977). The variability of AOAC methods of analysis as used in analytical pharmaceutical chemistry. *Journal of the Association of Official Analytical Chemists*, **60**, 1355–63.

Kaldor, J.M. (1991). Modeling complex exposure histories in epidemiological studies. In *Statistical Models for Longitudinal Studies of Health* (ed. J.H. Dwyer, M. Feinleib, P. Lippert, and H. Hoffmeister), pp. 332–48. Oxford University Press, New York.

Krämer, U., Koch, T., Ranft, U., Ring, J., and Berhendt, H. (2000).Traffic-related air pollution is associated with atopy in children living in urban areas. *Epidemiology*, **11**, 64–70.

Mace, A.E, (1964). *Sample-size Determination*, pp. 35–37, 69–70. Reinhold, New York.

Nicholson, W.J. (1989). Airborne mineral fibre levels in the non-occupational environment. In *Non-occupational Exposure to Mineral Fibres* (ed. J. Bignon, J. Peto, and R. Saracci), IARC Scientific Publication No.90, pp. 239–61. International Agency for Research on Cancer, Lyon.

National Research Council (1985). *Epidemiology and Air Pollution*. National Academy Press, Washington, DC.

Paul, A.A. and Southgate, D.A.T. (1978). *McCance and Widdowson's The Composition of Food* (4th edn), p. 31. North-Holland, Amsterdam.

Preston, D.L. and Pierce, D.A. (1987). *The Effects of Changes in Dosimetry on Cancer Mortality Risk Estimates in the Atomic Bomb Survivors*. Radiation Effects Research Foundation Technical Report 9–87, Radiation Effects Research Foundation, Hiroshima.

Rajhans, G.S. and Sullivan, J.L. (1981). *Asbestos Sampling and Analysis*. Ann Arbor Science, Ann Arbor, MI.

Roach, S.A. (1966). A more rational basis for air sampling. *American Industrial Hygiene Association Journal*, **27**, 1–12.

Saracci, R., Simonato, L., Acheson, E.D., *et al*. (1984). Mortality and cancer incidence of workers in the man-made vitreous fibres producing industry: an international investigation at thirteen European plants. *British Journal of Industrial Medicine*, **41**, 425–36.

Siemiatycki, J.(1996). Exposure assessment in community-based studies of occupational cancer. *Occupational Hygiene*, **3**, 41–58.

Simonato, L., Fletcher, A.C., Cherrie, J.W., *et al*. (1987). The International Agency for Research on Cancer historical cohort study of MMMF production workers in seven European countries: extension of the follow-up. *Annals of Occupational Hygiene*, **31**, 603–23.

Snedecor, G.W., and Cochran, W.G. (1980). *Statistical Methods* (7th edn), pp. 171–4. Iowa State University Press, Ames, IA.

Stewart, P.A., Blair, A., Cubit, D.A., *et al*. (1986). Estimating historical exposures to formaldehyde in a retrospective mortality study. *Applied Industrial Hygiene*, **1**, 34–41.

Thain, W. (1980). *Monitoring Toxic Gases in the Atmosphere for Hygiene and Pollution Control*, pp. 91–8. Pergamon Press, Oxford.

Tielemans, E., Kupper, L.L.,Kromhout, H.,Heederik, D., and Houba, R. (1998). Individual-based and group-based occupational exposure assessment: some equations to evaluate different strategies. *Annals of Occupational Hygiene*, **42**, 115–19.

Whitaker, T.B. and Dickens, J.W. (1974). Variability of aflatoxin test results. *Journal of the American Oil Chemists' Society*, **51**, 214–18.

Woitowitz, H.J., Schake, G., and Woitowitz, R. (1970). Ranking estimation of the dust exposure and industrial-medical epidemiology. *Staub Reinhaltung der Luft*, **30**, 15 (English translation).

Zanobetti, A., Schwartz, J., Gryparis, A., *et al*. (2003). The temporal pattern of respiratory and heart disease mortality in response to air pollution. *Environmental Health Perspectives*, **111**, 1188–93.

11

Response rates and their maximization

The only correct method of handling persons lost to
follow-up is not to have any.
(Dorn 1950)

Introduction

The emphasis of this book thus far has been on accurate measurement of
exposures in individuals, to reduce bias in the results of an epidemiological
study due to measurement error. However, the relationship between exposure
and outcome in an epidemiological study can also be biased if the exposure
measurements in study participants do not accurately reflect the distribution
of exposures in the actual population(s) of interest. This causes *selection bias*,
which is bias in the risk ratio (or other measure of association between the
exposure and disease) 'due to systematic differences in the characteristics
between those who take part in a study and those who do not' (Last 2001).

This chapter is directed at certain aspects of selection bias. Selection bias can
be caused by faulty study design, such as choice of the wrong sampling frame,
wrong eligibility criteria, or the wrong comparison group; these topics are
covered well in most textbooks on epidemiological methods and are not
discussed further here. Selection bias can also be caused by non-participation of
eligible individuals in a case–control study or by loss to follow-up of participants in a prospective study; this is due (in either type of study) to failure to
reach the subject or subject refusal. This *non-response* leads to a type of selection bias called *response bias*. Because these sources of bias occur during the
data collection phase of an epidemiological study, we have included a discussion of them in this chapter. Non-response to specific questions (item non-
response) and loss of subjects to a study because of their death before study
contact or their inability to participate are also sources of selection bias; these
are covered in earlier chapters of this book.

In this chapter, we define response rates, examine factors associated with non-response, describe the effects of selection bias, and provide strategies that can be used to maximize response rates.

Calculating response rates and other participation rates

The method of calculation of response rates and other participation rates is not standard in epidemiology. Moreover, the number of published epidemiological studies which do not report a response or participation rate is surprisingly large: 56 per cent of case–control studies published in 2003 in nine high-impact epidemiology and medical journals did not report a participation rate (Morton *et al.* 2006). Response rates should be reported in all studies, particularly the recruitment response rate in case–control or cross-sectional studies and the follow-up rate in cohort studies as these are essential inputs to the judgement of the methodological adequacy of the study

To compute a response rate, one needs the outcome, or *final disposition*, for each unit in the sampling frame. The *sampling frame* is a list of units (individuals, addresses, or randomly generated telephone numbers) from which all eligible individuals would ideally be included in the study. For simplicity, we assume that one unit (e.g. an address) can yield either one or no eligible subjects. We also assume that the study has a screening step before study participation to determine basic study eligibility (e.g. age range, sex, geographic area). This leads to just four final disposition codes:

P = number who *participated* in the study (screened for eligibility, were eligible, and participated)

R = number who *refused* (screened for eligibility, were eligible, and refused study)

I = number who were *ineligible* (screened for eligibility and were ineligible)

U = number with *unknown* eligibility (never reached or refused screening).

We define the *response rate* as the proportion of those in the sampling frame who were eligible for the study, who participated in the study. (It should be noted that although the term response rate is commonly used, it is in fact a proportion, not a rate over time.) Since one does not know the number of those with unknown eligibility who would have been eligible, it must be estimated:

E = *estimated* number of *eligibles* among those with unknown eligibility.

Then the response rate (proportion) can be estimated as follows:

response proportion = $P/(P + R + E)$.

Estimating E is the primary challenge of computing a response rate. In the simplest situation, $E = U \times e$, where e, the proportion of those with unknown eligibility who would have been eligible, is typically an educated guess. Most often, the number with unknown eligibility needs to be broken into subgroups with separate disposition codes (see American Association for Public Opinion Research (www.aapor.org/uploads/standarddefs_4.pdf) for examples). Then one can use separate estimates of e based on the reason for unknown eligibility to estimate E. For example, in random digit dialling recruitment, those with unknown eligibility would include a group for whom it was known that the phone number was for a household (either through the content of the answering machine message or by speaking to someone), but the household was never screened (either a person was never reached or the person answering the phone refused screening). Then one could reasonably estimate e for that group to be the same as the proportion of household phone numbers who agreed to be screened, who were eligible. For other components of U (e.g. phone numbers that were never answered after multiple attempts), a lower estimate of e would be appropriate, because some proportion of these would be telephone booths or non-working numbers. Other sources may be helpful in the estimation of e for various groups. Brick *et al.* (2002) have estimated eligibility proportions of undetermined telephone numbers, and Harvey *et al.* (2003) and White *et al.* (2004) have estimated eligibility proportions of non-responders to population-based mailed surveys.

Those ineligible by a final set of criteria which are only known after participation (e.g. exclusion of those with the history of disease under study or other medical conditions) can be ignored for the above calculation. The response rate computed by ignoring the final eligibility criteria is correct under the assumption that the proportion who would have remained eligible after the final exclusions is the same for all those eligible by the screening criteria, whether they participated or not.

Separate response rates should be reported for each sampling frame (e.g. for cases and for controls). Information about the major reasons for refusal, for unknown eligibility, and for ineligibility, and their associated numbers, should also be given to allow full assessment of the validity of the study (Olson *et al.* 2002). The study description should also include details of the sampling frame, as selection bias can also be introduced because of incomplete coverage of the sampling frame of the target population.

Some researchers report a cooperation rate rather than a response rate. The *cooperation rate (proportion)* is the participation proportion among the known eligibles:

cooperation proportion $= P/(P + R)$.

The above equation is *not* a good estimate of the response rate; to be a good estimate, all individuals on the sampling frame who were not reached or who refused screening for eligibility would have to be ineligible, which is very unlikely. The cooperation rate *overestimates* the response rate, and reporting it as a response rate is misleading as to the validity of the study.

Finally, the *completion rate (proportion)* is the proportion of all units in the sampling frame who were eligible and participated:

$$\text{completion proportion} = P/(P + R + I + U).$$

This rate is an *underestimate* of the response rate because not all units on the sampling frame represent eligible individuals. It is typically only reported when there is no pre-screening for eligibility (e.g. in large-scale mailings).

For longitudinal cohort studies, the follow-up rate should be reported in addition to the baseline response rate, because the response bias due to failure to follow up all enrolled participants is generally greater than the bias due to losses at baseline (see section on selection bias below). In the simple example of exposure collected at baseline and disease status collected at several follow-up points, the *follow-up rate (proportion)* could be computed as the proportion of eligible cohort members, for whom endpoint information was collected at the most recent follow-up. The follow-up rate could also be computed as the proportion of the follow-up time (person-years) which was successfully followed to ascertain the endpoints; this gives 'partial credit' for those followed up for several years who later dropped out or were lost to follow-up.

Factors associated with non-response

Time trends in response rates

There is evidence that response rates have become increasingly poor with time, particularly in the USA. In a review of 82 North American case–control studies, Olson (2001) reported a non-significant decline of 0.4 percentage points per year in response rates from 1972 to 1996 in control groups, with no decline in response rates among the cases. However, Morton *et al.* (2006) found much larger declines in participation rates (response rates or cooperation rates) over the period 1970–2003 among 143 studies reviewed: declines of 0.9 percentage points per year for cohort studies, 1.1 percentage points per year for cross-sectional studies, and 1.3 and 1.9 percentage points per year for cases and controls, respectively, in population-based case–control studies. When the population-based case–control studies were limited to those conducted after 1990, there was an alarming decline of 3.3 percentage points per year for cases and 5.2 percentage points per year for controls! In the 30-year University of Michigan Survey of Consumer Attitudes, participation began to decline (by about 1 percentage point per year) after 1990 (Curtin *et al.* 2000). That group and others have also noted that the number of phone calls for each completed interview and the proportion of interviews requiring refusal conversion have almost doubled over time (Curtin *et al.* 2000; Rogers *et al.* 2004).

The reasons for the fall in response rates and the increased effort needed to recruit respondents are poorly understood. Relevant variables which have varied with time that may affect the proportion of people likely to respond to surveys include:

- an increasing number of surveys being conducted, particularly telephone surveys, leading to individuals being contacted many times in a year
- an increasing incidence of 'false surveys' (telemarketing campaigns disguised as opinion surveys), although such marketing calls have been reduced in the USA with the implementation of the National Do Not Call Registry in 2003
- an increase in prevalence of the opinion that surveys are too long and that being interviewed is an unpleasant experience (Schleifer 1986)
- technological changes that allow individuals to screen their calls via answering machines or caller identification systems
- an increase in the proportion of studies which require more extensive participation, such as contributing a blood sample (Morton *et al.* 2006).

Case–control differences in response rates

It is easy to understand that cases would generally be more motivated to participate in a study of their medical condition than controls. Three studies have found a 4–12 percentage point lower response rate among controls compared with cases (Stang *et al.*1999; Olson 2001; Morton *et al.* 2006). Furthermore, as noted above, there has also been a greater decline in participation over the last several decades among controls compared with cases in case–control studies.

Other characteristics associated with non-response

A review of studies of the characteristics of respondents and non-respondents in medical studies is summarized in Table 11.1. The results from theses studies have been obtained in a number of different ways. Some involved direct comparisons of those who responded with those who did not, either by comparison of survey respondent characteristics with census data or by follow-up surveys of subjects who had been surveyed before. A number of comparisons have been made between early and late responders to surveys, or between those who responded with little prompting and those who required much persuasion. The assumption made is that those who are persuaded to respond with difficulty are intermediate in their characteristics between those who respond readily and those who do not respond at all.

The results of these different approaches have been quite consistent in pointing to the same demographic variables being associated with non-response. Moreover, the same characteristics of non-respondents have been reported over five decades of research and across a range of countries. Most of the studies reviewed found that participation in health-related studies is lower among men and among those not currently married. Studies have reported that both those in young adulthood and the elderly are less likely to participate; Moorman *et al.* (1999) found that this was due primarily to difficulty in contacting those in the youngest age groups and study refusals in the older age groups. Several studies observed lower participation among non-whites in the USA, and there is limited evidence that minorities or immigrants in other

Table 11.1 Summary of results of studies comparing characteristics of respondents and non-respondents in medical studies[a]

Factor	Characteristics of non-respondents
Sex	Male
Marital status	Not married
Age	Younger and older than middle-aged
Race	Non-white
Educational status	Lower
Occupational status	Lower or unemployed
Smoking status	Smoker
Alcohol drinking	More excess intake
Present health	Poorer
Future mortality	Higher
Use of medical care	Lower
Presence of specific health conditions	Inconsistent

[a] Robins (1963), Hochstim (1967), Loewenstein *et al.* (1969), Burgess and Tierney (1970), Kaplan and Cole (1970), Comstock and Helsing (1973), Oakes *et al.* (1973), Wilhelmsen *et al.* (1976), Criqui *et al.* (1978), Greenlick *et al.* (1979), Barton *et al.* (1980), De Maio (1980), Weeks *et al.* (1983), Wu and Brown (1983), Siemiatycki and Campbell (1984), Vernon *et al.* (1984), Brambilla and McKinlay (1987), Cottler *et al.* (1987), Walker *et al.* (1987), Bull *et al.* (1988), Iversen and Sabroe (1988), Wingo *et al.* (1988), Benfante *et al.* (1989), Shahar *et al.* (1996), Etter and Perneger (1997), Holt *et al.* (1997), Moorman *et al.* (1999), Une *et al.* (2000), Korkeila *et al.* (2001), Barchielli and Balzi (2002), Jacomb *et al.* (2002), Purdie *et al.* (2002), Thomas *et al.* (2002), Angus *et al.* (2003), Brogger *et al.* (2003), Caetano *et al.* (2003), Van Loon *et al.* (2003), Voigt *et al.* (2003), Pirzada *et al.* (2004).

countries also have lower response rates (Cartwright 1986; Purdie *et al.* 2002). There is a consistent pattern of association between various indicators of low socio-economic status and non-response, including lower education, higher unemployment, lower job status, and residence in lower-income areas.

Most studies report that those with more unhealthy behaviours are more likely to be non-respondents. Several studies have found that current smoking and higher alcohol intake are associated with non-response, and at least one study reported that those who exercise less tend to be non-respondents (Van Loon *et al.* 2003).

A number of studies have examined the association of non-response with measures of health status, and the relationship is not straightforward. Non-response has been fairly consistently associated with poor current health status as measured by global measures of health, such as disability and time away from work due to illness. Consistent with this, there is clear evidence that non-respondents to health studies have a higher mortality than those who respond (Wilhelmsen *et al.* 1976; Walker *et al.* 1987; Benfante *et al.* 1989; Une *et al.* 2000; Barchielli and Balzi 2002). However, several of these reports compared responders to invitations to be screened in a clinic for entry into a study with non-responders (Benfante *et al.*1989; Walker *et al.*1987). This type of study may be particularly vulnerable to lower participation by those who are in poor health. In contrast, respondents tend to be higher users of medical care, perhaps because those who are interested in health issues take advantage of more healthcare visits and also are more interested in health studies. Finally, there is no clear pattern of the relation of specific health conditions to survey response, except if the survey is clearly about the condition, in which case the condition will probably be more common among respondents (Gill *et al.* 2000), similar to the response differences between cases and controls discussed above.

There is limited evidence that those who can relate most to the topic of the study tend to participate. A study of sexuality found that respondents had less conservative sexual attitudes, an earlier age of sexual intercourse, and higher rates of smoking and alcohol use than non-respondents (Dunne *et al.* 1997). The latter two factors contrast with what the large majority of studies on non-respondents have reported, and may be due to the topic of the survey. A survey on healthcare experiences yielded respondents who were in poorer health than non-respondents (Fowler *et al.* 2002). This discrepant finding from the general association of poorer health with non-response may have been due to the aim of the survey. Finally, as noted above, less healthy people tend to participate less, except if the research topic is explicitly on their health condition.

Selection bias

Effect of selection bias

The effect of selection bias due to non-response on rate ratios in epidemiological studies has been discussed by a number of authors (Greenland 1977; Criqui 1979; Criqui *et al.* 1979; Austin *et al.* 1981; Kleinbaum *et al.* 1981). Criqui (1979) showed that bias in the rate ratio would be most likely to occur if there was 'combined risk factor and disease response bias'.

To make this more explicit, assume that the distribution of the target population by exposure and disease status is as shown on the left-hand side of Figure 11.1, with the true target population odds ratio denoted by OR_P. Because of non-participation of some selected subjects, only a subset of the target population become study participants, i.e. a subset of A become a, a subset of B become b, etc. The participation can be expressed as four participation rates: P_a, P_b, P_c, and P_d represent, respectively, the response proportions in those with the exposure and the disease, those with the exposure but without the disease, those without the exposure but with the disease, and those without the exposure and without the disease. P_a is computed as a/A, P_b as b/B, etc.

It can be shown quite simply (Austin *et al.* 1981) that the crude odds ratio OR_R for the association between an exposure and a disease derived from the respondents is related to the crude odds ratio OR_P in the target population as follows:

$$OR_R = (P_a P_d / P_b P_c) \times OR_P. \qquad [11.1]$$

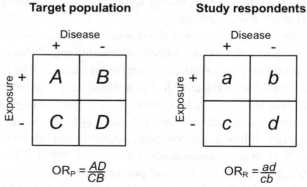

Figure 11.1 The effects of non-response on the numbers of individuals in a study and the odds ratio: a is a subset of A, b is a subset of B, etc.; OR_P is the odds ratio in the target population and OR_R is the odds ratio among study respondents.

If the values of P_a, P_b, P_c, and P_d are known, the true population odds ratio can be estimated from the observed odds ratio by solving Equation 11.1 for OR_P. Unfortunately, it is very difficult to obtain estimates of the four response proportions because the researcher usually cannot ascertain the exposure and disease status of non-respondents.

However, some generalities about the likelihood of selection bias can be made. Equation 11.1 shows that, provided that the response proportion depends only on the exposure status and is not influenced by disease status, i.e. $P_a = P_b$ and $P_c = P_d$, variation in the response proportion by exposure status will not bias OR_R. For example, if 90 per cent of those with the exposure and 70 per cent of those without the exposure participate, but participation is not influenced by the disease outcome, then the odds ratio will not have section bias. Similarly, if response proportions vary by disease status, but are not influenced by exposure status, i.e. $P_a = P_c$ and $P_b = P_d$, then variation in the response proportion by disease status will not bias OR_R. When both exposure and disease influence participation, but these occur independently (i.e. a multiplicative effect of a response proportion for exposure status times one for disease status), then $P_a P_d / P_b P_c = 1$ and the odds ratio will also not be subject to response bias. However, when the selection probabilities are jointly dependent on exposure and disease status, i.e. when $P_a P_d / P_b P_c \neq 1$, there is selection bias, i.e. $OR_P \neq OR_R$. Since the term $P_a P_d / P_b P_c$ can be greater or less than 1, selection bias can have any effect on the observed odds ratio based on the study respondents: OR_R can be biased toward the null in comparison to the population odds ratio OR_P, biased away from the null, or cross over the null value of 1 (i.e. the study results can show the exposure to be protective when it is in fact a risk factor).

Since the four participation rates are rarely known, selection bias should be suspected when participation rates could be influenced by both disease and exposure. Response bias is more likely in case–control and cross-sectional studies than in cohort studies because the potential participants in these studies probably know both their exposure and their disease status before study entry. Cases may participate because of their desire to contribute to knowledge about their disease regardless of their exposures, and only refuse because of poor health. Control participation may be more influenced by exposure status; for example, controls who are most interested in health issues and therefore have healthier lifestyles may be most likely to participate. Thus the prevalence of certain unhealthy behaviours (e.g. smoking) would be less in participating controls than in the target control population, leading to these behaviours spuriously appearing to be risk factors for the disease. Therefore there is often great potential for participation in case–control and cross-sectional studies to be influenced jointly by exposure and disease status, which will lead to response bias in the odds ratio. Equal response rates for cases and controls do not imply a low response bias. For example, a 75 per cent response rate for both cases and controls would lead to a large response bias if all non-participating cases were unexposed and all non-participating controls were exposed. As shown above, response bias depends on the four participation probabilities.

In a cohort study, initial participation rates are unlikely to be influenced jointly by exposure and by disease because future disease occurrence is unknown at study entry, although symptoms or a strong risk factor for the disease (e.g. family history) could influence interest in joining a study. Nonetheless, the potential for selection bias due to failures during initial recruitment is much less in cohort studies than in case–control or cross-sectional studies. However, in cohort studies, the likelihood that the researcher can successfully follow-up cohort members may be influenced by both exposure and disease, and this can lead to selection bias.

Evidence of selection bias due to non-response

As discussed in the section above on factors associated with non-response, it is clear that both disease status and at least some exposures, such as smoking and alcohol use, influence participation in health studies. However, the important issue is whether there are *joint* (non-independent) effects of exposure and disease on participation, which leads to selection bias in the risk ratio for the exposure–disease association.

Several studies provide empirical evidence that selection bias is a major problem in cross-sectional and case–control studies, and its magnitude. In a study by Criqui *et al.* (1978), data on six risk factors for cardiovascular disease (family history of heart attack, stroke, and diabetes, past history of hyperlipidaemia and hypertension, and present cigarette use) and history of four diseases (heart attack, heart failure, stroke, and diabetes) were obtained from respondents and also from a sample of 60 per cent of the non-respondents (weighted to represent all non-respondents). This permitted estimation of the magnitude of selection bias using estimates of P_a, P_b, P_c, and P_d for each of the risk factor–disease combinations. Values of the selection probability ratio $P_a P_d / P_b P_c$ varied from 0.83 to 1.63. Thus, appreciable bias was observed in some odds ratios even though the overall response rate was high (82 per cent). Similarly, Maclure and Hankinson (1990) used medical records and interviews to obtain information on non-respondents in a case–control study of renal cancer. The selection probability ratio ranged from 0.65 to 1.4 for a range of risk factors. This degree of selection bias suggests that a population odds ratio of 2 would yield an observed odds ratio based on the respondents of 1.3–2.8. However, other epidemiological studies have found little evidence of selection bias (Giovannucci *et al.* 1993; Krieger and Nishri 1997).

Methods to reduce selection bias

Findings reported in the material covered suggest that selection bias can be reduced by:

+ choice of study design (e.g. by a prospective cohort design)
+ not emphasizing the particular exposure under study when recruiting participants, particularly in case–control studies.

Selection bias due to non-response can also be minimized by:

+ achieving high response rates in case-control or cross-sectional studies
+ achieving high follow-up rates for disease outcomes in cohort studies.

These are important, because the higher the response rate in case–control studies or the follow-up rate in cohort studies, the lower is the potential for severe selection bias. Methods to maximize response rates and follow-up rates are covered in the remainder of this chapter.

Maximization of response rates

Choice of measurement method

A number of comparisons have been made, in epidemiological or health-related studies, of response rates achievable by the three main methods of obtaining data directly from respondents: face-to-face interview, telephone interview, and mailed self-administered questionnaire (Siemiatycki 1979; Battistutta *et al.* 1983; Weeks *et al.* 1983; Rolnick *et al.* 1989). Hox and de Leeuw (1994) conducted a meta-analysis of 45 studies from a wider range of academic fields which compared the response to these three methods. Most of the studies reviewed were conducted by assigning random samples of the study population to each method of data collection. They found the highest response rates for face-to-face interviews (70 per cent), followed by telephone interviews (67 per cent), with the lowest response to mailed surveys (61 per cent). However, direct comparison of methods is difficult because response rates depend strongly on the intensity of follow-up of non-respondents. For example, mail surveys to the general population typically require at least three mailings to achieve response rates as high as 60 per cent. The summary response rates in the Hox–de Leeuw meta-analysis are those achieved after multiple attempts to contact the participants using methods such as those described below.

Maximizing response to mail surveys

The strategies recommended for the maximization of response rates to mail surveys, as well as those for telephone and face-to-face surveys discussed below, are a combination of empirically supported techniques, experience, and intuition. No one technique has a large effect on response, but use of multiple techniques should lead to considerable improvement in response rates.

Factors which may increase response rates in mail surveys have been reviewed by Baumgartner and Heberlein (1984), Fox *et al.* (1988), Dillman (2000), and Edwards *et al.* (2002). They are summarized in Table 11.2. Edwards *et al.* (2002) conducted a comprehensive meta-analysis of 292 trials of methods to increase response rates to mailed questionnaires, and also quantified the effects of each method by the odds ratio of response. Those factors listed as having empirical support in Table 11.2 are the factors in the meta-analysis which had an odds ratio of at least 1.15, were statistically significant, and were

Table 11.2 Factors which may increase response rates in mail surveys

Empirically supported [a]

    A salient topic [b]

    University sponsorship

    Advance notice that a questionnaire will be sent [b]

    Avoidance of 'opt out' postcard

    Personalization of correspondence

    Multiple mailings/contacts

    Inclusion of a questionnaire with later mailings

    Special class (e.g. certified) mailings (typically used for non-responders to multiple mailings) [b]

    Stamped return envelope (versus business reply)

    A shorter questionnaire [b]

    A monetary incentive [b]

    An incentive included with the questionnaire (versus on return) [b]

    A non-monetary incentive

Recommended

    Blanket publicity (for very large mailings)

    Carefully constructed cover letter explaining importance of respondent to the survey

    Letter signed by patient's usual medical practitioner rather than researcher

[a] Factors in the meta-analysis by Edwards *et al.* (2002) which had odds ratios of response of 1.15 or greater, $p \leq 0.05$, and were based on at least two studies.

[b] Factors in the meta-analysis by Edwards *et al.* (2002) which had odds ratios of response of 1.5 or greater, $p \leq 0.05$, and were based on at least two studies.

based on at least two studies. Those factors with the largest impact on response (odds ratio of 1.50 or greater) are indicated by superscript 'b'.

Topic and sponsor of survey

Baumgartner and Heberlein (1984) found that surveys on highly salient topics can achieve response rates about 30 percentage points higher than those on non-salient topics. Similarly, the meta-analysis by Edwards *et al.* (2002) found that a more interesting versus a less interesting questionnaire doubled the odds of response. Clearly, it is important to bring out the salience of the survey topic as strongly as possible in the introductory letter. For example, Walter *et al.* (1988) found that the response to a letter seeking participation of controls in a case–control study increased from 74 to 85 per cent when the letter, which initially referred to a 'study of health and environmental/lifestyle risk factors', was changed to refer to a 'study of cancer and the environment' and indicated that it involved 'questions about the relationship between environmental factors and cancer'. This increased response can presumably be attributed to the increased salience of cancer and, perhaps, the effects of the environment on cancer to the subjects.

However, as noted above, the topic should be presented to the potential subjects in broad terms so as not to increase the salience for a specific group. Specifically, in case–control studies, it is important not to emphasize the specific exposures under study, as this could lead to more interest and thus greater participation by exposed controls, leading to selection bias.

There is consistent evidence that surveys conducted under the auspices of universities or government agencies achieve higher response rates than those conducted by commercial survey organizations (Baumgartner and Heberlein 1984; Fox *et al.* 1988; Edwards *et al.* 2002). Thus where several organizations are involved in a survey, the stationery used for the cover letter should be that of the organization thought likely to bring the greatest response.

Advance letter and blanket publicity

Advance notice that a questionnaire will be sent increases response rates (Spry *et al.* 1989; Edwards *et al.* 2002), with an odds ratio of response of 1.5 reported in the review by Edwards *et al.* (2002). This advance notice should be by mail rather than by telephone because a telephone call provides a means for the subject to refuse. The advance letter should be brief, state that an important survey will arrive in a few days, identify the research organization, state the study's purpose, and request cooperation in completing the survey.

For surveys that will be mailed to very large numbers of people, advance publicity may improve response rates. This can take the form of newspaper articles, or radio or television appearances.

Consent

Advance contacts should neither ask potential participants for specific consent to participate nor provide a way for them to decline to participate. Providing a means for individuals to opt out of the study, such as a return postcard, decreases response rates (odds ratio of response = 0.76) (Edwards *et al.* 2002). Such 'opt out' postcards should not be included in the advance letter or with the mailed questionnaire. A requirement for prior advance consent, i.e. an 'opt in' procedure, can have an even greater adverse effect on response rates. In a study in Scotland, conducted after a new confidentiality protocol required subjects to give prior consent by mail before being sent a mailed health survey, only 25 per cent of those contacted provided the advance consent (Angus *et al.* 2003). The response rate (the proportion of the sampling frame who both provided consent and completed the survey) was 20 per cent, compared with response rates of 70–80 per cent for earlier similar health surveys sent to the same population. This large difference was due in part to another restriction: researchers were not allowed to send multiple mailings to non-respondents in the consent step. It may also have been due to less of a sense of contribution from mailing back a consent form than from completing a questionnaire, or by a reluctance of people to commit to completing a questionnaire that they have not seen.

It is likely that requiring signed consent at the time of completion of a self-administered questionnaire also reduces response rates (as it does for interviews, discussed below), because some people are reluctant to provide their signature for any reason. A reasonable justification can be made to institutional ethics review boards that voluntary completion of a mailed questionnaire can be considered implied consent, without requiring the subject to sign a formal consent form.

Personalized and carefully constructed cover letter

Personalization of correspondence has also been shown to increase response rates by a small amount (Edwards *et al.* 2002). Personalization generally means that the recipient's name and address are in the heading, and the salutation says 'Dear Mr' or 'Ms' with the participant's last name. The rationale of personalization is to distinguish the questionnaire from 'junk mail', which may be even more important as the prevalence of junk mail increases. The sponsoring organization's normal business stationery (or a close facsimile) should be used. The letter should be signed personally by the study investigator using a blue pen (to distinguish it from a scanned image), and there is some evidence that response rates are improved if the signatory has a title (Kanuk and Berenson 1975). When possible and relevant, the letter should be signed by the subject's usual medical practitioner rather than by the researcher, as this also improves response (Smith *et al.* 1985).

The content of the cover letter needs to serve two purposes. First, it should motivate the potential participant to participate. Secondly, it needs to provide sufficient information about the study to allow an informed decision about whether he/she should respond. Human subject review boards typically review study materials to make sure that the latter goal is being met. (More information about ethical issues in epidemiological research is covered in Chapter 12.)

Research on the value of including motivational content in the cover letter has been disappointing. Randomized trials testing messages about the benefit of participation to the respondent, the benefit to the sponsor, or the benefit to society versus other messages have not shown that any of these appeals increase response rates (Edwards *et al.* 2002). Nonetheless, it seems appropriate to discuss the importance of the study to society and the importance of the respondent to the study.

The key elements of a cover letter are listed in Table 11.3, and a sample letter is shown in Figure 11.2. Dillman (2000) suggests that a short first paragraph should say what is being requested, the second paragraph why and how the

Table 11.3 Types of information included in covering letters with mailed questionnaires or in introductory statements when soliciting interviews[a]

Recommended

A statement about what is being requested

A statement of what the study is about and its usefulness

A statement of why the subject is important to the study

A description of participation commitment (e.g. interview length for telephone and in-person interviews, other study procedures, and future contacts)

A promise of confidentiality

An explanation that participation is voluntary

Reference to the incentive (if any)

A statement of whom to call if questions arise

An expression of appreciation

Optional

Number of subjects

How participants were selected

Sponsor (research organization and/or organization providing funding)

The statement 'I am not selling anything' or 'I am not calling for a contribution' (for telephone introductions)

Reference to more information on an attached question and answer sheet, brochure, or consent form (to keep cover letter to one page)

[a] Bourque and Fielder (1995), Dillman (2000), Fowler (2002), de Leeuw (2004).

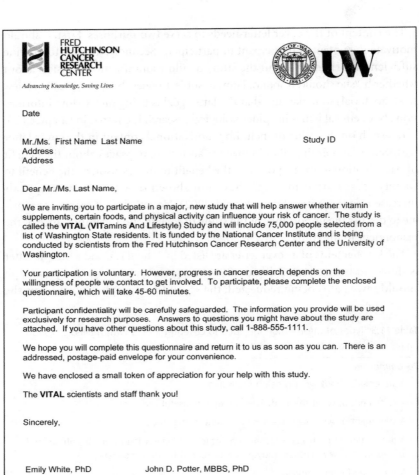

Figure 11.2 Sample cover letter requesting participation in a mailed survey. (VITAL Study, Fred Hutchinson Cancer Research Center, Emily White PhD, with permission.)

participant was selected, and the third the usefulness of the survey. The fourth paragraph should cover confidentiality and the voluntary nature of participation. Finally, the letter should mention any incentive, the willingness and method of having the researcher answer participants' questions, and should end with an expression of appreciation. Including a deadline for return of the questionnaire is not needed, as it has no effect on response rates (Edwards *et al.* 2002).

Cover letters should be limited to one page. In order to do this while fully informing the subject about the study, the letter may need to refer the subject to a question and answer page, the consent form, or a brochure about the study. A sample question and answer page is provided in Figure 11.3.

Questions and Answers about the VITamins And Lifestyle (VITAL) Study

What kinds of questions will this study answer? Because this is such a large study, we will be able to answer many questions about ways to reduce the risk of getting cancer and other diseases. Here are just a few examples:

- What vitamins or other supplements are beneficial and which ones are not?
- What types of food are most healthful: low fat, whole grains, dairy products?
- We know that exercise reduces your chance of heart disease, but does it reduce your risk of cancer?

Who is eligible for the study? You are – if this letter is addressed to you and you are age 50-75. You are eligible even if you have had a major disease, such as cancer.

How was I selected for this study? You were selected from a list of Washington State residents.

Why is it important for me to participate in this study? Only a small percent of Washington State residents was selected. For the results to be accurate, it is important that almost everyone selected for this study agrees to participate. Your responses to this questionnaire are VITAL!

What kind of future contacts will occur? If you complete this questionnaire, we will contact you by mail every 2 years. Some participants will be contacted about special studies in the future. These additional parts of the study are important, but are not required. If you complete the questionnaire enclosed, you will be part of the VITAL study. Of course, you may withdraw from the study at any time.

Can you tell me more about how you will follow participants in this study? If you participate, we will follow your health using the Washington State cancer registry, Washington State vital records, and other records that are approved for research. Changes of address will be followed using US Post Office records.

How can I be sure that my answers will be confidential? All the information you provide is strictly confidential as required by law and will be used exclusively for scientific purposes. Only research staff will have access to any identifying information, and your name can never be used in publications from this study. Your participation is voluntary and you may skip questions that you do not want to answer. Concerns regarding your rights as a research participant should be directed to our Institutional Review Administrator, Karen Smith, at 206-555-5000. **If you have questions about the study, please call our toll-free project line at 1-888-555-1111.**

Can I find out about the results of the study? Although we cannot directly inform our participants about the results of this study, we will publish our new findings about cancer risk. Your participation may not necessarily help you directly, however it will help future generations make more informed health choices.

Will I be asked for contributions of money? The VITAL study will never ask you for money, nor will we give our mailing list to anyone soliciting money or selling products. It is the contribution of your time, by completing this questionnaire that is valuable to us.

FRED HUTCHINSON CANCER RESEARCH CENTER
Advancing Knowledge, Saving Lives

Figure 11.3 Sample question and answer page included with a cover letter. (VITAL Study, Fred Hutchinson Cancer Research Center, Emily White PhD, with permission.)

Multiple contacts

A programme of multiple contacts is probably the single most important strategy for increasing response rates in mail surveys. Dillman (2000) recommends the following five steps and their timing.

1. A brief pre-notice letter sent a few days prior to the questionnaire, as described above.

2. A mailing of the questionnaire with a cover letter explaining why response is important.

3. About a week after the questionnaire is first mailed, a postcard should be sent to all subjects to thank those who have responded and to remind those who have not. (A sealed letter may be preferable for most epidemiological studies.) This brief correspondence should note that a questionnaire was sent, thank those who have already returned it, and request that the others complete it. It should give a short statement about why response is important and provide a phone number to call to obtain a new questionnaire if it was never received or has been misplaced.

4. A follow-up questionnaire and letter sent to non-respondents about three weeks after the first questionnaire. This letter should be similar but not identical to the original cover letter. It should explicitly state that 'your questionnaire has not yet been received' and restate in different words the importance of their participation.

5. A final contact, which can take the form of (a) a third mailing of a cover letter and questionnaire about three weeks after the second questionnaire by a special delivery mode such as overnight/priority mail or certified/recorded delivery, or (b) a telephone call reminder about a week after the last questionnaire was mailed. To have the greatest potential to maximize response rates, the telephone call should allow completion of the questionnaire by telephone interview.

As shown in Table 11.2, several of these steps have empirical support for improving response rates. Randomized trials have shown an increase in response rates with pre-contact of participants and with multiple mailings (Edwards *et al.* 2002). Trials have also shown that including the questionnaire in follow-up contacts (versus a follow-up reminder only) improves response (Edwards *et al.* 2002). Nonetheless, the third 'thank you/reminder' step above, which does not include a questionnaire, is recommended because it is inexpensive and may save costs of future mailings to non-respondents (Becker *et al.* 2000). Specialized delivery methods have a large effect on response, with an odds ratio of response of 2.2 in the meta-analysis by Edwards *et al.* (2002). However, because of their costs, their use often needs to be limited to the final mailing. Interestingly, Gibson *et al.* (1999) found that response rates were higher on a third mailing when it was by US certified mail (28 per cent) than by the more expensive US priority mail (22 per cent). However, certified mail may require recipients to travel to their post office to sign for the packet if they are not at home when it was to be delivered, which adds to subject burden.

Stamped return envelope

A mailed questionnaire packet should always include an addressed postage-paid envelope in which to return the completed questionnaire. A return envelope with real stamps increases response rates compared with a 'business reply paid' or franked envelope (Fox *et al.* 1988; Shiono and Klebanoff 1991; Edwards *et al.* 2002). The stamp may have a token value similar to a small incentive.

Questionnaire length and appearance

Response rates are higher for shorter questionnaires (Edwards *et al.* 2002). Response rates appear to decrease progressively after about four or five pages (Iglesias *et al.* 2000; Edwards *et al.* 2004). However, this limit is often not attainable in epidemiological surveys.

Dillman (2000) suggests that attractively formatted questionnaires have a modest impact on response rates. Questionnaire design is discussed in Chapter 6. Colored questionnaires do not appear to increase response rates (Etter *et al.* 2002, Edwards *et al.* 2002).

Incentives

Incentives improve response rates, with monetary incentives clearly superior to other types of incentives. In the Edwards *et al.* (2002) review of 49 studies of monetary incentives, the summary odds ratio of response was 2.0 for a monetary incentive versus no incentive, suggesting that this is one of the most effective ways to increase response rates.

Inclusion of the incentive with the questionnaire has a substantially greater impact on response than a promise of the incentive when the questionnaire is returned (Edwards *et al.* 2002). The appeal of the incentive to participants is probably not that they are being economically compensated for their effort (which a few dollars would not adequately do), rather, the incentive may be interpreted as a goodwill gesture that the respondent reciprocates by completing the questionnaire (Dillman 2000).

Monetary incentives can be costly in large studies and do not need to be sent to every potential participant or in every mailing. Dillman (2000) suggests including the incentive only with the first mailing of the questionnaire. Another approach is to include the incentive only with the second mailing of the questionnaire to non-respondents. It may also be inappropriate to send money to cases in a case–control study, since cases generally want to contribute to a study of their condition and may even be offended by an offer of money. As noted below, cash incentives sent to cases in a case–control telephone interview study reduced response (Coogan and Rosenburg 2004).

The monetary incentive need not be large. As recently as the 1990s or early 2000s, even one US dollar increased response rates. Gibson *et al.* (1999) found higher response rates among those sent $1 (48 per cent) or $2 (50 per cent) with the first mailing versus those sent no incentive (37 per cent). Doody *et al.* (2003) sent monetary incentives to non-responders only and reported response rates of 17 per cent for no incentive, 25 per cent for $1, and 29 per cent for $2. Parkes *et al.* (2000) reported a response rate of 62 per cent with no incentive, 73 per cent with a $2 incentive, and 77 per cent with $5.

While most studies of monetary incentives have used cash, Dillman (2000) suggests the use of cheques. He has found that cheques work about as well as cash in increasing response, and may save money. Fewer than 30 per cent of non-respondents will cash their cheques and only 80 per cent of respondents do so. However, the administrative costs of writing and handling cheques need to be considered.

Other incentives that have been used include an offer of a report of the results of the survey, a pen or pencil, a coffee coupon, a lottery ticket, or inclusion in some other kind of prize draw. Edwards *et al.* (2002) reviewed 45 studies of non-monetary incentives, and reported that such incentives modestly increase response rates on average (odds ratio of response = 1.2). Two randomized trials (White *et al.* 2005) of including a pen or pencil versus nothing with a second mailing of a questionnaire to non-responders found a 15–19 percentage point increase in the response rate to that mailing, perhaps because the pen or pencil is a facilitating factor, as well as a token of appreciation.

Maximizing response to telephone and in-person interviews

The factors that increase response in telephone and face-to-face interviews have received a great deal less attention than those influencing response to mail surveys, probably because of a perception that mail surveys are more in need of response-maximization strategies. However, many of the principles outlined above for mail surveys can be applied to telephone and face-to-face interviews.

Factors that have been shown empirically to increase response rates in interviews are summarized in Table 11.4, along with approaches that are recommended based on experience. Methods for increasing response to telephone

Table 11.4 Factors that may increase response rates in telephone and in-person interviews

Empirically supported

   Advance letter or postcard

   Avoidance of pre-interview consent procedures or 'opt out' postcard

   Incentive with pre-contact letter (for telephone interviews only)

   Experienced interviewers

   Personalized approach on telephone contact

   Delay in household screening

   Brief household screening procedures with immediate approach to interview selected respondent (random digit dialling telephone interviews)

   Multiple attempts to contact

   Callbacks to households or individuals who initially fail to participate

Recommended

   Careful selection and training of interviewers

   Persuasive introduction (carefully constructed text and interviewers' responses to participants' concerns)

   Termination of interviewers with high refusal rates

   Availability of verification of interviewers' credentials

   Avoidance of explicit refusals

   Use of particularly experienced interviewers to follow up near refusals

   Follow up by other modes of contact and interview (mail, telephone, home visit)

and in-person interviews are combined in this section, because recruitment for in-person interviews often begins with a telephone call to secure and schedule the interview. Therefore the approaches to increase responses rates are similar.

Advance letter

An advance letter increases the response to telephone surveys when the name and address of the subject is known (Dillman *et al.* 1976; Smith *et al.* 1995; Iredell *et al.* 2004). Recent studies suggest that an advance letter or postcard increases response rates by about 15 percentage points at a low cost (Smith *et al.* 1995; Iredell *et al.* 2004). These results probably also apply to in-person interview studies in which the initial contact is by telephone; therefore advance letters are recommended for in-person as well as telephone interviews.

Dillman (1978) suggests that an advance letter eliminates the element of surprise and provides tangible evidence that the interviewer is legitimately associated with a research organization. The advance letter for a telephone interview should advise that the subject will be called soon, provide a brief description of the study topic and its importance, give an indication of how long the interview will take, offer the possibility of requesting a call-back at a later time if the call comes at an inconvenient time, express appreciation to the participants, and provide an option of calling the study director for more information (Dillman 1978). For in-person interviews, the letter is similar, except that it explains that an interviewer will call to set up a convenient time and place for the interview. Letters to controls in case–control studies should explicitly say that healthy people are needed in the study. Otherwise, the letter could cause health concerns, for example in a woman who had a mammogram immediately before receiving an invitation to participate in a case–control study of breast cancer.

Consent

Participation rates are reduced if the advance contact provides a direct method to decline the interview (e.g. an 'opt out' postcard) or requires oral or signed consent prior to the first telephone contact by the study staff (Mueller *et al.* 1986; Nelson *et al.* 2002). In a 15-site US health survey, the response rate was 58 per cent at sites where advance permission was not required before the telephone interview, but was substantially lower in the areas that required oral advance consent (39 per cent) and the areas that required written advance consent (27 per cent) (Nelson *et al.* 2002). Even a request for signed consent at the beginning of an interview has been shown to reduce response rates (Bradburn and Sudman 1979). Thus, if necessary at all, the request for consent should be made at the end of the interview, provided of course that this approach is approved by the relevant ethical review committee. This approach may be particularly useful when the study involves both an interview and the collection of a blood sample, where signed consent is required only for the blood sample.

Incentives

The evidence for the effectiveness of monetary incentives in improving response to telephone interviews is similar to that for mailed surveys. Specifically, promises of payment do not improve response rates (Ward *et al.* 1984; Singer *et al.* 2000), while inclusion of a monetary incentive in a pre-contact letter does (Singer *et al.* 2000; Patten *et al.* 2003; Coogan and Rosenberg 2004). Patten *et al.* (2003) found that response rates increased from 58 to 73 per cent when a $5 (Canadian) incentive was included in the pre-contact letter for a health interview, and Coogan and Rosenburg (2004) reported an increase from 44 to 56 per cent when US $5 was included in the introductory letter to controls in a case–control study. It is noteworthy that in the latter study, the response rate among *cases* receiving the incentive was 64 per cent versus 68 per cent in the non-incentive group. While this difference was not statistically significant, it suggests that monetary incentives do not work and may even hurt response among cases. It is possible that some cases who would participate to increase knowledge about their disease feel insulted by the offer of money.

Incentives are not generally recommended for face-to-face interviews except when something additional is being asked of the subject, for example completion of a diary or submission to some form of physical examination or test. A US $10 honorarium was found to increase response to requests for a physical examination in the US Health Examination Survey (Bryant *et al.* 1975). However, a US $10 or $20 unconditional payment prior to securing an interview did not improve response rates in a US Census Bureau household survey (Davern *et al.* 2003).

Interviewer characteristics

Hartge *et al.* (1984) noted that, in their experience of random digit dialling surveys, the highest response rates were obtained by experienced interviewers. Male and female interviewers do not differ in response rates when level of experience is controlled (Groves and Lyberg 1988). Matching interviewers to respondents on race may increase study participation (Moorman *et al.* 1999).

There is evidence that interviewers who are perceived as competent and confident obtain better response rates than those who are not (Oksenberg and Cannell 1988; Fowler 2002). In studies of female interviewers, higher response rates were associated with a tone that was perceived as more positive, more competent, and higher in social class (Oksenberg *et al.*1986). Additionally, an interviewer speaking with a higher pitch, a greater variation in pitch, louder, faster, and more distinctly increased subject participation. Interviewers should exhibit an assertive manner which conveys that there is no doubt that the participant will cooperate with the study, yet they need to be sensitive to and respond to the concerns of the participant. Interview response rates should be carefully monitored, and interviewers with low response rates should be retrained or replaced.

Personalized approach

Dillman *et al.* (1976) found that when approaching a named participant, response rates were higher when the opening introduction was personalized ('Hello. Is this Mr/Mrs *(first and last name)*?') than when an impersonal opening introduction was given ('This is *(interviewer's name)* at Washington State University in Pullman and I'm calling for our Social Research Centre.').

The respondent's name will be known in most epidemiological studies, although not when subjects are being obtained by random digit dialling.

Persuasive introduction and avoidance of explicit refusals

Most refusals occur at the end of the introduction. While there is little empirical data to guide the construction of the introduction, clearly great care should be taken. Elements that should be included in the introduction are listed in Table 11.3. Dillman (1978) recommends that the introduction begin by ascertaining that the correct number or correct person has been reached. The interviewer should then introduce him/herself and the sponsoring organization. A statement of the purpose of the call, the importance of the respondent to the study, and the expected duration of the interview should then be given. Finally, the interviewer should offer to answer any questions that the subject may have and solicit participation by saying 'Okay?'

Telephone calls from strangers are often assumed to be solicitations. One study found that adding 'I am not selling anything' near the beginning of a telephone introduction increased the cooperation rate by 2 per cent (de Leeuw 2004). For calls in which the interviewer states that he/she is from a university or research institute, it might be more appropriate to state 'I am not calling for a contribution'.

Simply reading a predefined script is not sufficient to obtain high response rates. Interviewers need to interact personally with each potential respondent and provide appropriate responses to his/her concerns about participation. Table 7.1 (Chapter 7) lists questions commonly asked by potential participants, and interviewers need to be trained in how to respond.

The interviewer should end the call if an explicit refusal seems imminent. For example, if the interviewee insists that he/she is too busy even to schedule an interview for another day, the interviewer should end the conversation (*refusal aversion*). This allows a call-back by a more experienced interviewer at a time that may be more convenient for the respondent.

Verification of the interviewer's credentials

Interviewers arriving at participants' homes should carry a form of identification from the sponsoring institution. Because the telephone interviewer is unable to offer visible proof of his/her identity and association with the sponsoring organization, he/she should, if challenged, offer the respondent the option of calling a number to verify his/her credentials and then be transferred back to the interviewer.

Delay in household screening

When the sampling frame is of households, each household must usually be screened first to identify any eligible participant(s). A better response rate has been reported when personal information was sought first about the telephone answerer, and then about other household members, than when information about the whole household was sought first (Groves and Lyberg 1988). This result is consistent with the views of many interviewers that the household roster (the information needed for selection of an appropriate respondent from the household) is one of the most difficult sets of information to obtain.

Immediate interview of selected subject in random digit dialling

Harlow and Hartge (1983) reported a very high response rate (91 per cent) in a random digit dialling study when the selected subject was asked for an interview by telephone immediately after the household had been screened for eligible respondents. In a small experiment comparing this approach with the more usual approach of obtaining the full name and address of the eligible individual during screening and sending a preliminary letter to the selected subject, the immediate interview approach achieved a 16 per cent higher response rate. In random digit dialling, refusal to cooperate occurs most commonly at the stage of household screening, and it was thought that elimination of the need to ask for full name and address contributed to the high response rate of the direct approach.

Multiple attempts at contact

Multiple attempts to contact potential participants need to be made in order to have high response rates. Rogers *et al.* (2004) reported that between 1991 and 2003, the mean number of contacts per participant needed to achieve a final outcome in epidemiological studies in Utah (USA) increased from eight to 14, including phone calls, letters, and in-person visits. Phone call attempts should be made both in the evening and during weekends. Call-backs to non-responders a month or two later will reduce the proportion of telephones that are unanswered at the end of a study. For example, a second set of up to 11 calls a month later to those never reached increased response rates by 9 percentage points in a telephone health survey (Kristal *et al.* 1993). A careful record should be kept of calls made and their disposition (e.g. no answer, busy signal, etc.) so that the call strategy can be carefully monitored.

Often when the phone is not answered, an answering machine is reached. Leaving a message about the study and promising a call-back improved response rates by 20 percentage points among controls in a case–control study (Koepsell *et al.* 1996).

Multiple modes of contact and/or interview

Response rates to interviews can be increased by attempting to contact the participant (and perhaps conduct the interview) by multiple modes: mail, telephone, and home visit. The mail may catch an elusive but otherwise willing respondent, and a home visit may reach the participant or provide information about the reasons for non-contact (e.g. by asking the neighbours) which will lead to later contact. Similarly, for participants reluctant to participate in an in-person interview, offering them the option of a telephone interview may persuade them to participate.

Call-backs to near refusals

Call-backs by another, usually more experienced, interviewer to households or individuals which initially failed to cooperate can result in interviews in 25–40 per cent of cases (Groves and Lyberg 1988). These calls are usually made 6–12 months after the initial call. This second-round success probably results from a different person answering the telephone, the call coming at a more convenient time for the respondent, or the superior skills of the second interviewer. These are called *refusal conversions* in the field of survey research; however, they are only made to those classified as 'near' or 'soft refusal' (e.g. people who state that they are too busy to participate now). Ethical review committees generally do not allow call-backs to explicit 'hard refusals' (e.g. people who state that they do not want to be contacted again).

Maximizing response to collection of biological samples

There have been few studies on methods to enhance participation in the components of epidemiological studies which require collection of biological samples. A study by Colt *et al.* (2005) compared a cover letter with full disclosure that the study would include an interview and an optional blood draw and saliva sample with a cover letter which described the study as comprising an interview plus an optional 'second component'. There were no differences within the case or control groups in the interview rate by the type of cover letter received. However, participation in the blood draw was 11 per cent higher for cases and 7 per cent higher for controls who received the full disclosure letter. Thus full disclosure appears to be the best approach to maximize participation in all parts of the study.

For self-collected specimens, having study staff personally supply the collection kits to participants may lead to substantially higher response than mailing collection kits. Courtier *et al.* (2002) found a 20 per cent higher response to faecal sample collection when kits were personally delivered. For mailed self-collected specimens, a one-step approach in which the consent form is sent with the collection kit may be preferable to a two-step approach in which the consent form is mailed first and the collection kit is sent only if the consent form is returned. In two studies in which self-collected oral cells or fluid were requested by mail, a one-step approach led to a non-significantly higher response than a two-step approach (Morris *et al.* 2002; Cozier *et al.* 2004).

Some of the other approaches described above, such as multiple contacts and use of incentives, should also enhance agreement to provide biological specimens. The monetary incentive for biological samples would be higher than the token amount given for completing a questionnaire (e.g. about US $10–20 for a blood draw). However, as noted above, it may not be appropriate to offer money to cases in a case–control study.

Maximizing follow-up participation in longitudinal studies

As discussed in the section on selection bias above, in a cohort study, failure to obtain follow-up endpoint information from all members of the cohort is the main source of selection bias, rather than non-response at recruitment. Loss to follow-up may occur because some study subjects have decided not to participate any longer (drop-outs) or because the investigator has lost track of some participants. Methods of maximizing retention in longitudinal studies have been reviewed by Hunt and White (1998); they are listed in Table 11.5 and are discussed below.

Enrolment and baseline activities to enhance retention

Retention efforts begin during recruitment. Study staff should clearly communicate expectations of participation, including the frequency, duration, and types of follow-up visits or contacts that will occur. Before enrolment in the study, potential participants should be assessed for their willingness to participate. If the potential participant's future cooperation is questionable, he/she should not be enrolled. Specifically, investigators should not continue to reschedule no-shows or provide multiple attempts to enroll the participant. Also, before formal enrolment, participants should be required to complete the types of task that will be required during the follow-up phase, similar to a 'run-in' phase before randomization in a clinical trial. For example, if the participants are expected to complete questionnaires or come in for physical examinations throughout the study, these tasks should be part of the pre-enrolment baseline requirements. For example, in the Women's Health Initiative, a 12-year observational study of 100 000 women, expectations were clearly reviewed with potential cohort members during the consent process, and enrolment did not occur unless all baseline study components were completed (McTiernan *et al.* 1995).

Another activity that should be completed at baseline is the collection of information to aid in future follow-up. In longitudinal studies, useful items include the participant's full name including middle initial, address, phone

Table 11.5 Strategies to maximize retention in longitudinal studies[a]

Enrolment, consent, and baseline activities

   Screen potential participants for willingness to participate over the long term

   Fully inform participants of time commitment and requirements of study

   Have participants complete a set of tasks at baseline before enrolment

   Collect participant tracing information, such as address, phone number, Social Security or healthcare number, date of birth

   Collect names and telephone numbers of personal contacts

Continued contact and bonding

   Regular contacts with participant, at least every 6–24 months

   Create study logo and theme

   Send newsletters, study updates and/or holiday cards

   Provide small tokens of appreciation with study logo

Staff characteristics

   Well-trained and enthusiastic

   Respond promptly to questions or problems

   Flexible in terms of scheduling visits and other participant needs

Avoidance of complete study withdrawal

   Allow limited participation (e.g. by mail or telephone)

   Strive to collect primary outcomes, at a minimum

[a] Adapted from Hunt and White (1998).

numbers (home, mobile, and work), email address, birth date, and healthcare or population identification number (e.g. Social Security number in the USA). The names, addresses, and phone numbers of one or two friends or relatives not living with the participant who are likely to know his/her whereabouts are also important. Optional items which might aid in future contact are the name of the participant's spouse, name of the primary physician, place of birth, and, for women, maiden name. Those items that can change (e.g. address) should be updated periodically.

Continued contact and bonding

Once a participant has been enrolled, frequent contact (by mail, phone, or in person) with participants should be maintained. The frequency of follow-up contact in longitudinal epidemiological studies has generally been in the range of 6–24 months. While this depends on the frequency needed to collect accurate exposure and outcome data, contact every 6–24 months is generally needed to check current addresses and to maintain the participant's interest in the study.

Participants in a longitudinal study need to identify with the study and become committed to active involvement. Given *et al.* (1990) suggest creation of a study logo and theme, and use of these in letters, envelopes, questionnaires, and other communications to establish a connection with the study. Newsletters with updates on study progress and holiday cards have been used as bonding tools, as well as to provide an opportunity to obtain address correction information from the US Postal Service through use of a 'Change Service Requested' instruction on the mailed piece. Small gift incentives are often used in longitudinal studies to express appreciation for the participant's involvement and to remind them of their participation throughout the year. In the Family Caregiver's Study, participants were given coffee mugs, desk calendars, clocks, and ballpoint pens embossed with the study's logo (Given *et al.* 1990).

Retention is also enhanced by regular personal contact with study staff who reiterate the importance of the study and demonstrate their enthusiasm and commitment to the project. In a study that evaluated retention in the Framingham Children's Study, Marmor *et al.* (1991) found that staff characteristics, including their attitudes, responses to questions and problems, and scheduling flexibility, to be among the factors most important in keeping participants in the study.

Finally, many of the techniques discussed above and listed in Tables 11.2 and 11.4 can also be used to enhance continued participation of cohort members in completing questionnaires and interviews.

Collection of minimal information rather than allowing complete study withdrawal

When cohort members are reluctant to continue with full participation during the follow-up period, collection of information on the primary outcomes should be continued, at a minimum. An example comes from the Oxford Family Planning Association contraceptive study, in which 17 000 women received annual clinic follow-up examinations for 10 years. Women who stopped attending the clinic were sent a mailed questionnaire annually and, if this was not returned, were interviewed by telephone or during a home visit in an attempt to collect data on the primary outcomes (Zondervan *et al.* 1996).

Tracing hard to find (or 'lost') participants

In case–control and cross-sectional studies, the researcher must first locate each member of the sampling frame to solicit his/her participation. In longitudinal cohort studies, the researcher must find each enrolled cohort member to request follow-up information. Thus failure to locate subjects is a source of

Table 11.6 Strategies for locating participants who are hard to find[a,b]

Search for participant's current telephone number and address

Check telephone books, directory assistance, and/or on-line directories

Seek new address through whatever facilities may exist through a local postal service (e.g. in the USA, send letter to last known address using 'address service requested'); include a phone number to call, a form to verify or update address, and postage-paid envelope

Send certified letter to participant's last known address

For samples defined by occupation, healthcare source (e.g. health maintenance organization), or other source, contact the organization or appropriate professional licensing group

Submit search to postal system (e.g. US National Change of Address (NCOA) system, request residential phone service options as well as move information)

Check local and national registers

National Health Services/health insurance records

Driver's license registries

Marriage/divorce records (for new addresses/change of last name among women)

Voter registration records/electoral rolls

Public utility companies

Taxation and real estate records

Military Locator Service

Other national registries (e.g. population registries) where available

State and national death records (e.g. in the USA, Social Security Death Index and National Death Index)

Contact others

Contact (by telephone and/or mail) relatives or personal contacts of participants

Contact participant's physician

Contact participant's employer or employee pension company

For someone with an unusual last name, telephone others with the same name living in the same area

Contact current residents and/or neighbours of last known address; this can be aided by use of reverse directories (including on-line services (e.g. Polk, Cole's) which list household names organized by address)

Contact landlords or managers of rental properties

If a property has been sold, contact the real estate agency to obtain a new address

Use commercial tracing services

Use commercial background check services

Use credit bureaux (not legal in USA)

Table 11.6 (continued) Strategies for locating participants who are hard to find[a,b]

Additional strategies for high-risk populations

    Contact welfare and other social service agencies

    Contact drug treatment programmes, prisons, and parole officers

    Visit neighbourhood meeting places, such as bars, barber shops, and churches

[a] Generally listed from cheapest/easiest to most difficult/most expensive. All options may not be available/acceptable in all areas, and some options require explicit permission from study participants. Legality is agency and research institution specific.

[b] Adapted from Hunt and White (1998)

selection bias for all types of epidemiological study. The only way to reduce this source of non-response is through intensive efforts to locate each member.

Strategies that can be used to trace participants have been reviewed by Nordberg (1992) and by Hunt and White (1998). These are discussed below and summarized in Table 11.6. Since multiple approaches must often be employed before the participant can be located, it is usual to pursue the simpler, least expensive approaches first, and then to resort to the more difficult or expensive approaches. Furthermore, many of the options listed in Table 11.6 and discussed below vary in their availability by geographic area. Also, some options may require specific permission from study participants based on policies that vary depending on the country, the research institution, and the agency supplying the tracing information.

Activities to locate lost or hard to find participants should continue until the participant's location and/or vital status have been ascertained, or until search strategies have been exhausted. Even if contact is not established during initial attempts, further attempts to locate the participant after several months or years may be successful.

Search for participant's current telephone number and address

Initial attempts to locate a hard to find participant usually begin with mail, telephone, and/or email contacts. If the participant is employed, he/she could be contacted at work as well as at home. Among those participants not initially reachable, some will be available weeks or even months later, as would be the case with retired persons who may live elsewhere for several months during the year.

For participants whose phone number or address has changed, sources of new numbers and addresses include telephone books, directory assistance, or online directories. For sampling frames defined by occupation (e.g. a professional licensing group), healthcare source (e.g. a health maintenance organization), or other source, the original source of the names and addresses may have updated information.

Early mailed attempts often consist of sending the participant a letter requesting that he/she contact the study. Include a phone number to call, a form to verify or update address, and a postage-paid envelope. As with all mailings, the envelope should indicate a request for address correction from the post office. In the USA, this is achieved with a first-class mailing noting 'address service requested,' by which the mailing is forwarded to the participant and the study is provided notice of the new address. If no response is received to initial attempts and the known address is believed to be correct, a certified letter can be sent to the participant's last known address requesting that he/she contact the study.

The US National Change of Address (NCOA) linkage system

For large files of names and addresses (e.g. in longitudinal cohort studies), an attempt should be made to update addresses before mailings. In the USA, the postal service developed the National Change of Address (NCOA) linkage system (www.USPS.com/ncsc/addressservices/ moveupdate/changeaddress.htm) to reduce the amount of undeliverable commercial mail; this system can be useful for tracking the addresses of study members. The NCOA system accumulates all change-of-address data from almost the entire country and provides a file with this information on a regular basis to licensed private companies. To update study participant addresses, a file of current participant names and addresses is submitted to an NCOA licensee who, for a minimal fee, will search for matches on the NCOA file. If the change of address indicates that an individual has moved, a new address is provided if there is an exact match on first name, last name, and previous address, whereas if the change of address indicates a household move, all that is required is a match on last name and previous address. The NCOA licensee can also provide codes for moves without a forwarding address and codes indicating close but imperfect matches to indicate that the person might have moved. However, NCOA will not provide the new address for these. The researcher can then try to contact those individuals to verify their address or obtain a new address. NCOA can also provide phone numbers for participants.

Local, state, and national registers

Other state, local, and national sources which may provide current address information include Department of Motor Vehicles files, voter registration records, public utility records, healthcare or health insurance records, marriage records (for last name changes), and taxation records.

Tracing of subjects also involves ascertaining vital status, since some subjects who cannot be located have in fact died. All US states and almost all countries have death records that can be accessed by researchers.

The US National Death Index and the US Social Security Death Index

In the USA, the vital status of all study participants or only those who are 'lost' can be ascertained using the *National Death Index* (NDI). The NDI is an electronic file of all deaths occurring in the USA since 1979, established by the National Center for Health Statistics (www.cdc.gov/nchs/ndi.htm). For a fee, the NDI service will attempt to match study members with the death file.

Linkages are made based on matching certain sets of items on both the study file and the death records. Matching criteria are based on Social Security number, first name or initial, middle initial, last name, month, day, and year (±1) of birth, and father's surname. All possible matches are reported to the user; having additional identifiers, such as sex, last known age alive, race, marital status, state of birth, and state of residence, increases the chance of a valid match. (Note that women who have never worked often share a Social Security number with their husband.) The NDI provides the investigator with the date of death, the state in which the death occurred, and, for an additional fee, the cause of death codes. The main limitation of this system is that deaths for each calendar year are not available for searches until about 16 months after the end of that year, i.e. 16–28 months after the death occurred. Also, because of the cost structure (a processing fee plus a per record fee), NDI searches are usually only cost effective if done on hundreds or thousands of subjects at once.

Several studies have found the quality of results provided by the National Death Index to be quite good (Wentworth *et al.* 1983; Stampfer *et al.* 1984; Boyle and Decouflé 1990; Calle and Terrell 1993). For example, Stampfer *et al.* (1984) found that 96.5 per cent of known deaths in a cohort of women were successfully matched by National Death Index, and Wentworth *et al.* (1983) reported 98.4 per cent successful matches in a cohort of men. Quality improves if a Social Security number is available; a middle initial also adds to the likelihood of an accurate match. Ascertainment of full and accurate information at the beginning of the cohort study is extremely important to enhance the likelihood that a valid match will be made. When complete and accurate member data are available, the majority of those not matched by the NDI can be considered to be alive as of the most recent date for which the NDI has been updated.

The US *Social Security Death Index* (SSDI) is a file of deaths that is made available to certain organizations. These organizations (often genealogical services) then provide online searches, usually free of charge. Searches are generally based on name, Social Security number, birth date, and/or state of residence. The search returns possible matches, with date of death and city of last residence. The SSDI death records are not complete, in that they only include deaths (since 1962) for those who had a Social Security number and whose death was reported to the Social Security Administration. Sesso *et al.* (2000) found that 95 per cent of definite deaths identified by NDI were found on a web-based SSDI search. Although this file is less complete than the National Death Index, searches can be done individually and immediately when a subject is lost, searches are free, and the SSDI records are generally more up to date than the NDI.

Contact others who may be knowledgeable about participant's whereabouts

In a longitudinal study, the personal contacts provided by the participant at baseline can be contacted by phone or by mail to obtain updated address and phone number information on the participant, and to confirm that he/she is not deceased. These contacts include the participant's spouse, friends or relatives not living with the participant, physician, employer, or pension company. For someone with an unusual last name, other people who live in the same area with the same last name could be called, as they may be related to the missing participant and have information on his/her whereabouts. If these contacts are unwilling to provide the new phone number or address of the participant, they may be willing to contact the participant and ask him/her to call the study office. If attempts at contacting personal contacts are unsuccessful, others who might be able to provide a new address or phone number include former neighbours, the current resident at the participant's last known address (using city directories), or the real estate agency who sold the participant's home.

Tracing services

Certain organizations specialize in providing background information on individuals, and these companies can be helpful for tracing study subjects. These organizations include commercial companies which specialize in doing background checks before employment or before leasing a residence, or organizations which conduct genealogical searches. In the USA, credit bureaux can no longer be used to locate individuals, but these agencies may be available in other countries.

Tracing high-risk participants

Creative strategies must often be employed when tracing hard-to-reach and high-risk segments of the population. The St Louis Effort to Reduce the Spread of AIDS study used several innovative methods to trace intravenous drug users, such as contacting parole officers, prisons, and drug treatment programmes (Cottler *et al.* 1996). Additional strategies for locating cohort members from high-risk populations include contacting governmental and non-governmental welfare and social service agencies, or visiting homeless shelters and popular meeting places, such as bars, barbershops, and churches.

Summary

Selection bias is bias in the risk ratio (or other measure of association between exposure and disease) that is due to differences in the characteristics between those who take part in a study and those who are eligible for the study but do not participate. Response bias is a type of selection bias that is due to non-participation of some eligible individuals in a case–control study or loss to follow-up of some participants in a prospective study. The non-response in either type of study can be due to failure to reach the subject or subject refusal.

Selection bias occurs when disease and exposure have a joint (non-independent) effect on an eligible person's likelihood of participation in the study. The effect of selection bias due to non-response on the odds ratio of disease in a population can be estimated from:

$$OR_R = (P_a P_d / P_b P_c) \times OR_P$$

where OR_R is the odds ratio in the respondents, OR_P is the odds ratio in the target population, and P_a, P_b, P_c, and P_d are respectively the response proportions in those with the risk factor and the disease, those with the risk factor but without the disease, those without the risk factor but with the disease, and those without the risk factor and without the disease. Since the four participation proportions are rarely known, selection bias should be suspected whenever exposure and disease may jointly influence participation.

Efforts to achieve high response rates in case–control or cross-sectional studies and high follow-up rates in cohort studies are important ways to minimize response bias. The response rate (the number of study participants/estimated eligible individuals in the sampling frame) should be carefully estimated. Response rates should always be reported in publications from epidemiological studies, so that the results can be interpreted in light of the methodological quality of the study.

There is evidence that response rates in population surveys in the USA have fallen over the past several decades, with large declines since 1990. Non-respondents are more likely to be male, not married, younger or older than middle aged, non-white, and of lower socio-economic status, and to have poorer health behaviours, such as cigarette smoking and excess alcohol intake. They also tend to have poorer health and use less medical care. There is evidence that respondents tend to be those who most relate to the exposures or health condition being studied (if these are known when deciding whether to participate); for example, cases have higher participation than controls in case–control studies.

Response rates tend to be highest for face-to-face interviews, intermediate for telephone interviews, and least for mailed questionnaires.

A variety of techniques can be used to maximize response rates in different types of epidemiological studies. They include:

- advance notice of contact, but without required advanced consent
- a carefully constructed introductory letter or statement, with wording which may enhance the interest in the study topic to potential respondents
- personalized mail or phone approach
- experienced interviewers perceived as sounding confident and competent
- a monetary incentive (except to cases in case–controls studies) or a non-monetary incentive
- stamped return envelopes (versus business reply) in mailed surveys
- avoidance of signed consent procedures for mailed surveys or at the beginning of interviews
- multiple attempts to contact potential participants by multiple means: telephone, mail, certified mail, in person
- avoidance of explicit refusals by potential subjects, and further approach by highly experienced interviewers to those who do not participate initially.

Retention in longitudinal cohort studies can be enhanced by a 'run-in' phase before enrolment, frequent contact with the study, and enthusiastic and responsive staff, as well as by the applicable techniques listed above.

Strategies should be adopted to locate study subjects who are initially hard to find, including online searches and use of local and national registers. In cohort studies this is enhanced by collecting information at baseline that will aid later follow-up, including the names and contact information of friends or relatives who do not live with the participant.

References

Angus, V.C., Entwistle, V.A., Emslie, M.J., Walker, K.A., and Andrew, J.E. (2003). The requirement for prior consent to participate on survey response rates: a population-based survey in Grampian. *Biomedical Central Health Services Research*, **3**, 21.

Austin, M.A., Criqui, M.H., Barrett-Connor, E., and Holdbrook, M.J. (1981). The effect of response bias on the odds ratio. *American Journal of Epidemiology*, **114**, 137–43.

Barchielli, A. and Balzi, D. (2002). Nine-year follow-up of a survey on smoking habits in Florence (Italy): higher mortality among non-responders. *International Journal of Epidemiology*, **31**, 1038–42.

Barton, J., Bain, C., Hennekens, C.H., *et al.* (1980). Characteristics of respondents and non-respondents to a mailed questionnaire. *American Journal of Public Health*, **70**, 823–5.

Battistutta, D., Byth, K., Norton, R., and Rose, G. (1983). Response rates: a comparison of mail, telephone and personal interview strategies for an Australian population. *Community Health Studies*, **7**, 309–13.

Baumgartner, R.M., and Heberlein, T. A. (1984). Recent research on mailed questionnaire response rates. In *Making Effective Use of Mailed Questionnaires* (ed. D.C. Lockhart), pp. 65–76. Jossey-Bass, San Francisco, CA.

Becker, H., Cookston, J., and Kulberg, V. (2000). Mailed survey follow-ups. Are postcard reminders more cost-effective than second questionnaires? *Western Journal of Nursing Research*, **22**, 642–7.

Benfante, R., Reed, D., MacLean, C., and Kagan, A. (1989). Response bias in the Honolulu Heart Program. *American Journal of Epidemiology*, **130**, 1088–1100.

Bourque, L. B., and Fielder, E.P. (1995). *How to Conduct Self-Administered and Mail Surveys.* Sage, Thousand Oaks, CA.

Boyle, C.A., and Decouflé, P. (1990). National sources of vital status information: extent of coverage and possible selectivity in reporting. *American Journal of Epidemiology*, **131**, 160–8.

Bradburn, N.M., and Sudman, S. (1979). *Improving Interview Method and Questionnaire Design.* Jossey-Bass, San Francisco, CA.

Brambilla, D.J., and McKinlay, S.M. (1987). A comparison of responses to mailed question-naires and telephone interviews in a mixed mode health survey. *American Journal of Epidemiology*, **126**, 962–71.

Brick, J.M., Montaquila, J., and Scheuren, F. (2002). Estimating residency rates for undeter-mined telephone numbers. *Public Opinion Quarterly*, **66**, 18–39.

Brogger, J., Bakke, P., Eide, G.E., and Gulsvik, A. (2003). Contribution of follow-up of nonresponders to prevalence and risk estimates: a Norwegian respiratory health survey. *American Journal of Epidemiology*, **157**, 558–66.

Bryant, E.E., Kovar, M.G., and Miller, H. (1975). A study of the effect of remuneration upon responses in the health and nutrition examination survey. In *Vital and Health Statistics*, Series 2, No 67. Department of Health, Education, and Welfare, Washington DC

Bull, S.B., Pederson, L.L., Ashley, M.J., and Lefcoe, N.M. (1988). Intensity of follow-up. Effects on estimates in a population telephone survey with an extension of Kish's (1965) approach. *American Journal of Epidemiology*, **127**, 552–61.

Burgess, A.M. and Tierney, J.T. (1970). Bias due to non-response in a mail survey of Rhode Island physician's smoking habits,1968. *New England Journal of Medicine*, **282**, 908.

Caetano, R., Ramisetty-Mikler, S., and McGrath, C. (2003). Characteristics of non-respon-dents in a US national longitudinal survey on drinking and intimate partner violence. *Addiction*, **98**, 791–7.

Calle, E.E. and Terrell, D.D. (1993). Utility of the National Death Index for ascertainment of mortality among Cancer Prevention Study II participants. *American Journal of Epidemiology*, **137**, 235–41.

Cartwright, A. (1986). Who responds to postal questionnaires? *Journal of Epidemiology and Community Health*, **40**, 267–73.

Colt, J.S., Wacholder, S., Schwartz, K., Davis, F., Graubard, B., and Chow, W.H. (2005). Response rates in a case–control study: effect of disclosure of biologic sample collection in the initial contact letter. *Annals of Epidemiology*, **15**, 700–4.

Comstock, G.W., and Helsing, K. (1973). Characteristics of respondents and non-respondents to a questionnaire for estimating community mood. *American Journal of Epidemiology*, **97**, 233–9.

Coogan, P.F., and Rosenberg, L. (2004). Impact of a financial incentive on case and control participation in a telephone interview. *American Journal of Epidemiology*, **160**, 295–8.

Cottler, L.B., Zipp, J.F., Robins, L.N., and Spitznagel, E.L. (1987). Difficult to recruit respondents and their effect on prevalence estimates in an epidemiologic survey. *American Journal of Epidemiology*, **125**, 329–39.

Cottler, L.B., Compton, W.M., Ben-Abdallah, A., Horne, M., and Claverie, D. (1996). Achieving a 96.6 percent follow-up rate in a longitudinal study of drug abusers *Drug Alcohol Depend*, **41**, 209–17.

Courtier, R., Casamitjana, M., Macia, F., *et al.* (2002). Participation in a colorectal cancer screening programme: influence of the method of contacting the target population. *European Journal of Cancer Prevention*, **11**, 209–13.

Cozier, Y.C., Palmer, J.R., and Rosenberg, L. (2004). Comparison of methods for collection of DNA samples by mail in the Black Women's Health Study. *Annals of Epidemiology*, **14**, 117–22.

Criqui, M.H. (1979). Response bias and risk ratios in epidemiologic studies. *American Journal of Epidemiology*, **109**, 394–9.

Criqui, M.H., Barrett-Connor, E., and Austin, M. A. (1978). Differences between respondents and non-respondents in a population-based cardiovascular disease study. *American Journal of Epidemiology*, **108**, 367–72.

Criqui, M.H., Austin, M.A., and Barrett-Connor, E. (1979). The effects of non-response on risk ratios in a cardiovascular disease study. *Journal of Chronic Diseases*, **32**, 633–8.

Curtin, R., Presser, S., and Singer, E. (2000). The effects of response rate changes on the index of consumer sentiment. *Public Opinion Quarterly*, **64**, 413–28.

Davern, M., Rockwood, T.H., Sherrod, R., and Campbell, S. (2003). Prepaid monetary incentives and data quality in face-to-face interviews: data from the 1996 Survey of Income and Program Participation Incentive Experiment. *Public Opinion Quarterly*, **67**, 139–47.

de Leeuw, E. D. (2004). I am not selling anything: 29 experiments in telephone introductions. *International Journal of Public Opinion Research*, **16**, 464–73.

De Maio, T.J. (1980). Refusals: who, where and why. *Public Opinion Quarterly*, **44**, 223–33.

Dillman, D.A. (1978). *Mail and Telephone Surveys*. Wiley, New York.

Dillman, D.A. (2000). *Mail and Internet Surveys* (2nd edn). Wiley, New York.

Dillman, D.A., Gallegos, J.G., and Frey, J.H. (1976). Reducing refusal rates for telephone interviews. *Public Opinion Quarterly*, **40**, 66–78.

Doody, N.M., Sigurdson, A.S., Kampa, D., *et al.* (2003). Randomized trial of financial incentives and delivery methods for improving response to a mailed questionnaire. *American Journal of Epidemiology*, **157**, 643–51.

Dorn, H.F. (1950). Methods of analysis for follow-up studies. *Human Biology*, **22**, 238–48.

Dunne, M.P., Martin, N.G., Bailey, J.M., *et al.* (1997). Participation bias in a sexuality survey: psychological and behavioural characteristics of responders and non-responders. *International Journal of Epidemiology*, **26**, 844–54.

Edwards, P., Roberts, I., Clarke, M., *et al.* (2002). Increasing response rates to postal questionnaires: systematic review. *British Medical Journal*, **324**, 1183–85.

Edwards, P., Roberts, I., Sandercock, P., and Frost, C. (2004). Follow-up by mail in clinical trials: does questionnaire length matter? *Control Clinical Trials*, **25**, 31–52.

Etter, J. F., Cucherat, M., and Perneger, T. V. (2002). Questionnaire color and response rates to mailed surveys. A randomized trial and a meta-analysis. *Evaluation and the Health Professions*, **25**, 185–99.

Etter, J.F., and Perneger, T.V. (1997). Analysis of non-response bias in a mailed health survey. *Journal of Clinical Epidemiology*, **50**, 1123–8.

Fowler, F.J. (2002). *survey research methods* (3rd edn). Sage, Thousand Oaks, CA.

Fowler, F.J., Gallagher, P.M., Stringfellow, V.L., Zaslavsky, A.M., Thompson, J.W., and Cleary, P.D. (2002). Using telephone interviews to reduce nonresponse bias to mail surveys of health plan members. *Medical Care*, **40**, 190-200.

Fox, R.J., Crask, M.R., and Jong Hoon, K. (1988). Mail survey response rate. A meta-analysis of selected techniques for inducing response. *Public Opinion Quarterly*, **52**, 467–91.

Gibson, P.J., Koepsell, T.D., Diehr, P., and Hale, C. (1999). Increasing response rates for mailed surveys of Medicaid clients and other low-income populations. *American Journal of Epidemiology*, **149**, 1057–62.

Gill, D., Merlin, K., Plunkett, A., Jolley, D., and Marks, R. (2000). Population-based surveys on the frequency of common skin diseases in adults. Is there a risk of response bias? *Clinical and Experimental Dermatology*, **25**, 62–6.

Giovannucci, E., Stampfer, M.J., Colditz, G.A., *et al.* (1993). Recall and selection bias in reporting past alcohol consumption among breast cancer cases. *Cancer Causes and Control*, **4**, 441–8.

Given, B.A., Keilman, L.J., Collins, C., and Given, C.W. (1990). Strategies to minimize attrition in longitudinal studies. *Nursing Research*, **39**, 184–6.

Greenland, S. (1977). Response and follow-up bias in cohort studies. *American Journal of Epidemiology*, **106**, 184–7.

Greenlick, M.R., Bailey, J.W., Wild, J., and Grover, J. (1979). Characteristics of men most likely to respond to an invitation to be screened. *American Journal of Public Health*, **69**, 1011–15.

Groves, R.N., and Lyberg, L.E. (1988). An overview of non-response issues in telephone surveys. In: *Telephone Survey Methodology* (ed. R.M. Groves, P.P. Biemer, L.E. Lyberg, J.T. Massey, W.L. Nicholls, and J. Waksberg), pp. 191–211. Wiley, New York.

Harlow, B.L., and Hartge, P. (1983). Telephone household screening and interviewing. *American Journal of Epidemiology*, **117**, 632–3.

Hartge, P., Brinton, L.A., Rosenthal, J.F., Cahill, J.I., Hoover, R.N., and Waksberg, J. (1984). Random digit dialing in selecting a population-based control group. *American Journal of Epidemiology*, **120**, 825–33.

Harvey, B.J., Wilkins, A.L., Hawker, G.A., *et al.* (2003). Using publicly available directories to trace survey nonresponders and calculate adjusted response rates. *American Journal of Epidemiology*, **158**, 1007–11.

Hochstim, J.R. (1967). A critical comparison of three strategies of collecting data from households. *Journal of American Statistical Association*, **62**, 976–82.

Holt, V.L., Martin, D.P., and LoGerfo, J.P. (1997). Correlates and effect of non-response in a postpartum survey of obstetrical care quality. *Journal of Clinical Epidemiology*, **50**, 1117–22.

Hox, J.J., and de Leeuw, E.D. (1994). A comparison of non-response in mail, telephone, and face-to-face surveys. *Quality and Quantity*, **28**, 329–344.

Hunt, J.R., and White, E. (1998). Retaining and tracking cohort study members. *Epidemiologic Reviews*, **20**, 57–70.

Iglesias, C., and Torgerson, D. (2000). Does length of questionnaire matter? A randomised trial of response rates to a mailed questionnaire. *Journal of Health Services Research Policy*, **5**, 219–21.

Iredell, H., Shaw, T., Howat, P., James, R., and Granich, J. (2004). Introductory postcards: do they increase response rate in a telephone survey of older persons? *Health Education Research*, **19**, 159–64.

Iversen, L. and Sabroe, S. (1988). Participation in a follow-up study of health among unemployed and employed people after a company closedown: drop outs and selection bias. *Journal of Epidemiology and Community Health*, **42**, 396–401.

Jacomb, P.A., Jorm, A.F., Korten, A.E., Christensen, H., and Henderson, A. S. (2002). Predictors of refusal to participate: a longitudinal health survey of the elderly in Australia. *BMC Public Health*, **2**, 4.

Kanuk, L. and Berenson, C. (1975). Mail surveys and response rates: a literature review. *Journal of Marketing Research*, **12**, 440–53.

Kaplan, S., and Cole, P. (1970). Factors affecting response to postal questionnaires. *British Journal of Preventive and Social Medicine*, **24**, 245–7.

Kleinbaum, D.G., Morgernstern, H., and Kupper, L.L. (1981). Selection bias in epidemiologic studies. *American Journal of Epidemiology*, **113**, 452–63.

Koepsell, T.D., McGuire, V., Longstreth W.T., Jr, Nelson, L.M., and van Belle, G. (1996). Randomized trial of leaving messages on telephone answering machines for control recruitment in an epidemiologic study. *American Journal of Epidemiology*, **144**, 704–6.

Korkeila, K., Suominen, S., Ahvenainen, J., *et al.* (2001). Non-response and related factors in a nation-wide health survey. *European Journal of Epidemiology*, **17**, 991–9.

Krieger, N., and Nishri, E.D. (1997). The effect of nonresponse on estimation of relative risk in a case–control study. *Annals of Epidemiology*, **7**, 194–9.

Kristal, A.R., White, E., Davis, J.R., *et al.* (1993). The effects of enhanced calling efforts on response rates, estimates of health behavior, and costs in a telephone health survey using random-digit dialing. *Public Health Reports*, **108**, 372–79.

Last, J.M. (2001). *A Dictionary of Epidemiology* (4th edn). Oxford University Press.

Loewenstein, R., Colombotos, J., and Elinson, J. (1969). Interviews hardest to obtain in an urban health survey. *Milbank Memorial Fund Quarterly*, **47**, 195–200.

Maclure, M., and Hankinson, S. (1990). Analysis of selection bias in a case–control study of renal adenocarcinoma. *Epidemiology*, **1**, 441–7.

McTiernan, A., Rossouw, J., and Manson, J.E. (1995). Informed consent in the Women's Health Initiative Clinical Trial and Observational Study. *Journal of Women's Health*, **4**, 519–28.

Marmor, J.K., Oliveria, S.A., Donahue, R.P., *et al.* (1991). Factors encouraging cohort maintenance in a longitudinal study. *Journal of Clinical Epidemiology*, **44**, 531–5.

Moorman, P.G., Newman, B., Millikan, R.C., Tse, C.K., and Sandler, D.P. (1999). Participation rates in a case–control study: the impact of age, race, and race of interviewer. *Annals of Epidemiology*, **9**, 188–95.

Morris, M.C., Edmunds, W.J., Miller, E., and Brown, D.W. (2002). Oral fluid collection by post: a pilot study of two approaches. *Public Health*, **116**, 113–19.

Morton, L.M., Cahill, J., and Hartze, P. (2006). Reporting participation in epidemiology studies: a survey of practice. *American Journal of Epidemiology*, **163**, 197–203.

Mueller, B.A., McTiernan, A., and Daling, J.R. (1986). Level of response in epidemiologic studies using the card-back system to contact subjects. *American Journal of Public Health*, **76**, 1331–2.

Nelson, K., Garcia, R.E., Brown, J., *et al.* (2002). Do patient consent procedures affect participation rates in health services research? *Medical Care*, **40**, 283–8.

Nordberg, P.M. (1992). Leave no stone unturned. *American Journal of Epidemiology*, **136**, 1160–6.

Oakes, T.W., Friedman, G.D., and Seltzer, E.E. (1973). Mail survey response by health status of smokers, non-smokers, and ex-smokers. *American Journal of Epidemiology*, **98**, 50–5.

Oksenberg, L. and Cannell, C. (1988). Effects of interviewer vocal characteristics on non-response. In *Telephone Survey Methodology* (ed. R.M. Groves, P.P. Biemer, L.E. Lyberg, J.T. Massey, W.L. Nicholls, and J. Waksberg), pp. 257–69. Wiley, New York.

Oksenberg, L., Coleman, L., and Cannell, C.F. (1986). Interviewers' voices and refusal rates in telephone surveys. *Public Opinion Quarterly*, **50**, 97–111.

Olson, S. H. (2001). Reported participation in case–control studies: changes over time. *American Journal of Epidemiology*, **154**, 574–81.

Olson, S.H., Voigt, L.F., Begg, C.B., and Weiss, N.S. (2002). Reporting participation in case–control studies. *Epidemiology*, **13**, 123–6.

Parkes, R., Kreiger, N., James, B., and Johnson, K.C. (2000). Effects on subject response of information brochures and small cash incentives in a mail-based case–control study. *Annals of Epidemiology*, **10**, 117–24.

Patten, S.B., Li, F.X., Cook, T., Hilsden, R.J., and Sutherland, L.R. (2003). Irritable bowel syndrome. Are incentives useful for improving survey response rates? *Journal of Clinical Epidemiology*, **56**, 256–61.

Pirzada, A., Yan, L.L., Garside, D.B., Schiffer, L., Dyer, A.R., and Daviglus, M.L. (2004). Response rates to a questionnaire 26 years after baseline examination with minimal interim participant contact and baseline differences between respondents and nonrespondents. *American Journal of Epidemiology*, **159**, 94–101.

Purdie, D.M., Dunne, M.P., Boyle, F.M., Cook, M.D., and Najman, J.M. (2002). Health and demographic characteristics of respondents in an Australian national sexuality survey: comparison with population norms. *Journal of Epidemiology in Community Health*, **56**, 748–53.

Robins, L.N. (1963). The reluctant respondent. *Public Opinion Quarterly*, **27**, 276–86.

Rogers, A., Murtaugh, M.A., Edwards, S., and Slattery, M.L. (2004). Contacting controls: Are we working harder for similar response rates, and does it make a difference? *American Journal of Epidemiology*, **160**, 85–90.

Rolnick, S.J., Gross, C.J., Garrard, J., and Gibson, R.W. (1989). A comparison of response rate, data quality, and cost in the collection of data on sexual history and personal behaviours. Mail survey approaches and in-person interviews. *American Journal of Epidemiology*, **129**, 1052–61.

Schleifer, S. (1986). Trends in attitudes toward participation in survey research. *Public Opinion Quarterly*, **50**, 17–26.

Sesso, H. D., Paffenbarger, R.S., and Lee, I.M. (2000). Comparison of National Death Index and World Wide Web death searches. *American Journal of Epidemiology*, **152**, 107–11.

Shahar, E., Folsom, A.R., and Jackson, R. (1996). The effect of nonresponse on prevalence estimates for a referent population: insights from a population-based cohort study. Atherosclerosis Risk in Communities (ARIC) Study Investigators. *Annals of Epidemiology*, **6**, 498–506.

Shiono, P.H., and Klebanoff, M.A. (1991). The effect of two mailing strategies on the response to a survey of physicians. *American Journal of Epidemiology*, **134**, 539–42.

Siemiatycki, J. (1979). A comparison of mail, telephone, and home interview strategies for household health surveys. *American Journal of Public Health*, **69**, 238–45.

Siemiatycki, J. and Campbell, S. (1984). Non-response bias and early versus all responders in mail and telephone surveys. *American Journal of Epidemiology*, **120**, 291–301.

Singer, E., Van Hoewyk, J., and Maher, M.P. (2000). Experiments with incentives in telephone surveys. *Public Opinion Quarterly*, **64**, 171–88.

Smith, W., Chey, T., Jalaludin, B., Salkeld, G., and Capon, T. (1995). Increasing response rates in telephone surveys: a randomized trial. *Journal of Public Health Medicine*, **17**, 33–8.

Smith, W.E.S., Crombie, I.K., Campion, P.D., and Knox, J.D.E. (1985). Comparison of response rates to a postal questionnaire from a general practice research unit. *British Medical Journal*, **291**, 1483–5.

Spry, V.M., Hovell, M.F., Sallis, J.G., Hofstetter, C.R., Elder, J.P., and Molgaard, C.A. (1989). Recruiting survey respondents to mailed surveys: controlled trials of incentives and prompts. *American Journal of Epidemiology*, **130**, 166–72.

Stampfer, M.J., Willett, W.C., Speizer, F.E., *et al.* (1984). Test of the National Death Index. *American Journal of Epidemiology*, **119**, 837–9.

Stang, A., Ahrens, W., and Jockel, K.H. (1999). Control response proportions in population-based case–control studies in Germany. *Epidemiology*, **10**, 181–3.

Thomas, M.C., Walker, M., Lennon, L.T., *et al.* (2002). Non-attendance at re-examination 20 years after screening in the British Regional Heart Study. *Journal of Public Health Medicine*, **24**, 285–91.

Une, H., Miyazaki, M., and Momose, Y. (2000). Comparison of mortality between respondents and non-respondents in a mail survey. *Journal of Epidemiology*, **10**, 136–9.

Van Loon, A.J., Tijhuis, M., Picavet, H.S., Surtees, P.G., and Ormel, J. (2003). Survey non-response in the Netherlands: effects on prevalence estimates and associations. *Annals of Epidemiology*, **13**, 105–10.

Vernon, S.W., Roberts, R.E., and Lee, E.S. (1984). Ethnic status and participation in longitudinal health surveys. *American Journal of Epidemiology*, **119**, 99–113.

Voigt, L.F., Koepsell, T.D., and Daling, J.R. (2003). Characteristics of telephone survey respondents according to willingness to participate. *American Journal of Epidemiology*, **157**, 66–73.

Walker, M., Shaper, A.G., and Cook, D.G. (1987). Non-participation and mortality in a prospective study of cardiovascular disease. *Journal of Epidemiology and Community Health*, **41**, 295–9.

Walter, S.D., Marrett, L.D., and Mishkel, N. (1988). Effect of contact letter on control response rates in cancer studies. *American Journal of Epidemiology*, **127**, 691–4.

Ward, E.M., Kramer, S., and Meadows, A. T. (1984). The efficacy of random digit dialing in selecting matched controls for a case–control study of pediatric cancer. *American Journal of Epidemiology*, **120**, 582–91.

Weeks, M.F., Kulka, R.A., Lessler, J.T., and Whitemore, R.W. (1983). Personal versus telephone surveys for collecting household health data at the local level. *American Journal of Public Health*, **73**, 1389–94.

Wentworth, D.N., Neaton, J.D., and Rasmussen, W.L. (1983). An evaluation of the Social Security Administration master beneficiary record file and the National Death Index in the ascertainment of vital status. *American Journal of Public Health*, **73**, 1270–4.

White, E., Patterson, R.E., Kristal, A.R., Thornquist, M., King, I.B., and Shattuck, A.L. (2004). VITamins And Lifestyle cohort study: study design and characteristics of supplement users. *American Journal of Epidemiology*, **159**, 83–93.

White, E., Carney, P.A., and Shattuck, A.L. (2005). Increasing response to mailed questionnaires by including a pen/pencil. *American Journal of Epidemiology*, **162**, 261–6.

Wilhelmsen, L., Ljunberg, S., Wedel, H., and Werko, L. (1976). A comparison between participants and non-participants in a primary preventive trial. *Journal of Chronic Diseases*, **29**, 331–9.

Wingo, P.A., Ory, H.W., Layde, P.M., and Lee, N.C. (1988). The Cancer and Steroid Hormone Study Group. The evaluation of the data collection process for a multicenter, population-based, case–control design. *American Journal of Epidemiology*, **128**, 206–17.

Wu, M., and Brown, B.W. (1983). Detection and evaluation of bias in a postal survey of the health of dental personnel. In *Methods and Issues in Occupational and Environmental Epidemiology* (ed. L. Chiazze, F.E. Lundin, and D. Watkins), pp. 133–42. Ann Arbor Science, Ann Arbor, MI.

Zondervan, K.T., Carpenter, L.M., Painter, R., and Vessey, M.P. (1996). Oral contraceptives and cervical cancer: further findings from the Oxford Family Planning Association contraceptive study. *British Journal of Cancer*, **73**, 1291–7.

12

Ethical issues

It may be accepted as a maxim that a poorly or
improperly designed study involving human subjects …
is by definition unethical. Moreover, when a study is in
itself scientifically invalid, all other ethical
considerations become irrelevant. There is no point in
obtaining 'informed consent' to perform a useless
study.
(Attributed to David Rutstein by Silverman 1986)

Introduction

Ethics are rules or principles that govern right conduct. In the research
context, 'right conduct' may be defined in terms of what is right for science,
what is right for the subject of the research, or what is right for society at large.
Ethics based on social benefit and scientific merit are potentially in conflict
with ethics that protect the rights of research subjects. A highly informative
and therefore socially valuable investigation which is conducted according to
sound scientific principles may carry unacceptable hazards to the subjects.
Removal of the hazards may render the investigation less satisfactory, or even
worthless scientifically, and therefore less useful, or even useless, socially.
Resolution of this conflict between ethics will almost always involve compromise and lead to a result which is less than wholly desirable when measured
against some scale of values.

The atrocities committed in the name of medical science during the Second
World War, the resulting Nuremberg trials, the Nuremberg Code which arose
from them, and the Declaration of Helsinki, adopted by the World Medical
Association in 1964 and revised several times, most recently in 2000 (CIOMS
2002), have placed the ethical emphasis in biomedical research on protection
of the rights of individual subjects. The implications of these rights for a
specific research project can be analysed in the light of three general principles
that need to be satisfied (Beauchamp and Childress 2001).

1. *Autonomy*: the right of a person to self-governance has to be recognized and the person entitled to autonomous decisions free of imposed limitations.

2. *Non-maleficence and beneficence*: possible harms and wrongs to persons should be minimized ('do not harm') and possible benefits maximized ('do good').

3. *Justice*: persons considered to be alike should be treated alike and persons who are considered different can be treated in ways that acknowledge their difference.

Full and simultaneous satisfaction of each of these three principles is rarely, if ever, achievable and the purpose of the ethical analysis of a research project is to arrive at a practicable compromise between them. This chapter aims to outline how the problems arising in particular in exposure measurement in epidemiology can be examined and how compromises between the three principles can be achieved in a variety of cases.

Human rights and epidemiological research

The United Nations Universal Declaration of Basic Human rights is probably the most widely accepted statement of its kind. Those articles of it which are relevant to the participation of human subjects in epidemiological research are listed in Table 12.1. Articles 1 and 3 declare the right of freedom of the individual to decide whether or not to participate in research. Articles 3 and 5

Table 12.1 Articles of the United Nations Universal Declaration of Basic Human Rights that are relevant to the participation of human subjects in epidemiological research[a]

Article 1
All human beings are born free and equal in dignity and rights. They are endowed with reason and conscience and should act towards one another in a spirit of brotherhood.

Article 3
Everyone has the right to life, liberty and security of person.

Article 5
No one shall be subjected to torture or to cruel, inhuman or degrading treatment or punishment.

Article 12
No one shall be subjected to arbitrary interference with his privacy, family, home or correspondence, nor to attacks upon his honour and reputation. Everyone has the right to the protection of the law against such interference or attacks.

[a] See Reynolds (1979).

declare the right of freedom from harm during the course of experimentation, and Article 12 declares the right of personal privacy.

The Nuremberg Code and the Declaration of Helsinki (Reynolds 1979) were aimed at protecting these rights by establishing a code of practice to be followed in biomedical research. They dealt mainly with the provision of informed consent, protection of the subject against physical injury, and the freedom of the subject to withdraw from the research at any time. The Nuremberg Code also made some cogent points about the quality of the research that might justify limitation of the rights of human subjects (Table 12.2). It is clear from these statements that the justification of the research in social terms and the quality of the methods whereby it is to be conducted must form a part of the judgement as to whether or not it is ethical. Poor-quality research is unethical if it presents any threat at all to human rights, including simple inconvenience to the persons, and perhaps even if it presents no such threat but wastes resources. This concept is also embodied in guideline 1 of the *International Ethical Guidelines for Biomedical Research Involving Human Subjects* published by the Council for International Organizations in Medical Sciences (CIOMS 2002): '...scientifically invalid research is unethical in that it exposes research subjects to risks without possible benefit [of knowledge] ...'.

These statements imply that judgements of the scientific quality and ethical acceptability of research should go hand in hand. This conjunction may be difficult to achieve in practice, at least by means of one committee, because of the different types of people required for each judgement (May 1975; Denham *et al.* 1979). For the research practitioner, they imply an ethical obligation to pursue excellence in research and thus, for example, to seek peer review of the objectives and methods of the research, in addition to seeking ethical review of the safeguards provided for human rights. They lead to the

Table 12.2 Elements of the Nuremberg Code that deal with the quality of research in balance with the rights of human subjects

Article 2
The experiment should be such as to yield fruitful results for the good of society, unprocurable by other methods or means of study, and not random and unnecessary in nature.

Article 3
The experiment should be so designed and based on the results of animal experimentation and a knowledge of the natural history of disease or other problem under study that the anticipated results will justify the performance of the experiment.

almost absolute requirements that all research on humans be conducted according to written protocols; without a written protocol the quality and ethical nature of the research cannot be assured or judged by persons other than the investigators.

An ethical duty also logically arises, although it is not often clearly recognized, to publish the results of all research carried out on human subjects whatever those results may be. If research is conducted which potentially impinges on the rights of human subjects, then the counterbalancing 'greater good' to society will not be realized unless the data are published. Also, it may be argued that, given the application-oriented rather than purely biological character of most epidemiological research, the epidemiologist has an ethical duty not to regard the publication of results as an end it itself, with no concern for any action that may appear to be needed in their light. This is of crucial importance in developing countries where the research epidemiologist also often has wider public health responsibilities. But even in developed countries the duty can be considered to arise '... to speak as experts on behalf of the public health' (Rose 1989).

The conduct of epidemiological research, and specifically the measurement of exposure, may raise a number of problems relevant to the rights of research subjects. The three areas in which problems are mostly likely to arise are:

+ free and informed consent to participate in research
+ protection of personal privacy and confidentiality of personal data
+ risk of physical or psychological harm.

Free and informed consent

The use of unreasonable pressure to elicit the cooperation of research subjects may violate the right to autonomy and Articles 1 and 3 of the United Nations Declaration (Table 12.1). High response rates are necessary if unbiased data are to be obtained. However, the use of multiple methods of approach to subjects, as recommended in Chapter 11, may be considered by some to be unreasonable pressure. At least one ethics committee ruled that more than one postal reminder or a follow-up home visit were ethically unacceptable in a survey conducted initially by mail (Allen and Waters 1982). The use of financial incentives to obtain cooperation may also be considered by some to represent unreasonable pressure, although it is an effective way of increasing response (Chapter 11) and thus increasing the validity of the study.

There is a clear conflict between the autonomy principle prescribing that subjects should be completely free to choose whether or not to participate in research and the ethical need, in most epidemiological studies, to ensure that a high participation rate is obtained for the sake of scientific validity. Where participation in the research presents minimal risk of harm to subjects, it seems reasonable to permit, within reason, the use of methods of recruitment that maximize response. The issue of 'minimal risk' is dealt with in greater detail below.

Subjects may also be given incomplete information about the research. However, what constitutes 'incomplete' information may not be clear cut or absolute and, like what constitutes 'unreasonable pressure', may be influenced by other ethical considerations. For example, it is common in case–control studies that the research hypotheses are not outlined in detail so as to avoid bias in the recall of exposures. In a case–control study of malignant melanoma, both cases and controls were told only that they were participating in a study of 'environment, lifestyle and health' (Holman and Armstrong 1984). It was hoped, thereby, to make the study equally salient to cases and controls. In a randomized controlled trial of vegetarian diet in the control of mild hypertension, subjects were all given 50 mg of vitamin C daily and told that the aim of the study was to determine the effect of vitamin C on blood pressure in interaction with dietary change (Margetts *et al.* 1985). This was intended to create a uniform placebo response across the experimental and control diets because of the impossibility of keeping the subjects blind to the dietary change. It is doubtful whether, in either of these examples, it would have been ethically more appropriate to inform the subjects of all details of the research at the risk of prejudicing the scientific validity of the studies, itself a prerequisite for an ethically acceptable investigation.

A similar but much more delicate issue of incomplete information arises if subjects are asked to donate biological samples to be stored for future measurements of exposures (e.g. of genetic polymorphisms) which cannot be specified as their relevance will only emerge from new scientific hypotheses, not currently known. Clearly, under these circumstances, the very 'informed' nature of the consent is called into question. One approach taken has been to seek consent that is relatively broad, but confined to the context of the present study. For example, in seeking consent to use DNA collected in a case–control study of non-Hodgkin lymphoma for genetic testing, subjects were asked to give their consent to 'DNA testing for mutations of and variations in genes that may be associated with lymphoma' (Purdue *et al.* 2007).

Privacy and confidentiality

Privacy has been defined, with survey research in mind, as 'the freedom of the individual to choose for himself the time and circumstances under which and the extent to which his attitudes, beliefs, behaviour and opinions are to be shared or withheld from others' (Rubehausen and Brim 1966). More generally, privacy implies that the individual has the right to decide whether and how any information regarding his/her person is used. This does not apply to information publicly available, for example in a telephone directory. Invasion of privacy may violate the principle of autonomy and Article 12 of the United Nations Declaration; it may also violate the principle of non-maleficence and Articles 1 and 3 of the United Nations Declaration to the extent that it may produce actual damage to the person. In exposure measurements, autonomy is fully preserved only if subjects interviewed by telephone or in person are contacted in advance by letter to obtain consent. However, such an approach may substantially reduce participation rates and so threaten the validity of the research.

Confidentiality is automatically preserved if epidemiological studies are restricted to the use of data that cannot be identified with the individuals to whom it relates. However, such a restriction greatly limits the capacity of epidemiology to provide answers to socially important questions (Gordis *et al.* 1977). When personal data provided by the subject within a confidential relationship are passed to a third party for research purpose, confidentiality can be protected by obtaining the subject's consent. However, obtaining consent may be logistically difficult, particularly in large studies. It may indeed be impossible if, for example, the subjects must first be identified in order to be traced or if they are already dead. Thus, again, it can be seen that the epidemiologist's ethical duty to individual subjects is in conflict with his/her ethical duty to the wider community to conduct valid research.

Physical or psychological damage

The occurrence of injury in the course of research potentially violates the principle of non-maleficence and Articles 1, 3, and 5 of the United Nations Declaration. The possibility of physical injury is much less common in epidemiology than in most areas of biomedical research. However, physically invasive procedures are used for the measurement of exposure to agents of disease, for example sampling of blood or tissue for measurement of the concentration of chemicals or detection of the results of chemical exposure. Psychological injury is also a possibility, especially when subjects are required to recall events that are embarrassing (e.g. details of sexual history or of socially undesirable behaviours) or that they would prefer to suppress. The sharing of this information with the investigator may also lead to anxiety about the potential effects of any subsequent breach of confidentiality. Occasionally, research brings to light information about subjects that they might prefer not to know and prefer others not to know (e.g. presence of antibodies to human immunodeficiency syndrome) and thus may cause them substantial distress.

In a mail survey of 128 participants in a case–control study of cervical neoplasia, conducted up to 12 months after interview, Savitz *et al.* (1986) found that 24 per cent of subjects were 'bothered' in some way by the interview questions. Of these, 30 per cent were bothered by questions on sexual partners, 6 per cent by questions on sexually transmitted disease, and 5 per cent by questions on pregnancies. Fifteen per cent recalled a desire to stop the interview during its course and, in retrospect, 3 per cent regretted their participation. On the positive side, 90 per cent were very happy or somewhat happy about their participation. Similar results were obtained in a follow-up survey of women with breast cancer who had participated in a prior health interview about mastectomy (Funch and Marshall 1981). While the topics of both these research projects were sensitive ones to women and might, perhaps, have generated more than average numbers of adverse feelings, they do indicate the potential of epidemiological research to cause some psychological distress.

As well as individuals, groups of subjects may incur damage if, for example, a group is found to have a high prevalence of a socially stigmatizing condition such as alcoholism or mental diseases. If this possibility is envisaged, it may be advisable to have individual consent supplemented by a community consultation (CIOMS 2002).

Ethical practice in epidemiological research

It is not uncommon for particular professional groups to establish an ethical code of their own. Specific guidelines have been drafted for epidemiologists in several countries over the last several decades (Fluss *et al.* 1990) and are now available in most countries where an epidemiological scientific society exists. At the international level, the International Epidemiological Association has prepared a *Good Epidemiological Practice* document (IEA 2007). In addition to the core ethical concern of protection of the rights of subjects involved in epidemiological research, the code encompasses issues such as publication policies and duties arising from collaborative work.

Biomedical research workers, including epidemiologists, are coming more and more to be judged by ethical codes laid down by governments and research funding bodies. Probably the most influential of these codes is that mandated by the US Department of Health and Human Services for research that it funds (USDHHS 2005). Institutions in which such research is conducted are required to have an institutional review board which operates according to the principles laid down by the Department. This board reviews and approves or disapproves, on ethical grounds, all research proposing the use of human subjects. The US Department of Health and Human Services exempts certain types of research from its requirements, but it is doubtful whether much aetiological research in epidemiology would be covered by these exemptions (except for research based solely on analysis of publicly available data), and the wisest course for epidemiologists is to seek institutional review board approval for most if not all of their research. Similar procedures have come into operation in many countries during the last two decades.

Internationally, the best established set of guidelines are the *International Ethical Guidelines for Biomedical Research Involving Human Subjects* prepared by the Council for International Organizations of Medical Sciences (CIOMS 2002). As well as covering the general principles articulated in Helsinki II, these guidelines give special attention to ethical problems which may arise in the conduct of research in developing countries under sponsorship from international agencies or developed countries. These guidelines have been complemented by a separate set specifically devoted to epidemiological research (*International Guidelines for Ethical Review of Epidemiological Studies* (CIOMS 1991)) which are currently under revision (CIOMS 2007).

We summarize below, under eight headings, our advice on how an ethically acceptable balance may be achieved between the rights of individuals and the wider good of society as pursued through epidemiological research. This advice reflects the documents cited above, as well as our personal experience at national and international levels as researchers, members of committees dealing with ethical issues, and citizens with our own subjective values.

Written protocols

All epidemiological research should be conducted according to written protocols which specifically address ethical issues.

The basis for this recommendation has already been outlined. In summary, neither the investigator nor anyone else can be assured of the justification, scientific quality, or ethical propriety of a proposed research programme unless it has been thought through sufficiently to be put down on paper.

Ethics committees

All protocols for epidemiological research involving human subjects should be passed by a properly constituted institutional review board or ethics committee.

This practice provides protection from the natural tendency of investigators to view their research in a more favourable light than others might view it. Pragmatically, it is no longer possible in most countries to obtain funds for research from funding bodies unless the protocol has been approved by an ethics committee.

The submission to the ethics committee should:

- state the aims of the research and whether or not the protocol has passed scientific peer review (for an optimal assessment this should be the case)
- clearly identify the subjects in terms of their numbers, age, sex, state of health, other demographic characteristics, if different from the general population, as well as with respect to any reduced or impaired capacity of providing informed and free consent, as for children, those mentally impaired, prisoners, etc.
- describe the research procedures with details of any intervention proposed and emphasis on anything likely to have adverse consequences, such as physically or psychologically invasive procedures or administration of a drug or other potentially harmful substance
- describe how the results of the research will be made public and whether or not the information generated by the research and concerning each individual subject will be communicated to the subject
- list any potential benefits of the research to the subjects and to society
- state whether any commercial benefits may derive from the research and to whom these may accrue
- describe how the confidentiality of information about the subjects will be preserved
- state whether or not subjects will be remunerated and to what extent
- describe in detail the information about the research that will be given to participants, by whom and how it will be given, and in which form the consent will be obtained; any document to be signed by the subject should be included and special procedures described for obtaining permission by guardians if subjects with reduced or impaired capacity to provide informed and free consent are involved.

Investigators' ethical responsibility

The investigators should in any case assure themselves that a particular research programme involving human subjects contains adequate safeguards for the rights of those subjects and that these are put into effect throughout all stages of the investigation.

Ultimately, the ethical responsibility for the research and for what happens to the subjects involved lies with the investigators themselves. They do not absolve themselves of this responsibility when they have a protocol passed by an institutional review board or ethics committee, nor even when they can produce a pack of signed informed consent forms.

Subject's consent

Consent must be obtained from each research subject for their direct participation in epidemiological research.

In giving information prior to obtaining consent, all information that may be material to a subject's decision to participate should be given. It should include:

- a clear explanation, in terms that the subject can understand, of the purposes of the study and the procedures to be followed
- a description of any discomfort and possible hazards involved, including those that might materialize in the future from the use of information or biological specimens provided by the subject
- a statement on whether any information generated by the research and concerning the subject will or will not be communicated to him or her
- an accurate statement of the potential benefits to them and to society
- a statement, when applicable, of the commercial benefits that may derive from the research and to whom they may accrue
- a description of the procedures adopted to preserve the confidentiality of information on the subject
- a statement on whether or not the subject will be remunerated and to what extent
- a statement that they are free to withdraw their participation at any time
- a statement, when relevant, that their future interests will not be prejudiced in any way by refusal to participate
- an offer to answer any questions that they may have.

The information given to potential subjects is usually in the form of a written consent statement, to be signed by the participant. The participant may be given a copy for his/her records.

For 'minimal risk research' the requirement for both complete information and written consent may be waived provided that any information important to the subjects is given to them after their participation has ended. Since 1981, the US Department of Health and Human Services (USDHHS 1981, 2005) has defined 'minimal risk research' as research that offers anticipated risks of harm that are not greater, considering probability and magnitude, than those ordinarily encountered in daily life or during the performance of routine physical or psychological examinations or tests. The US code (USDHHS 1981, 2005) permits both 'fully informed' and 'written' consent provisions to be waived for projects judged by an institutional review board to be minimal risk. Most epidemiological research which only requires participation in an interview or completion of a self-administered questionnaire probably qualifies as minimal risk research, although what 'risks ordinarily encountered in daily life' means in practice is open to wide subjective interpretation.

Waiver of the requirement to obtain written consent is important to some epidemiological research. For example, there are logistic problems in obtaining written consent to a telephone interview, especially if the subject has been selected by a process such as random digit dialling. In addition, a requirement for signed consent reduces the participation rate in otherwise apparently harmless research (Chapter 11). However, lack of a requirement for written documentation of consent does not absolve the investigator from providing the subject with information about the research. Thus the protocol should still specify what information will be provided and how it will be given when written consent is not going to be obtained. Generally subjects in a minimal risk study can be given the information about the study listed above in a cover letter or verbally (e.g. for telephone interviews). It seems reasonable to assume that if a subject then completes the questionnaire or interview, he/she has consented to the procedure.

In some studies, information may be provided and consent obtained in two steps: initially, say, for interview and, subsequently, for taking a blood sample. This procedure may be justified to obtain the highest possible rate of participation in the interview, unimpeded by subjects' disinclination to have a blood sample taken. Special care should be taken, if this approach is adopted, to explain to the subjects that they are at liberty to refuse to participate in the second or any subsequent phase of the study.

It is usually not feasible in community-based intervention trials to obtain consent to the intervention from each individual member of the community. The decision whether or not to permit or undertake the research will, in these circumstances, usually lie with the responsible public health authority. However, all possible means should be used to inform the community concerned of the aims and nature of the research, and any possible hazards or inconvenience. If feasible, dissenting individuals should have the option of not participating (CIOMS 1991).

Obtaining consent for research on children requires special attention. It is axiomatic that children should never be the subjects of research that could equally well be done in adults. On the other hand, participation of children may be necessary for research into prevention or treatment of diseases of childhood (CIOMS 2002). When children are the subjects of research, both their own agreement (assent) and the permission of a parent of other legal guardian should be obtained. While the capacity of children to assent will be influenced by age and understanding, their willing cooperation should be sought after they have been informed of the purposes and nature of the research and any possible discomfort or inconvenience. The amount of information given, and whether or not written permission will be sought from the parent or guardian, will be determined by the considerations outlined above.

Special considerations regarding consent are also necessary for research involving people with impaired mental capacity. It has been argued for such persons that '... it is extremely unlikely whether valid third party consent can be given for procedures which are not essential for the preservation of life or health, such as ... participation in medical research projects of no direct benefit to the patient' (Hayes and Hayes 1983). A similar argument might be made with respect to research involving highly unsophisticated 'third world' populations, individuals from which may have little prospect of understanding any explanation of a research project (Jamrozik 1984).

As noted above, there may be situations when it is important to the scientific validity of an investigation that the subjects are not provided with complete information about the purposes of the study at the time of their participation. If no alternatives to this choice exist, the attention of the ethics committee that reviews the protocol should be drawn to it and to the reasons for it. For example, in a case–control study of the relationship between birth defects and prenatal use of a particular drug, it would be wrong to give the name of the drug in question when explaining the purpose of the study to the participating mothers. Disclosure of the name of the drug would be likely to lead to both recruitment into the study of a higher proportion of mothers exposed to the drug than mothers not exposed, and to more assiduous recall of exposure by the mothers of malformed children than by mothers of healthy children. These effects could produce a positive and potentially spurious association between the drug and birth defects (NHMRC 1985). It is doubtful whether in this case it would be necessary to go back to the subjects after the study is terminated and explain the true purpose. In other situations, however, it may be important to go back to the subjects after their participation has ended and disclose the previous hidden information (CPHPR 1982). For example, participants in a randomized controlled trial should be advised, after the code has been broken, of what treatment they received.

An ethically thorny issue has emerged in the last two decades with the development of long-term cohort studies aimed at exploring the role of such factors as nutrition or genetics on adult health. An essential component of these studies is the collection of biological specimens to be stored in bio-repositories for future determinations of genetic, nutritional, or other biomarkers which cannot be specified at the time of the collection. This feature clashes directly with the requirement of 'informed' consent to the use of the specimens, a dilemma that has not found any generally accepted solution. For example, the Council of Europe (2006) states:

> General rule. Research on biological materials should only be undertaken if it is within the scope of the consent given by the person concerned. The person concerned may place restrictions on the use of his or her biological materials.

However, this begs the key question of what may be adequate information enabling the person to place restrictions on the consent. A compromise solution to the dilemma may consist of a specific consent to the collection of the specimens for long-term storage within the frame of an investigation defined in relatively broad terms (e.g. on nutrition, genetics, and health) coupled with an authorization to an ethics committee to decide in the future whether a particular biomarker study is permissible, and upon what conditions; this neither prescribes nor excludes the condition of going back to the subjects and asking them for explicit consent to given tests on the specimens. This solution was adopted by, for example, the ethics committee chaired by one of us at an international research institution and was supported by national or local ethics committees in several European countries. Other solutions along similar lines have recently been proposed (Caulfield *et al.* 2003).

Access to personally identifiable data sources

Access to medical or other records, or to biological specimens collected for clinical purposes and carrying the identification of the subjects, may be obtained without the prior consent of the subjects provided that a number of conditions are met.

The conditions that should be met include the following:

♦ the access is essential to achievement of the objectives of the research

♦ no alternative sources of data are available for the specific research purposes; this separates the use of biological specimens for research related to the health conditions for which they were collected in clinical practice from the potential use of such specimens as a cheaply available material for any kind of test—an ethically unjustifiable use

♦ a requirement for consent would render the research logistically or economically impracticable or would crucially prejudice its scientific value

- the consent of the custodian of the records or specimens is obtained
- the data obtained from record abstraction or analyses on biological specimens are the minimum necessary to achievement of the objectives of the research
- the data are protected against disclosure to persons not immediately involved in the research
- the data are not used for new research without the further consent of the custodian of the records and further ethical review
- the study has been approved by an independent ethics committee.

Access to confidential data is essential to the conduct of much epidemiological research (Gordis and Gold 1980; MRC 1985). Accepting that, the issue becomes whether or not access should be permitted without the knowledge and consent of the record subject. The implied requirement is that the consent of subjects be obtained for access to records when this course is practicable and does not threaten the success of the research. However, obtaining consent would be impracticable in many situations (Gordis and Gold 1980), and a requirement to obtain it would prevent much potentially important research.

The view of most legal authorities and government commissions that have considered the matter has been that the consent of the record subjects to the disclosure of information about them for research purposes need not be obtained provided that certain conditions such as those listed above are met (Armstrong 1984). (However, it should be stressed that legal and ethical requirements are different in nature and do not necessarily coincide in practice).

In the USA, there are national regulations about the use of medical information. In response to the Health Insurance Portability and Accountability Act 1996 (HIPAA), the US Department of Health and Human Services issued regulations entitled *Standards for Privacy of Individually Identifiable Health Information*, known as the Privacy Rule, which were implemented in 2003. The Privacy Rule defines certain data that come from hospitals, health plans, or healthcare providers as personal health information. Personal health information can only be released for research purposes under certain circumstances; for example, the subject has granted specific written permission, the information released has no personal identifiers, or certain waivers have been obtained (see http: http://privacyruleandresearch.nih.gov/clin_research.asp).

Confidentiality of personally identifiable data

The confidentiality of personally identifiable data and biological specimens obtained in the course of epidemiological research should be protected in such a way as to render its disclosure to the detriment of the subject an extremely remote possibility.

If confidential data are to be protected adequately, it is important that investigators think through the safeguards required and prepare a written code of practice for the protection of confidential data. Briefly, such a code might include the following provisions.

(a) All persons who have access to name-identified research data or biological specimens during the course of their work sign a declaration that they will respect the confidentiality of the data with which they work.

(b) As far as possible, the records containing research information (whether on paper or in computer storage media), as well as the biological specimens and the corresponding personal identifiers, are kept physically and logically separate and are linkable only by mean of a common non-personal identifier such as a record number, which may in turn be encrypted using a key.

(c) Records containing personal identifiers are kept under lock and key when not being worked on or, in the case of computer records, under an equivalent level of security.

(d) The personal identifiers are retained only as long as it is necessary to achieve the objectives of the research; this extends over decades for long-term prospective studies.

(e) Disposal of identified records is carried out with strict attention to security.

(f) Research results are never published in a form that would permit the identification of any individual subject.

While the destruction of personal identifiers as soon as the objectives of the research have been achieved obviously protects confidentiality, it may often lead to the loss of future opportunities for the efficient conduct of worthwhile research.

Many epidemiological studies have as their starting point data obtained in an earlier study to which the original personal identifiers can still be linked. For example, Newman *et al.* (1986) reported on the relationship of body weight and dietary fat intake to survival after diagnosis of breast cancer by follow-up of patients with breast cancer interviewed 5–7 years earlier in a case–control study of aetiology. Such follow-up studies are frequently not envisaged when the original data are being collected, and would not be possible if the personal identifying data were to be destroyed when no longer needed for the original study. However, if identifiers are to be retained beyond their period of actual use, their retention should be justified specifically in the protocol, the manner in which they are to be stored should be stated, and both should be approved (or otherwise) by the ethics committee.

Within the 27 countries of the European Union, an *ad hoc* directive (European Commission 1995) laid down the criteria for personal data protection within a country and for transfer of data between countries. The directive permits the individual states to reinforce the protection requirements, a clause which has translated, not unusually, in the hands of data custodians into an impediment to data access without the consent of the subjects, even when this was obviously impossible, for example because the subjects were dead.

It may not be possible in all jurisdictions for epidemiologists to guarantee that personal data in their care can be protected against disclosure in court, a circumstance highlighting a potential conflict between ethical and legal obligations. However, in one example the US Court of Appeals protected women in a study of the toxic shock syndrome from the disclosure of their identities to another party to the court proceedings, the manufacturers of one of the allegedly offending tampons (Curran 1986). In some states of Australia there exist amendments to the Health Act that provide protection against use in court of data about identifiable individuals collected in the course of an approved research project. This kind of protection for research data should be sought whenever possible.

Permission to approach subjects

An approach to subjects identified through non-public records should only be made with the permission of the record custodian or whomever else the custodian should nominate.

An approach to patients with a particular disease identified through medical records is probably the most common circumstance in which epidemiological research involves an approach to subjects identified through non-public records. In this situation, permission to the approach should be obtained from the doctor responsible for the patients' care at the time the record was made, an appropriate successor to that doctor, or the medical superintendent or other appropriate authority in the hospital in which the record is held. This permission is necessary for a number of reasons.

(a) It is a matter of common courtesy.

(b) It is the doctor responsible for care of the patient who is most likely to know whether an approach to the patient will cause emotional distress or other harm.

(c) Pragmatically, if this permission is not obtained, it is likely that future access to the records in which the subjects were identified will be denied.

Objections may be raised that doctors do not 'own' their patients and should not be allowed to deny patients their right to participate in worthwhile research. In practice, doctors rarely deny access to their patients. Also, there are data indicating that patients favour requesting the doctor's permission; a study on the causes of breast, ovarian, and endometrial cancers showed that 50 per cent of women considered that the request for access had been a necessary step (Boring et al. 1984).

Communication of research results

If, in the course of epidemiological research, information is obtained about a subject that necessitates some courses of action in the subject's interests, that course should be taken after due consultation with the subject.

This recommendation is usually applied when a previously unsuspected disease or physiological or biochemical risk factor for disease is discovered during the course of, for example, a prevalence survey or the collection of data on risk factors for an aetiological study. The investigator has an obligation to inform the subject of the finding, to explain its significance to him/her, to recommend an appropriate course of action, and to make reasonable efforts to ensure that this course is followed, provided that the subject consents. A common approach, when a risk factor such as high blood pressure or hypercholesterolaemia is found, would be to refer the subject to his/her usual medical practitioner.

This type of communication concerning medically controllable factors may be regarded only as a minimum, and the question might also be raised as to whether epidemiologists have an ethical duty to advise subjects regarding known hazardous or behavioural exposures that may be ascertained during data collection. For example, should smokers who participate in epidemiological research be advised, as part of the research programme, to give up smoking? What responsibility does an epidemiologist have towards a person who drinks in excess of, say, 40 g of alcohol a day? In these situations the subject him/herself may be seen as responsible for the exposure, and the risk associated with it is already known rather than uncovered by the study. The ethical questions that they raise have not been discussed to any substantial extent in epidemiology, although the duty to notify the subjects has been considered to exist in some cases. For example, in a survey of non-melanocytic skin cancer (Kricker et al. 1990), an attempt was made to do this by providing all subjects, regardless of their exposure, with an educational leaflet on exposure to the sun. The efficiency of this indiscriminate approach to providing information would need to be compared, in each specific instance, with a more selective approach which entails the added cost of identifying and targeting subjects with particular levels of the exposure.

Taking the obligation to inform one step further, it may be argued that members of an exposed population, be it an occupational group (ICOH 2002) or a town's population, have the right, not only as individuals but also as members of the group, to be informed about hazardous exposures uncovered during a research project so that they are in a position to take whatever protective action they deem appropriate. This duty towards the community in which a study is conducted, as well as the duty towards study subjects, has been considered in ethical guidelines for epidemiology (CIOMS 1991).

Clearly, there are problems in deciding whether or not to notify, the most important of which is the need to be confident that the risk is real and that notification does not lead to anxiety which is out of proportion to the size of the risk. At one extreme there is no point in notifying the subjects about the finding of a genetic polymorphism whose status as a risk factor or risk indicator is not yet established, while at the other extreme notification is probably required if a woman is found to be a carrier of the *BRCA1* gene mutation entailing a very high lifetime risk of a treatable condition like breast cancer. The case of a mutated gene causing a non-treatable (other than supportively) and fatal disease such as Huntington chorea is debatable. In this, as in most other situations discussed here, the key consideration is that the possible outcomes of the research must be part of the information provided to the subject before obtaining consent to participate in a study. The option of whether the subject wishes or not to be informed, and in which way, about findings directly relevant to his/her health should become part of the consent specifications.

The US National Heart Lung and Blood Institute convened a working group in 2004 to specifically address the issue of reporting genetic results to participants in research studies (available at http://www.nhlbi.nih.gov/meetings/ workshops/gene-results.htm). That group concluded that the conditions under which genetic test results should be reported to research participants are as follows.

1. The risk of disease associated with the genetic variant should be 'significant', i.e. a relative risk greater than 2.0.

2. The disease should have important health implications, i.e. substantial morbidity or reproductive implications.

3. Proven preventive or therapeutic interventions are available.

The working group also recommended that the decision about whether to report results back to participants and their physicians should not be made by the researcher alone, but in consultation with an ethics committee; that the results should be from a certified laboratory; and that the physicians should be given a one-page summary of what is known about the test and its implications.

Another consideration applies to the question of information when the study has disclosed a hazard to others rather than to the subject. This is a highly controversial issue which may give rise to dilemmas that are not soluble in any way without serious infringement of somebody's rights. This dilemma is exemplified by the person at high risk of human immunodeficiency virus infection who does not want to know whether he/she is seropositive for the virus and thus poses a potential serious hazard to his/her sexual partners.

Summary

The overriding ethical principle in the conduct of research on human subjects is that the rights of individual subjects should take precedence over the expected benefits to human knowledge or the community. This principle does not preclude research that may lead to some harm to subjects, provided that the subjects accept voluntarily, and with complete information, the possibility of harm. In addition, the principle can be modified when it may reasonably be judged that the probability of harm from the research is no greater than individuals assume daily as part of the normal activities of life.

The disclosure of confidential information about research subjects has the potential for harm. This is the main ethical risk that most epidemiological research carries and should be treated with the same seriousness as would any more direct threat of harm.

The epidemiologist's ethical duty to the subjects of research is in potential conflict with his/her wider duty to society to conduct research that is scientifically valid and has the potential to improve the health of the community. This conflict can be resolved by the investigator's accepting personal responsibility for ensuring ethical practice in epidemiological research and adopting appropriate policies for this practice. These policies should include:

- working only from written research protocols which specifically address ethical issues
- ensuring that all research protocols have been passed by an appropriate ethical review committee
- obtaining fully informed consent from subjects to their participation in research, except where the research is judged to present no more than minimal risk to the subject
- obtaining access to personally identifiable data sources without the subjects' consent only under carefully defined conditions

- making express and adequate provision for maintenance of the confidentiality of personally identifiable data
- obtaining the permission of the custodian of the records for an approach to subjects identified through non-public records
- ensuring that results obtained during the course of research that may have a bearing on the health or welfare of subjects are communicated to them.

It is important for investigators to appreciate that scientifically poor research is unethical because it entails hazards, however minimal, and inconvenience to human subjects and it wastes resources. Failure to publish the results of research in a readily accessible form is unethical for similar reasons.

References

Allen, P.A. and Waters, W.E. (1982). Development of an ethical committee and its effects on research design. *Lancet*, **i**, 1233–6.

Armstrong, B.K. (1984). Privacy and medical research. *Medical Journal of Australia*, **141**, 620–1.

Beauchamp, T.L. and Childress, J.F. (2001). *Principles of Biomedical Ethics* (5th edn). Oxford University Press, New York.

Boring, C.C., Brockman, E., Causey, N., Gregory, H.R., and Greenberg, R.S. (1984). Patient attitudes toward physician consent in epidemiological research. *American Journal of Public Health*, **74**, 1406–8.

Caulfield, T., Upshur, R.E.G., and Daar, A. (2003). DNA databanks and consent: a suggested policy option involving an authorization model. *BMC Medical Ethics*, **4**, 1. Available online at: http://www.biomedcentral.com/l 472–6939/4/l

CIOMS (Council for International Organizations of Medical Sciences) (1991). *International Guidelines for Ethical Review of Epidemiological Studies*. Council for International Organizations of Medical Sciences, Geneva.

CIOMS (Council for International Organizations of Medical Sciences) (2002). *International Ethical Guidelines for Biomedical Research Involving Human Subjects*. Council for International Organizations of Medical Sciences, Geneva.

CIOMS (Council for International Organizations of Medical Sciences) (2007). *International Ethical Guidelines for Epidemiological Studies: Draft*. Available online at: http://www.cioms.ch

Council of Europe (2006). *Recommendation Rec (2006) 4 of the Committee of Ministers to Member States on Research on Biological Materials of Human Origin*. Council of Europe, Strasbourg.

CPHPR (Committee for the Protection of Human Participants in Research) (1982). *Ethical Principles in the Conduct of Research with Human Participants*. American Psychological Association, Washington.

Curran, W.J. (1986). Protecting confidentiality in epidemiological investigations by the Centers for Disease Control. *New England Journal of Medicine*, **314**, 1027–8.

Denham, M.J., Foster, A., and Tyrrell, D.A.J. (1979). Work of a district ethical committee. *British Medical Journal*, **2**, 1042–5.

European Commission (1995). Directive 95/46/EC on the protection of individuals with regard to the processing of personal data and on the free movement of such data. *Official Journal of the European Communities*, No. 281, 31–50.

Fluss, S., Simon, F., and Gutteridge, F. (1990). A survey of policies and laws, pp. 7–9. Presented at the Conference on Development of International Ethical Guidelines for Epidemiological Research and Practice held by the Council for International Organizations of Medical Sciences, Geneva, November 1990.

Funch, D.O. and Marshall, J.R. (1981). Patients' attitudes following participation in a health outcome survey. *American Journal of Public Health*, **71**, 1396–8.

Gordis, L. and Gold, E. (1980). Privacy, confidentiality, and the use of medical records in research. *Science*, **207**, 153–6.

Gordis, L., Gold, E., and Seltser, R. (1977). Privacy protection in epidemiological and medical research: a challenge and responsibility. *American Journal of Epidemiology*, **105**, 163–8.

Hayes, S. and Hayes, R. (1983). Third-party consent to medical procedures. *Medical Journal of Australia*, **2**, 90–2.

Holman, C.D.J. and Armstrong, B.K. (1984). Pigmentary traits, ethnic origin, benign naevi and family history as risk factors for cutaneous malignant melanoma. *Journal of the National Cancer Institute*, **72**, 257–66.

ICOH (International Commission on Occupational Health) (2002). *International Code of Ethics for Health Professionals*. Available online at: http://www.icoh.org

IEA (International Epidemiological Association) (2007). *Discussion Documents. Good Epidemiological Practice(GEP)*. Available online at: http://www.ieaweb.org

Jamrozik, K. (1984). Ethical consideration in clinical research. *Papua New Guinea Medical Journal*, **27**, 4–6.

Kricker, A., English, D., Randell, P.L., *et al.* (1990). Skin cancer in Geraldton, Western Australia: a survey of incidence and prevalence. *Medical Journal of Australia*, **152**, 399–407.

Margetts, B.M., Beilin, L.J., Armstrong, B.K., and Vandongen, R. (1985). A randomized controlled trial of vegetarian diet in the treatment of hypertension. *Clinical Experiments in Pharmacology and Physiology*, **12**, 263–6.

May, W.W. (1975). The composition and function of ethical committees. *Journal of Medical Ethics*, **1**, 23–9.

MRC (Medical Research Council) (1985). Responsibility in the use of personal medical information for research: principles and guide to practice. *American Journal of Epidemiology*, **290**, 1120–4.

Newman, S.C., Miller, A.B., and Howe, G.R. (1986). A study of the effect of weight and dietary fat on breast cancer survival time. *American Journal of Epidemiology*, **123**, 767–74.

NHMRC (National health and Medical Research Council) (1985). *Report on Ethics in Epidemiological Research*. Australian Government Publishing Service, Canberra.

Purdue, M.P., Lan, Q., Kricker, A., *et al.* (2007). Polymorphisms in immune function genes and risk of non-Hodgkin lymphoma: findings from the New South Wales Non-Hodgkin Lymphoma Study. *Carcinogenesis*, **28**, 704–12.

Reynolds, P.D. (1979). *Ethical Dilemmas and Social Research*. Jossey-Bass, San Francisco, CA.

Rose, G. (1989). Ethics and public policy. In *Assessment of Inhalation Hazards* (ed. V. Mohr), pp.349–56. Springer-Verlag, Berlin.

Rubehausen, O.M. and Brimm, O.G., Jr (1966). Privacy and behavioral research. *American Psychologist*, **21**, 423–44.

Savitz, D.A., Hamman, R.F., Grace, C., and Stroo, K. (1986). Respondents' attitudes regarding participation in an epidemiological study. *American Journal of Epidemiology*, **123**, 362–6.

Silverman, W. (1986). *Human Experimentation*, p.156. Oxford University Press, New York.

USDHHS (US Department of Health and Human Services) (1981). Final regulations amending basic HHS policy for the protection of human research subjects. *Federal Register*, **46**, 8366–91.

USDHHS (US Department of Health and Human Services) (2005). *Code of Federal Regulations*. Title 45, *Public Welfare*. Part 46, *Protection of Human Subjects*. Available online at: http://www.hhs.gov/ohrp/humansubjects/guidance/45cfr46.htm

Index